Encyclopedia of Neuroimaging: Clinical Neuroscience
Volume II

Edited by **Miles Scott**

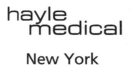

New York

Published by Hayle Medical,
30 West, 37th Street, Suite 612,
New York, NY 10018, USA
www.haylemedical.com

Encyclopedia of Neuroimaging: Clinical Neuroscience
Volume II
Edited by Miles Scott

International Standard Book Number: 978-1-63241-183-9 (Hardback)

Contents

Preface

The clinical neurosciences of neuroimaging are described in this all-inclusive book. The rate of technological advancement is stimulating increasingly comprehensive lines of enquiry in neuroscience, which displays no sign of slowing down in the distant future. However, it is unlikely that even the most powerful advocates of the cognitive neuroscience approach would maintain that developments in cognitive theory have kept in step with techniques-based advancements. There are numerous reasons for the failure of neuroimaging studies to satisfactorily resolve a number of most significant theoretical debates in the literature. For example, a crucial proportion of published functional magnetic resonance imaging (fMRI) studies are not well explained in cognitive theory, and this depicts a step away from the conventional approach in experimental psychology of systematically and technically building on (or chipping away at) present theoretical models using authentic methodologies. Unless, the experimental analysis design is set up within a vividly outlined theoretical framework, any inferences that are drawn are unlikely to be accepted as anything other than analytical. This book examines neuroimaging data in bipolar disorder, neuroimaging outcomes of brain training trials, somatosensory stimulation in functional neuroimaging, reinforcement learning and human brain.

All of the data presented henceforth, was collaborated in the wake of recent advancements in the field. The aim of this book is to present the diversified developments from across the globe in a comprehensible manner. The opinions expressed in each chapter belong solely to the contributing authors. Their interpretations of the topics are the integral part of this book, which I have carefully compiled for a better understanding of the readers.

At the end, I would like to thank all those who dedicated their time and efforts for the successful completion of this book. I also wish to convey my gratitude towards my friends and family who supported me at every step.

Editor

Neuroimaging Data in Bipolar Disorder: An Updated View

Bernardo Dell'Osso, Cristina Dobrea, Maria Carlotta Palazzo,
Laura Cremaschi, Chiara Arici, Beatrice Benatti and A. Carlo Altamura
Department of Psychiatry, University of Milan, Fondazione IRCCS Cà Granda,
Ospedale Maggiore Policlinico, Milano,
Italy

1. Introduction

BD is a prevalent mood disorder, often comorbid with other medical and psychiatric conditions and frequently misdiagnosed (Altamura et al., 2011a). Intense emotional states that occur in BD comprise manic, hypomanic, mixed or depressive episodes. According to the Diagnostic and Statistical Manual of Mental Disorders, IVth edition, text revision (DSM-IV-TR; American Psychiatric Association, 2000), BD spectrum ranges from cyclothymia to Bipolar I, Bipolar II Disorder and Not Otherwise Specified (NOS) forms. BD can also be conceptualized as a gradual change in mood scale, which ranges from severe depression to severe mania with an intermediate euthymic state or balanced mood.

Dysthymia is a chronic state of mild low mood occurring for a minimum of two years. At the other end of the scale there is hypomania and severe mania. An alternative and broader dimensional approach conceptualizes BD as a continuum, between unipolar depression, schizoaffective disorder (which is considered by some authors a subcategory of BD) and schizophrenia. This theory may be supported from a clinical point of view by the fact that, sometimes, during severe manic, mixed or depressive episodes, bipolar patients experience psychotic symptoms, such as hallucinations or delusions. It is also supported by the presence of morphometric alterations of frequent observation among major psychoses, such as enlarged ventricles and white matter volume reductions in the left and temporoparietal regions (Czobor et al., 2007).

In BD, symptomatic states are frequently associated with poor working functioning and social impairment. Bipolar patients, moreover, have higher suicide rates than the general population and among the highest of psychiatric patients. In a recent study on factors predicting suicide in BD, white race, family history of suicide, and previous cocaine abuse were considered predictive of suicidal behaviour (Cassidy, 2011). Usually BD develops in early adulthood/late teens, with an age of onset ranging from 15 to 50 years (Cassano et al., 2006).

International treatment guidelines for BD recommend the use of mood stabilizers - either in monotherapy or in association - as the gold standard in both acute and long-term therapy. The concept of stabilization, in fact, has been stressed as the ultimate objective of the treatment of BD, given the chronic and recurrent nature of the illness, which accounts for its significant levels of impairment and disability (Altamura et al., 2011b). Beyond the aforementioned core mood symptoms and clinical features of BD, over the last decade, neurocognitive dysfunction has been stressed as another nuclear dimension of BD and, possibly, a marker of its underlying pathophysiology (Lewandowski et al., 2010). There is accumulating evidence that individuals with BD have neurocognitive impairment that persists even during euthymia: the degree of impairment is more severe in patients with depressive symptoms, with functions associated with processing speed and attentional control being particularly implicated (Chaves et al., 2011; Van der Werf-Eldering et al., 2010). In addition, in older euthimic adults with BD, resting-state corticolimbic dysregulation was related to sustained attention deficits and inhibitory control, which could reflect the cumulative impact of repeated affective episodes upon cerebral metabolism and neurocognitive performance (Brooks et al., 2011). Cognitive impairment in BD is influenced by the severity of illness (Yates et al., 2010).

In addition, neuropsychological and imaging studies in BD suggested the presence of cognitive deficits and subtle magnetic resonance imaging (MRI) changes in limbic areas that may persist over euthymia. However, other studies are inconsistent with this claim. For example, a recent study did not identify any difference between BD patients and controls in levels of cognition over a two-year period, indicating that BD doesn't have a significant adverse impact on cognition (Delaloye et al., 2011).

Neuroimaging has recently gained an important role both in clinical practice and research of psychiatric disorders, including BD. Structural imaging techniques such as computed tomography (CT), magnetic resonance imaging (MRI) and magnetic resonance spectroscopy (MRS) have contributed to a deeper understanding of the structural changes in the brain in the context of psychiatric disorders. Positron Emission Tomography (PET), Single Photon Emission Computed Tomography (SPECT), Functional Magnetic Resonance Imaging (fMRI) and Diffusion Tensor Imaging (DTI) are techniques which measure changes in response to cognitive demand and/or connectivity between brain regions. As such, these approaches provide an opportunity for investigating the neural bases of behavioural and cognitive impairment in psychiatric populations, including BD.

2. Structural neuroimaging

2.1 Computed Tomography (CT)
In the last two decades, the first important data about neuroanatomic abnormalities in BD were obtained by means of CT. More recently, the widespread use of MRI has brought several advantages over CT, particularly in terms of higher resolution of images of subcortical regions (Steffens, 1998). Although a typical pattern of abnormality has not been identified yet (Supprian, 2004), several brain structures were found to be affected in patients with BD according to imaging studies.

CT provides excellent imaging data and rapid image acquisition at relatively low cost, it is widely available and more easily tolerated by patients, remaining the imaging modality of first choice in many clinical situations (Dougherty et al., 2004).

CT consists of a series of slices or tomograms. Its measurements are performed at the periphery of the body. The image of each slice is acquired by means of an X-ray source and detectors positioned at 180 degrees on the other side of the body. By spinning the source and the detectors on one plane of the head, data are collected from multiple angles. A computer then processes X-ray attenuation measured from different points and uses specific algorithms to create a structural image within the plane. Ionic and non-ionic intravenous

contrasts can be used to improve the visualization of certain normal or abnormal structures (Dougherty et al., 2004).
The measurement of total brain volume and ventricular volumes has been the aim of the first investigations using CT in psychiatric disorders. In this perspective, less consistent results have been found for affective disorders compared to schizophrenia and dementia (Beyer et al., 2002). The limited number of controlled CT studies focused on bipolar patients, in fact, showed heterogeneous findings. These include increased lateral ventricle size compared to controls (Andreasen et al., 1990; Nasrallah et al., 1982; Pearlson et al., 1984) or, in contrast, non significant differences between patients and controls (Dewan et al., 1988; Schlegel et al., 1987; Young et al., 1999). A larger third ventricle has been reported as well (Dewan et al., 1988; Schlegel et al., 1987). Studies on cortical alterations in BD revealed that there was no significant difference between patients and controls with respect to the level of cortical atrophy (Iacono et al., 1988; Rieder et al., 1983; Schlegel et al., 1987). However, a positive correlation between increased cortical sulcal widening and age of onset/age of first manic episode has been observed in bipolar patients in a subsequent study (Young et al., 1999). Volumetric changes in the cerebellum have been also reported, including higher rates of atrophy in bipolar patients (Nasrallah et al., 1982), even though the research of these abnormalities is limited.
In synthesis, some studies using CT in bipolar patients found an increased lateral ventricles size. In addition, cortical atrophy (which was not statistically different from controls), atrophy in the cerebellum as well as a larger third ventricle have also been reported.

2.2 Magnetic Resonance Imaging (MRI)

MRI takes advantage of the magnetic properties of the atomic constituents of the tissues in order to create an image of the different parts of the body. Every MRI scanner has a static magnet; its strength usually ranges from 1.5 to 3 Tesla. A steady magnetic field is generated as an electric current passes through the coils. In order to have a nuclear magnetic resonance signal, only atomic nuclei with unpaired protons and/or neutrons can be used. Medical MRI uses essentially hydrogen (^{1}H) as it is widely diffused in the human body and it has only one proton in its nucleus. Each proton has its own magnetic field or dipole moment, induced by the rotation around its axis. When an externally magnetic field is applied, protons' magnetic dipoles tend to align and to oscillate around the longitudinal axis of the applied field (this phenomenon is called precession) (Dougherty et al., 2004).
An horizontal radio frequency (RF) pulse is applied perpendicularly to the longitudinal axis of the external magnetic field with the aim to create a transverse component to the magnetization vector. This induces the generation of an electric current which is transduced into an MRI image. T1 is the "longitudinal" relaxation time and it indicates the time required to regain longitudinal magnetization following RF pulse. T2 is the "transverse" relaxation time that measures how long the resonating protons precess "in phase" following a 90° RF pulse. Due to the T1 and T2 relaxation properties in MRI, differentiation between various tissues in the body is possible (Jezzard et al., 2001).
Despite intensive research, to date no pathognomonic structural MRI finding has been correlated with affective disorders in general and to BD in particular. There are many heterogeneous data (Table 1) revealing a variety of structural alterations in bipolar patients (Dougherty et al., 2004). It must be considered, moreover, that some of these differences may be referred to the effects of medications (Van der Schot, 2009). For instance, chronic lithium treatment may prevent volume loss in treated patients because of its neuroprotective action

(Manji et al., 2000). Furthermore, genetic and/or environmental factors involved in BD may influence some brain abnormalities. In this perspective, decreases in white matter have been associated with the genetic risk of developing BD, whereas important environmental correlations have been found in relation to cortical gray matter volume (Van der Schot, 2009).

Brain abnormalities reported by fMRI studies in patients with BD include changes in cortical volumes, cerebral white matter, cortical and prefrontal gray matter. Enlargement of the ventricles, dimensional modifications of the amygdala, nuclei of the basal ganglia, corpus callosum and cerebellum have also been detected.

Main findings on lobar volumes concern frontal, temporal and insular cortex. Results on frontal lobes are quite discordant. In fact, they were found to be smaller (Coffman et al., 1990; Schlaepfer et al., 1994) or of the same size as controls (Strakowski et al., 1999). With respect to temporal lobes, no differences (Johnstone et al. 1989), bilateral reduction of volume (Altshuler et al., 1991) or loss of normal symmetry were found. Even in terms of loss of symmetry of the temporal lobes findings were sometimes discordant. In fact, a study reported a larger right temporal lobe than the left one in male bipolar patients (Swayze et al., 1992) and another study observed a larger left temporal lobe (Harvey et al., 1994). Voxel-based morphometric (VBM) MRI studies showed an increased gray matter in the insular cortex (Lochhead et al., 2004) or non significant differences in this region (McDonald et al., 2005; Nugent et al., 2006; Scherk et al., 2008a). An inverse correlation has been observed between the volume of the anterior insular cortex and the lifetime number of depressive episodes (Takahashy, 2010).

Bipolar patients, in particular those with late onset, were found to have a higher incidence of subcortical hypertensities (Dupont et al., 1990; Figiel et al., 1991; McDonald et al., 1991; Norris et al., 1997; Soares & Mann, 1997; Stoll et al., 2000; Swayze et al.,1990; Videbech, 1997). On the other hand, another study (Botteron & Figiel, 1997) identified an increased rate of white matter hyperintensity in relatively young individuals.

Lateral ventricular enlargement has been observed in BD and associated with multiple episodes of mania (Strakowski et al., 2002). A larger third ventricle was reported in elderly depressive patients and in cases of first manic episode (Strakowski et al., 1993). Likewise, correlations have been found between third ventricle volume and psychotic symptoms, advanced age, late onset of the disease, male gender and positive dexamethasone suppression test (Benabarre et al., 2002).

Studies on alterations of the amygdala in bipolar patients reported heterogeneous results, showing normal (Swayze et al., 1992), smaller (Pearlson et al., 1997) or larger volumes (Altshuler et al., 1998). More recent studies documented an increased volume in the right amygdala (Bremner et al., 2000), in bilateral amygdala in first episode subjects (Frodl et al., 2002) and loss of normal symmetry (Mervaala et al., 2000). The heterogeneity of the adult studies may be referred to the different age of subjects. It is still unclear, however, the positive correlation between increased amygdala volume and age (Usher, 2010).

A greater caudate volume as well as asymmetries among the structures of the basal ganglia were found in male bipolar patients (Aylward et al., 1994). Another study focused on the caudate volume in manic subjects in their first episode, reporting no significant differences vs healthy controls (Strakowski et al., 1999). The alterations may be attributed to a secondary effect of neuroleptic drugs (Benabarre et al., 2002). Studies examining alterations of the corpus callosum found volume reduction in bipolar patients, correlated with greater global neuropsychological dysfunction (Coffman et al., 1990). Finally, significant reduction of the cerebellar posterior vermis area was reported in patients with BD (DelBello et al., 1999).

Central nervous system structure involved	Main MRI alterations in BD
Frontal lobes	Reduced or unchanged volume
Temporal lobes	Reduced or unchanged volume Loss of the symmetry
Insular cortex	Increased gray matter or no changes
Subcortical areas	Increased hyperintensities
Lateral ventricles	Increased (association with number of episodes of mania)
Third ventricle	Increased
Amygdala	Larger, smaller or unchanged volume Loss of normal symmetry
Caudate nucleus	Increased or unchanged volume
Corpus callosum	Reduced volume
Cerebellar posterior vermis	Reduced

Table 1. Main MRI findings in BD.

2.3 Magnetic Resonance Spectroscopy

Magnetic Resonance Spectroscopy (MRS) is an MRI complement and serves as a non-invasive tool for tissue characterization. While MRI uses the signal from hydrogen protons to create a visual representation of the tissues, proton MRS (^{1}H- MRS) uses this information to determine the concentration of brain metabolites such as N-acetyl aspartate, choline, creatine and lactate in the examined tissue (Gujar et al., 2005).

MRS has been principally used for the diagnosis of some metabolic disorders, especially those of the central nervous system. MRS has not an optimal specificity, but in association with MRI and clinical data can be very helpful. Indeed, the main purpose of this technique is to obtain biochemical information from any part of the body in a non invasive way, i.e. not by means of radioactive tracers or electromagnetic radiation (Dougherty et al., 2004).

In psychiatry, MRS can be employed to assess the activity of different neurotransmitters, membrane and second messenger metabolism. The uniqueness of MRS is to provide an overview of the biochemical pathology of BD. Studies using proton MRS (^{1}H- MRS) reported increased glutamate and GLX (glutamate, GABA and glutamine) levels in the dorsolateral prefrontal cortex, frontal lobes, basal ganglia and gray matter of medication-free bipolar subjects and in patients with acute mania (Yildiz-Yesiloglu & Ankerst, 2006). Abnormal levels of N-acetyl aspartate, choline and myo-inositol have also been reported (Scherk et al., 2008b). N-acetyl aspartate seems to be reduced in the prefrontal cortex and hippocampus in bipolar individuals. Choline levels were found to be increased in the striatum and anterior cingulate cortex and can be normalized or decreased after treatment with antidepressants and lithium (Moore et al., 2000). Myo-inositol levels were increased in individuals with mania and euthymia and, on the contrary, reduced in bipolar depression.

Studies using phosphorus MRS (^{31}P- MRS) have found phase-specific alterations of phospholipid membranes, high energy phosphates and intracellular brain pH in BD. In particular, a number of investigations reported a reduced intracellular cerebral pH in bipolar subjects which has been associated with the increased levels of lactate observed in some ^{1}H- MRS studies. Both conditions are indicative of a shift from oxidative phosphorylation to glycolysis. There is also a ^{31}P- MRS based-report of decreased levels of phosphocreatine and of phosphomonoesters in BD (Kato et al., 1995).

Stork and Renshaw proposed a cohesive model that puts together the majority of MRS findings. They hypothesized that the impaired oxidative phopshorilation, the decreased cellular energy and the altered membrane metabolism could be due to an underlying altered mitochondrial metabolism in BD (Stork & Renshaw, 2005).

Main MRS findings in BD are synthetized in Table 2.

Technique		Main alterations
^{1}H- MRS	N- acetyl aspartate	Reduced levels
	Choline	Increased levels
	Glutamate, GABA and Glutamine	Increased levels
	Myo-inositol	Increased levels in mania and euthymia and reduced levels in bipolar depression
	Lactate	Increased levels
^{31}P- MRS	Phosphocreatine	Reduced levels
	Phosphomonoesters	Reduced levels
	Intracellular brain pH	Reduced levels

Table 2. Main MRS findings in BD.

3. Functional neuroimaging

The major limitation of structural neuroimaging techniques is that they are suitable for studying diseases associated with morphologic alterations, such as neurologic conditions. For this reason, they are only partially useful in psychiatric disorders which are characterized by behavioral abnormalities due to neurochemical impairment. In this perspective, PET (Abraham & Feng, 2011) and fMRI represent the gold standard for brain imaging aimed to assess cognitive performance (Glower, 2011). Electroencefalography, Event-Related Potentials and Magnetoencephalography are less specific and, therefore, mostly used to exclude neurological conditions in clinical practice or for research purposes (Cohen & Cuffin, 1983). Medication, drug or alcohol abuse and genetic/epigenetic influence represent major confounding factors (Nakama et al., 2011; Schulte et al., 2010). On the other side, following the biopsychosocial model for psychiatric disorders, functional neuroimaging could help understanding the complex interaction between environmental stressors, genetic risk and precipitating events in the plasticity of neural circuitry and consequently in clinical symptoms.

Functional neuroimaging attempts to explain psychiatric disorders by means of degenerative or developmental model of illness and/or in terms of hypometabolism. In fact, elevated activity of the hippocampus or of the ventral prefrontal cortex as well as dorsolateral prefrontal cortex hypofunction are recurrent themes in literature (Savitz & Drevets, 2009).

3.1 Positron Emission Tomography (PET) and Single Photon Emission Computed Tomography (SPECT)

PET imaging is a direct measure of a radioactive decay due to cerebral metabolism of a radioactive substance or radionuclide. Different body tissues are characterized by different consumption rates of radionuclides (Ter-Pogossian et al., 1975; Vyas et al., 2011). Radionuclides used in clinical practice are usually major compounds of biologic molecules (18-Fluorine in the form of 18-Fluorodeoxyglucose or FDG for measuring glucose metabolism, 15-Oxygen for measuring blood flow, 11-Carbon or 13-Nitrogen common in diagnostic PET procedures). The nuclide is introduced in the patient and the radioactive decay is measured (Phelps et al., 1975): in particular, the positron emitted by nuclides has a collision with electrons producing a gamma photon which is measured by the PET camera (Roncali & Cherry, 2011). PET can measure both blood flow and glucose metabolism, often used as surrogate measures of neuronal synaptic activity. A first line comparison is between the neuroligand uptake in target regions and reference area while a more complex analysis can compare blood flow or glucose uptake in the same subject in different states, i.e. while resting or during a cognitive performance. Both ways provide useful data for research and clinical analysis; anyway, a major limitation is the use of a radioactive nuclide. Specifically, targeted PET radioligands are used to investigate neurotransmitter systems (Weisel, 1989). Cerebral PET has its major use in neurological disease: excluding primary or secondary oncologic lesions, evaluation of dementia, confirming epilepsy or assessing the state in cerebrovascular disease (Cavalcanti et al., 2011; Mazzuca et al., 2011; Person et al., 2010; Quigley et al., 2010; Salas and Gonzales, 2011).

SPECT works capturing orbiting electrons without a positron-electron collision, but by means of an emission of a single photon by the SPECT nuclide. Main nuclides used in SPECT are 123-Iodine, 33-Technetium or 133-Xenon. Single photons are selected with the use of multiple collimators.

PET and SPECT studies in depressive disorders have shown that blood rate and flow are increased both in BD and in unipolar depression in the frontal lobes during depressive episodes. However, they are increased during mania in the dorsal cingulate cortex, striatal regions, and the nucleus accumbens, as well as in limbic structures of the temporal lobes and reduced in dorsolateral prefrontal cortex, possibly reflecting its loss of modulatory control over limbic structures (Gonul et al., 2009).

With respect to neurotransmitters, serotonin (5-HT) transporter was found to have an increased density in the thalamus (Laje et al., 2010), dorsal cingulate cortex, medial prefrontal cortex and insula of depressed BD patients. 5-HT has been implicated in mania as well: in particular, individuals with current mania had significantly lower 5-HT2 receptor binding potential in frontal, temporal, parietal and occipital cortical regions, with more prominent changes in the right cortical regions compared to controls (Yatham et al., 2010, 2002a, 2002b). With regards to 5-HT1A receptor, bipolar depressed patients were found to show higher 5-HT1A in raphe nuclei and forebrain (Sullivan et al., 2009). An interesting use of PET consists of assessing the role of serotonin in major depressive episodes comparing

BD vs unipolar depression. In fact, both unipolar and bipolar depression were associated with elevated 5-HT transporter binding in the insula, thalamus and striatum, but showed distinct abnormalities in the brainstem (Cannon et al., 2007).

With respect to dopamine, D1 receptor binding potentials were found to be reduced in frontal cortex, even though striatal D2 receptor density was normal in all phases of non-psychotic BD (Bauer, 2003; Suhara et al., 1992).

In synthesis, PET and SPECT studies have shown in BD a loss of modulatory control of the cortex over limbic structures, reflected by specific phase-dependent modifications of blood rate and flow. Alterations of neurotransmitters involved in the pathogenesis of BD have also been reported, particularly with respect to serotonin transporter, serotonin receptor density and dopamine receptor density.

3.2 Functional Magnetic Resonance Imaging (fMRI)

FMRI is the most used technique in brain mapping and in psychiatric research due to its non-invasive technology, wide availability, high spatial and temporal resolution and the lack of ionizing radiation that allows the clinician to repeat functional exams over time as well as in different phases of illness. FMRI, in fact, is suitable for studying bipolar patients' performances on the same cognitive tasks during depressed, manic or euthymic phases. It can also compare brain activity during symptom exacerbation as well as over periods of remission.

One limit of fMRI is that it gives limited information on subcortical structures. Spatial resolution remains anyway highly relevant for the study of psychiatric diseases, given the clear correlation between cortical dysfunction and many psychiatric symptoms. Another limit consists of the increased variance of the results obtained with this technique in psychiatric patients (Dougherty et al., 2004).

FMRI measures changes in blood flow in areas of the central nervous system (Konarsky et al., 2007). The hemodynamic response reflects neural activity in the brain or spinal cord as neurons have no reserve for oxygen or glucose and they need to rapidly increase blood flow when necessary. A Blood-oxygen-level dependent (BOLD) signal is measured by fMRI. From a physiological perspective, hemoglobin is diamagnetic when oxygenated (oxyhemoglobin) and paramagnetic when deoxygenated (deoxyhemoglobin) producing different signals that are higher when coming from activated areas. Actually, an increase in cerebral blood flow produces changes in oxygen consumption resulting in increased BOLD signals (Bandettini, 2003).

Studies with fMRI in bipolar patients showed various alterations of the activity in different regions of the cortico-limbic pathways responsible for emotional regulation: amygdala, thalamus, striatum, portions of the prefrontal cortex and anterior cingulated cortex. Studies, however, were limited by the small samples size and by the possible interference of the medication. The increased activation of amygdala, striatum and thalamus were the most constant findings among the different studies (Cerullo et al., 2009).

Increased amygdala and subcortical activity to emotional stimuli, in particular negative stimuli, as well as reduced activity of the prefrontal cortical regions during cognitive performances are common to all phases of BD, suggesting that they may be trait features of the disease (Phillips & Vieta, 2007). Other additional frontal and temporal regions were found to be activated, maybe as a compensatory mechanism (Townsed et al., 2010).

FMRI studies in bipolar patients also suggest the presence of phase-dependent abnormalities. In fact, bipolar depression is associated with attenuated bilateral orbitofrontal or elevated left orbitofrontal activity. Right dorsolateral prefrontal cortical activity was found to be reduced, while the increased left prefrontal activity seems to be a state marker of bipolar depression (Altshuler et al., 2008).

The few studies with fMRI on manic patients report an increased activity of the amygdala, insular cortex and subcortical areas in response to negative emotional stimuli. Ventral striatal activity was found to be elevated at rest and during motor tasks. On the other hand, ventral prefrontal activity was found to be attenuated during cognitive performances (Altshuler et al., 2005; Elliott et al., 2004). In addition, bilateral orbitofrontal attenuation has been reported in mania and may represent a trait feature of the disorder as it is also present during bipolar depression (Altshuler et al., 2008).

BD Phase	Central nervous system structures involved	Main fMRI alterations
Bipolar depression	Orbitofrontal cortex	Activity reduced bilaterally or increased on the left
	Prefrontal cortex	Reduced right activity; Increased left activity
Mania	Amygdala Insula Subcortical areas	Increased activity in response to negative stimuli
	Ventral prefrontal cortex	Reduced activity during cognitive performances
	Orbitofrontal cortex	Reduced activity bilaterally
Euthymia	Ventral prefrontal cortex Anterior cingulate gyrus	Reduced activity during attentional tasks
	Dorsolateral prefrontal cortex	Increased (i.e. during attentional tasks) or reduced activity (i.e. in response to fearful stimuli, during working memory tasks)
	Subcortical areas	Increased activity during performance or working memory tasks
	Amygdala	Increased activity in response to fearful stimuli
	Striatum	Increased activity in response to fearful stimuli; Significantly increased activity in response to reward stimuli

Table 3. Main fMRI findings in BD.

Findings on euthymic bipolar patients are more consistent and have pointed out reduced activity in dorsal, ventral prefrontal cortical regions and dorsal regions of the anterior cingulate gyrus during performance of attentional tasks. Dorsolateral prefrontal cortical activity was found to be, on the contrary, increased. Other studies have reported reduced dorsolateral prefrontal cortex activity in euthymic individuals during working memory and verbal encoding tasks (Deckersbach et al, 2006; Monks et al., 2004). Increases in activity within subcortical regions associated with emotion processing rather than working memory or attention have also been detected in remitted, euthymic individuals with BD during performance of a continuous performance task (Strakowski et al., 2004) and working memory task (Adler et al., 2004). Other studies investigated the response of the activity of these structures to fearful expressions in remitted bipolar patients. Results showed an increased activity in the amygdala and in the striatum and, on the other hand, a reduction of the dorsolateral prefrontal cortex activity (Phillips & Vieta, 2007). Of note, striatal activity in response to potentially rewarding stimuli was found to be significantly elevated. Other emotional stimuli led to decreased dorsolateral prefrontal cortical activity. These two patterns may underlie mood instabilities in euthymic patients, especially in those with comorbidities (Hassel et al., 2008).

In synthesis, fMRI findings in bipolar patients are heterogeneous: they may be present in all phases of BD and/or can be phase-dependent. Among the formers, the most significant data include an increased activity of the amygdala and of the subcortical areas to negative stimuli and a reduced activity of the prefrontal cortex during cognitive tasks. Bipolar depression has been associated with modifications of the activity of the orbitofrontal and prefrontal cortex. In mania, specific alterations include an increased activity of the striatum at rest and during motor tasks and a reduction of the prefrontal cortex activity during cognitive performances. There are several studies on euthymic patients showing modifications of the activity of the prefrontal cortex during attentional or working memory tasks. Structures implicated in the emotional processing seem to be involved as well: in fact, modifications of the activity of the amygdala, striatum and dorsolateral prefrontal cortex in response to different emotional stimuli have been reported.

3.3 Diffusion Tensor Imaging (DTI)

Diffusion tensor imaging (DTI) is an MRI application developed in order to investigate white matter connections between regions of interest. These connections provide information on functional activity between areas of the central nervous system. DTI is particularly useful to detect white matter lesions or dysfunction (Versace et al., 2008).

There are few studies with DTI in BD, most of them based on the promising results from MRI research showing microstructural alterations in white matter in various neocortical areas and in the corpus callosum. In particular, fractional anisotropy, the most sensitive DTI marker which reflects fiber density, axonal diameter and myelination in white matter, was found to be decreased significantly in the ventral part of the corpus callosum in patients with BD (Heller et al., 2011). Other interesting results coming from DTI revealed that gray matter concentration was reduced in BD in the right anterior insula, head of the caudate nucleus, nucleus accumbens, ventral putamen and frontal orbital cortex. Other studies pointed out that BD patients showed abnormalities within white matter tracts connecting the frontal cortex with the temporal and parietal cortices and the fronto-subcortical circuits (Lin et al., 2011). White matter abnormalities seem to persist by the time of remission even after the first manic episodes (Chan et al., 2010), suggesting that disruption of white matter cortical-subcortical networks as well as projection, associative and commissural tracts may be a hallmark of the illness (Heng et al., 2010) involving prefrontal and frontal regions, associative and commissural fibres.

Some recent studies reported that certain variants of BD may be due to an increased functional or effective connectivity between orbitofrontal and temporal pole structures in the dominant hemisphere. The orbitofrontal cortex codifies the value of different stimuli, allowing goal and sub-goal structuring. Moreover, it is involved in reward prediction. On the other hand, the temporal pole seems to be activated in basic semantic processes with person-emotion linkages associated with narrative. BD patients have a deficit of performance on visuospatial and constructional praxis which suggests an atypical localization of cognitive functions. This atypical localization and the hyperconnectivity between specific regions could be responsible for the enhanced creativity and writing ability observed in BD probands (McCrea, 2008).

Recently, abnormalities in perigenual anterior cingulate cortex-amygdala functional connectivity during emotional processing have been found in BD (Wang et al., 2009). Similar findings have been reported even in children and adolescents with BD, concluding that in these subjects significant white matter tract alterations were present in regions involved in emotional, behavioural and cognitive regulation. In addition, these results suggest that alterations in white matter are present early in the course of disease in familial BD (Barnea-Goraly et al., 2009; Kavafaris et al., 2009). An impaired fiber density in anterior corona radiata (as detected with a decreased fractional anisotropy) was detected in BD in pediatric age and in Attention Deficit and Hyperactivity Disorder suggesting a possible link between the two disorders (Pavuluri et al., 2008).

DTI studies can allow to detect a possible overlap between BD and schizophrenia. In fact, reduced integrity of the anterior limb of the internal capsule, uncinate fasciculus and anterior thalamic radiation regions is common to both schizophrenia and BD suggesting an overlap in white matter pathology, possibly relating to risk factors common to both disorders (Sussman et al., 2008).

Concerning antidepressants and mood stabilizers, these compounds seem to have neuroprotective effects and are not likely to explain white matter abnormalities, even though minor effects cannot be excluded (Bruno et al., 2008). Anyway, microstructural abnormality in the white matter has been associated with a low remission rate of major depression.

In synthesis, DTI provides information on functional connectivity between regions of the central nervous system. DTI studies on bipolar probands showed a reduced gray matter in areas such as putamen, caudate nucleus, nucleus acumbens, insula and orbitofrontal cortex. As concerns white matter, connections between orbitofrontal cortex, temporal, parietal corteces and the frontosubcortical circuits were found to be altered during mania and also over euthymia, as possible traits of BD. DTI findings have interesting implications on the association between BD and creativity. The hyperconnectivity between specific regions and the atypical localization of cognitive functions seem to be correlated to the enhanced creativity and writing ability of BD subjects. On the other hand, the atypical localization of cognitive functions could underlie the visuoconstructional praxis deficit present in BD.

4. Conclusions

Since the introduction of CT, researchers focused their efforts in elucidating the connection between psychiatric diseases and the presence of structural cerebral alterations through neuroimaging. CT pioneered this research without providing, however, a complete answer. Actually, a growing body of evidence has been accumulated in literature as newer techniques such as MRI and functional imaging (i.e., SPECT, PET, fMRI) have been introduced revealing much about the biological underpinnings of neuropsychiatric disorders. Neuroimaging research in BD has already produced several data documenting the involvement of different cortical and subcortical regions in different phases of the illness. In particular, published studies explored structural and functional abnormalities present in BD and tried to establish specific correlations with outcome (Moore et al., 2001; Wingo et al., 2009, Bearden, 2010) as well as difficult-to-treat conditions such as treatment resistant forms (Regenold et al., 2008).

The possibility to study cognitive function in BD through fMRI represents another major acquisition of neuroimaging in psychiatric research. The attainment of this goal can be facilitated by identifying biomarkers reflecting pathophysiologic processes in BD, namely impaired emotion regulation, impaired attention, and distractibility, which persist during depression and remission and are not common to unipolar depression (Phillips & Vieta, 2007).

5. References

Abraham T., Feng J. (2011). Evolution of brain imaging instrumentation. *Seminars in nuclear medicine*, Vol. 41, No.3, (May 2011), ISSN 0001-2998

Adler, C.M., Holland, S.K., Schmithorst, V., Tuchfarber, M.J., Strakowsky, S.M. (2004). Changes in neuronal activation in patients with bipolar disorder during performance of a working memory task. *Bipolar Disorders*, Vol.6, No.6, (December 2004), pp. 540–549, ISSN 1398-5647

Altamura, A.C., Serati, M., Albano, A., Paoli, R.A., Glick, I.D., & Dell'Osso, B. (2011). An epidemiologic and clinical overview of medical and psychopathological comorbidities in major psychoses. *European Archives of Psychiatry and Clinical Neuroscience*, (February 2011), epub ahead of print (a)

Altamura, A.C., Lietti, L., Dobrea, C., Benatti, B., Arici, C., & Dell'Osso, B. (2011). Mood stabilizers for patients with bipolar disorder: the state of the art. *Expert Review of Neurotherapeutics*, Vol.11, No.1, (January 2011), pp. 85-99, ISSN 1473-7175 (b)

Altshuler, L., Bookheimer, S., Townsend, J., Proenza, M.A., Sabb, F., Mintz, J., & Cohen, M.S. (2008). Regional brain changes in bipolar I depression: a functional magnetic resonance imaging study. *Bipolar Disorders*, Vol.10, No.6, (September 2008), pp. 708-17, ISSN 1398-5647

Altshuler, L., Bookheimer, S., Proenza, M.A., Townsend, J., Sabb, F., Firestine, A., Bartzokis, G., Mintz, J., Mazziotta, J., Cohen, M.S. (2005). Increased amygdala activation during mania: a functional magnetic resonance imaging study. *The American Journal of Psychiatry*, Vol.162, No.6, (June 2005), pp. 1211–1213, ISSN 0002-953X

Altshuler, L.L, Conrad, A., Hauser, P., Li, X.M., Guze, B.H., Denikoff, K., Tourtellotte, W., Post, R. (1991). Reduction of temporal lobe volume in bipolar disorder: A preliminary report of magnetic resonance imaging. *Archives of General Psychiatry*, Vol.48, No.5, (May 1991), pp. 482–483, ISSN 0003-990X

Altshuler, L.L., Bartzokis, G., Grieder, T., Curran, J., & Mintz, J. (1998). Amygdala enlargement in bipolar disorder and hippocampal reduction in schizophrenia: An MRI study demonstrating neuroanatomic specificity. *Archives of General Psychiatry*, Vol.55, No.7, (July 1998), pp. 663–664, ISSN 0003-990X

Andreasen, N.C., Swayze, V., Flaum, M., Alliger, R., & Cohen, G. (1990). Ventricular abnormalities in affective disorder: clinical and demographic correlates. *The American Journal of Psychiatry*, Vol.147, No.7, (July 1990), pp. 893-900, ISSN 0002-953X

Bandettini P.A. (2003). Functional MRI, In: *Handbook of Neuropsychology*, Vol. 9, J. Grafman and I.H. Robertson, ISBN 9780444503664, UK

Barnea-Goraly, N., Chang, K.D., Karchemskiy, A., Howe, M.E., & Reiss, A.L. (2009). Limbic and corpus callosum aberrations in adolescents with BD: a tract-based spatial statistics analysis. *Biological Psychiatry*, Vol.66, No.3, (August 2009), pp. 238-44, ISSN 0006-3223

Bauer, M., London, E.D., Silverman, D.H., Rasgon, N., Kirchheiner, J., & Whybrow, P.C. (2003). Thyroid, brain and mood modulation in affective disorder: insights from molecular research and functional brain imaging. *Pharmacopsychiatry*, Vol.36, Suppl.3, (November 2003), pp. 215-21, ISSN 0176-3679

Bearden, C.E., Woogen, M., & Glahn, D.C. (2010). Neurocognitive and Neuroimaging Predictors of Clinical Outcome in bipolar disorder. *Current Psychiatry Reports*, Vol.12, No.6, (December 2010), pp. 499–504, ISSN 1523-3812

Beyer, J.L., & Krishnan, K.R. (2002). Volumetric brain imaging findings in mood disorders. *Bipolar Disorders*, Vol.4, No.2, (April 2002), pp. 89-104, ISSN 1398-5647

Botteron, K.N., & Figiel, G.S. (1997). The neuromorphometry of affective disorders, In: *Brain Imaging in Clinical Psychiatry*, Krishnan, K.R., Doraiswamy, P.M.(Eds.), 145–184, M. Dekker, ISBN 0824798597 , New York, USA.

Bremner, J.D., Narayan, M., Anderson, E.R., Staib, L.H., Miller, H.L., Charney, D.S. (2000). Hippocampal volume reduction in major depression. *The American Journal of Psychiatry*, Vol.157, No.1, (January 2000), pp. 115–118, ISSN 0002-953X

Brooks, J.O., Bearden, C.E., Hoblyn, J.C., Woodard, S.A., & Ketter, T.A. (2010). Prefrontal and paralimbic metabolic dysregulation related to sustained attention in euthymic older adults with BD. *Bipolar Disorders*, Vol.12, No.8, (December 2010), pp. 866-74, ISSN 1398-5647

Bruno, S., Cercignani, M., & Ron, M.A. (2008). White matter abnormalities in bipolar disorder: a voxel-based diffusion tensor imaging study. *Bipolar Disorders*, Vol.10, No.4, (June 2008), pp. 460-8, ISSN 1398-5647

Cannon, D.M., Ichise, M., Rollis, D., Klaver, J.M., Gandhi, S.K., Charney, D.S., Manji, H.K., & Drevets, W.C. (2007). Elevated serotonin transporter binding in major depressive disorder assessed using positron emission tomography and [11C]DASB; comparison with bipolar disorder. *Biological Psychiatry*, Vol.62, No.8, (October 2007), pp. 870-877, ISSN 0006-3223

Cassano G.B., Tundo A. (2006). *Psicopatologia e clinica psichiatrica*. Edizione UTET. ISBN 8802071942. Torino, Italia.

Cassidy, F. (2011). Risk factors of attempted suicide in bipolar disorder. *Suicide and Life-Threatening Behavior*, Vol.41, No.1, (February 2011), pp. 6-11, ISSN 0363-0234

Cavalcanti Filho, J.L., de Souza Leão Lima, R., de Souza Machado Neto, L., Kayat Bittencourt, L., Domingues, R.C., & da Fonseca, L.M. (2011). PET/CT and vascular disease: Current concepts. *European Journal of Radiology*, (March 2011), epub ahead of print.

Cerullo, M.A., Adler, C.M., Delbello, M.P., & Strakowski, S.M. (2009). The functional neuroanatomy of bipolar disorder. *International Review of Psychiatry*, Vol.21, No.4, (2009), pp. 314-22, ISSN 0954-0261

Chan, W.Y., Yang, G.L., Chia, M.Y., Woon, P.S., Lee, J., Keefe, R., Sitoh, Y.Y., Nowinski, W.L., & Sim, K. (2010). Cortical and subcortical white matter abnormalities in adults with remitted first-episode mania revealed by Tract-Based Spatial Statistics. *Bipolar Disorders*, Vol.12, No.4, (June 2010), pp. 383-389, ISSN 1398-5647

Chaves, O.C., Lombardo, L.E., Bearden, C.E., Woolsey, M.D., Martinez, D.M., Barrett J., A., Miller, A.L., Velligan, D.I., & Glahn, D.C. (2011). Association of clinical symptoms and neurocognitive performance in bipolar disorder: a longitudinal study. *Bipolar Disorders*, Vol.13, No.1, (February 2011), pp. 118-23, ISSN 1398-5647

Coffman, J.A., Bornstein, R.A., Olson, S.C., Schwarzkopf, S.B., & Nasrallah, H.A. (1990). Cognitive impairment and cerebral structure by MRI in bipolar disorder. *Biological Psychiatry*, Vol. 27, No.11, (June 1990), pp. 1188–1196, ISSN 0006-3223

Cohen D., Cuffin B.N. (1983). Demonstration of useful differences between magnetoencephalogram and electroencephalogram. *Electroencephalography and Clinical Neurophysiology,* Vol. 56, No.1, (July 1983), pp.38-51, ISSN 0013-4694

Czobor, P., Jaeger, J., Berns, S.M., Gonzalez, C., & Loftus, S. (2007). Neuropsychological symptom dimensions in bipolar disorder and schizophrenia. *Bipolar disorders*, Vol.9, No.1-2, (February-March 2007), pp. 71-92, ISSN 1398-5647

Deckersbach, T., Dougherty, D.D., Savage, C., McMurrich, S., Fischman, A.J., Nierenberg, A., Sachs, G., & Rauch, S.L. (2006). Impaired recruitment of the dorsolateral prefrontal cortex and hippocampus during encoding in bipolar disorder. *Biological Psychiatry*, Vol.59, No.2, (January 2006)), pp. 138–146, ISSN 0006-3223

Delaloye, C., Moy, G., de Bilbao, F., Weber, K., Baudois, S., Haller, S., Xekardaki, A., Canuto, A., Giardini, U., Lövblad, K.O., Gold, G., & Giannakopoulos, P. (2011). Longitudinal analysis of cognitive performances and structural brain changes in late-life bipolar disorder. *International Journal of Geriatric Psychiatry*, (March 2011), epub ahead of print.

DelBello, M.P., Strakowski, S.M., Zimmermann, M.E., Hawkins, J.M., & Sax, K.W. (1999). MRI analysis of the cerebellum in bipolar disorder: a pilot study. *Neuropsychopharmacology*, Vol.21, No.1, (July 1999), pp. 63–68, ISSN 0893-133X

Dewan, M.J., Haldipur, C.V., Lane, E.E., Ispahani, A., Boucher, M.F., & Major, L.F. (1988). Bipolar affective disorder: I. Comprehensive quantitative computed tomography. *Acta Psychiatrica Scandinavica*, Vol.77, No.6, (June 1988), pp. 670-682, ISSN 0001-690X

Dougherty, D.D., Rauch, S.L., Rosenbaum, J.F. (2004). *Essentials of Neuroimaging for Clinical Practice.* American Psychiatric Publishing, ISBN 1-58562-079-3. Arlington, Virginia, USA

Elliott, R. (2004). Abnormal ventral frontal response during performance of an affective go/no go task in patients with mania. *Biological Psychiatry*, Vol.55, No.12, (June 2004), pp. 1163–1170, ISSN 0006-3223

Frodl, T., Meisenzahl, E., Zetzsche, T., Bottlelender, R., Born, C., Groll, C., Jäger, M., Leinsinger, G., Hahn, K., Möller, H.J. (2002). Enlargement of the amygdala in patients with a first episode of major depression. *Biological Psychiatry*, Vol.51, No.9, (May 2002), pp. 708–714, ISSN 0006-3223

Glover G.H. (2011). Overview of functional magnetic resonance imaging. *Neurosurgery Clinics of North America,* Vol.22, No.2, (April 2011), ISSN 1042-3680

Gonul, A.S., Coburn, K., & Kula, M. (2009). Cerebral blood flow, metabolic, receptor, and transporter changes in bipolar disorder: the role of PET and SPECT studies. *International Review of Psychiatry*, Vol.21, No.4, (2009), pp. 323-335, ISSN 0954-0261

Gujar, S.K., Maheshwari, S., Björkman-Burtscher, I., & Sundgren, P.C. (2005). Magnetic resonance spectroscopy. *J Neuroophthalmol*, Vol.25, No.3, (September 2005), pp. 217-226, ISSN 1070-8022

Haller, S., Xekardaki, A., Delaloye, C., Canuto, A., Lövblad, K.O., Gold, G., & Giannakopoulos, P. (2011). Combined analysis of grey matter voxel-based morphometry and white matter tract-based spatial statistics in late-life bipolar disorder. *Journal of Psychiatry Neuroscience*, Vol.36, No.1, (January 2011), pp 100140, ISSN 1180-4882

Harvey, I., Persaud, R., Ron, M.A., Baker, G., & Murray, R.M. (1994). Volumetric MRI measurements in bipolars compared with schizophrenics and healthy controls. *Psychological Medicine*, Vol.24, No.3, (August 1994), pp. 689–699, ISSN 0033-2917

Hassel, S., Almeida, J.R., Kerr, N., Nau, S., Ladouceur, C.D., Fissell, K., Kupfer, D.J., & Phillips, M.L. (2008). Elevated striatal and decreased dorsolateral prefrontal cortical activity in response to emotional stimuli in euthymic BD: no associations with psychotropic medication load. *Bipolar disorders*, Vol.10, No.8, (December 2008), pp. 916-927, ISSN 1398-5647

Heng, S., Song, A.W., Sim, K. (2010). White matter abnormalities in bipolar disorder: insights from diffusion tensor imaging studies. *Journal of Neural Transmission*, Vol.117, No.5, (May 2010), pp. 639-54, ISSN 0300-9564

Iacono, W.G., Smith, G.N., Moreau, M., Beiser, M., Fleming, J.A.E., Lin, T., & Flak, B. (1988). Ventricular and sulcal size at the onset of psychosis. *The American Journal of Psychiatry*, Vol.145, No.7, (July 1988), pp. 820–824, ISSN 0002-953X

Jezzard P., Matthews P.M., Smith S.M. (2001) *Functional MRI: An Introduction to Methods.* Oxford University Press, pp. 6-8, ISBN 0 19 263071 7, New York, USA

Johnstone, E.C., Owens, D.G., Crow, T.J., Frith, C.D., Alexandropolis, K., Bydder, G., & Colter, N. (1989). Temporal lobe structure as determined by nuclear magnetic resonance in schizophrenia and bipolar affective disorder. *Journal of Neurology, Neurosurgery & Psychiatry*, Vol.52, No.6, (June 1989), pp. 736-741, ISSN 0022-3050

Kafantaris, V., Kingsley, P., Ardekani, B., Saito, E., Lencz, T., Lim, K., & Szeszko, P. (2009). Lower orbital frontal white matter integrity in adolescents with bipolar I disorder. *Journal of the American Academy of Child & Adolescent Psychiatry*, Vol.48, No.1, (January 2009), pp. 79-86, ISSN 0021-9630

Kato, T., Shioiri, T., Murashita, J., Hamakawa, H., Inubushi, T., Takahashi, S. (1995). Lateralized abnormality of high-energy phosphate and bilateral reduction of phosphomonoester measured by phosphorus-31 magnetic resonance spectroscopy of the frontal lobes in schizophrenia. *Psychiatry Research*, Vol.61, No.3, (September 2005), pp. 151-160, ISSN 0022-3956

Konarski, J.Z., McIntyre, R.S., Soczynska, J.K., & Kennedy, S.H. (2007). Neuroimaging approaches in mood disorders: technique and clinical implications. *Annals of Clinical Psychiatry*, Vol.19, No.4, (October-December 2007), pp. 265-277, ISSN 1040-1237

Laje, G., Cannon, D.M., Allen, A.S., Klaver, J.M., Peck, S.A., Liu, X., Manji, H.K., Drevets, W.C., & McMahon, F.J. (2010). Genetic variation in HTR2A influences serotonin transporter binding potential as measured using PET and [11C]DASB. *International Journal of Neuropsychopharmacology*, Vol.13, No.6, (July 2010), pp. 715-724, ISSN 1461-1457

Lewandowski, K.E., Cohen, B.M., & Ongur, D. (2011). Evolution of neuropsychological dysfunction during the course of schizophrenia and bipolar disorder. *Psychological Medicine*, Vol.41, No.2, (February 2011), pp. 225-241, ISSN 0033-2917

Lim, K.O., Rosenbloom, M.J., Faustman, W.O., Sullivan, E.V., & Pfefferbaum, A. (1999). Cortical gray matter deficit in patients with bipolar disorder. *Schizophrenia Research*, Vol.40, No.3, (December 1999), pp. 219–227, ISSN 0920-9964

Lin, F., Wenig, S., Xie, B., Wu, G., & Lei, H. (2011). Abnormal frontal cortex white matter connections in bipolar disorder: A DTI tractography study. *Journal of Affective Disorders*, (January 2011), epub ahead of print.

Lochhead, R.A., Parsey, R.V., Oquendo, M.A., & Mann, J.J. (2004). Regional brain gray matter volume differences in patients with bipolar disorder as assessed by optimized voxel-based morphometry. *Biological Psychiatry*, Vol.55, No.12, (June 2004), pp. 1154–1162, ISSN 0006-3223

Manji, H.K., Moore, G.J., & Chen, G. (2000). Lithium up-regulates the cytoprotective protein Bcl-2 in the CNS in vivo: A role for neurotrophic and neuroprotective effects in manic depressive illness. *Journal of Clinical Psychiatry*, Vol.61, Suppl.9, (2000), pp. 82–96, ISSN 0160-6689

Mazzuca, M., Jambaque, I., Hertz-Pannier, L., Bouilleret, V., Archambaud, F., Caviness, V., Rodrigo, S., Dulac, O., & Chiron, C. (2011). 18F-FDG PET reveals frontotemporal dysfunction in children with fever-induced refractory epileptic encephalopathy. *The Journal of Nuclear Medicine*, Vol.52, No.1, (January 2011), pp. 40-47, ISSN 0161-5505

McCrea, S.M. (2008). Bipolar Disorder and neurophysiologic mechanisms. *Neuropsychiatric Disease and Treatment*, Vol.4, No.6, (December 2008), pp. 1129-53, ISSN 1176-6328

McDonald, W.M., Krishnan, K.R., Doraiswamy, P.M., & Blazer, D.G. (1991). Occurrence of subcortical hyperintensities in elderly subjects with mania. *Psychiatry Research*, Vol.40, No.4, (December 1991), pp. 211–220, ISSN 0022-3956

McDonald, C., Bullmore, E., Sham, P., Chitnis, X., Suckling, J., MacCabe, J., Walshe, M., & Murray, R.M. (2005). Regional volume deviations of brain structure in schizophrenia and psychotic bipolar disorder: computational morphometry study. *British Journal of Psychiatry*, Vol.186, (May 2005), pp. 369–377, ISSN 1472-1465

Mervaala, E., Fohr, J., Kononen, M., Valkonen-Korhonen, M., Vainio, P., Partanen, K., Partanen, J., Tiihonen, J., Viinamäki, H., Karjalainen, A.K., & Lehtonen, J. (2000). Quantitative MRI of the hippocampus and amygdala in severe depression. *Psychological Medicine*, Vol.30, No.1, (January 2000), pp. 117–125, ISSN 0033-2917

Monks, P.J., Thompson, J.M., Bullmore, E.T., Suckling, J., Brammer, M.J., Williams, S.C., Simmons, A., Giles, N., Lloyd, A.J., Harrison, C.L., Seal, M., Murray, R.M., Ferrier, I.N., Young, A.H., & Curtis, V.A. (2004). A functional MRI study of working memory task in euthymic bipolar disorder: evidence for task-specific dysfunction. *Bipolar Disorders*, Vol.6, No.6, (December 2004), pp. 550–564, ISSN 1398-5647

Moore, P., Shepherd, D., Eccleston, D., Macmillan, I.C., Goswami, U., McAllister, V.L., & Ferrier, I.N. (2001). Cerebral white matter lesions in bipolar affective disorder: relationship to outcome. *The British Journal of Psychiatry*, Vol.178, (February 2001), pp. 172–176, ISSN 0007-1250

Nakama H., Chang L., Fein G., Shimotsu R., Jiang C.S., Ernst T. (2011). Methamphetamine Users Show Greater than Normal Age-Related Cortical Grey Matter Loss. *Addiction*, (March 2011), epub ahead print.

Nasrallah, H.A., McCalley-Whitters, M., & Jacoby, C.G. (1982). Cortical atrophy in schizophrenia and mania: a comparative CT study. *The Journal of Clinical Psychiatry*, Vol.43, No.11, (November 1982), pp. 439-441, ISSN 0160-6689

Norris, S.D., Krishnan, K.R.R., & Ahearn, E. (1997). Structural changes in the brain of patients with bipolar affective disorder by MRI: a review of the literature. *Progress in Neuro-Psychopharmacology and Biological Psychiatry*, Vol.21, No.8, (November 1997), pp. 1323- 1337, ISSN 0278-5846

Nugent, A.C., Milham, M.P., Bain, E.E., Mah, L., Cannon, D.M., Marrett, S., Zarate, C.A., Pine, D.S., Price, J.L., & Drevets, W.C. (2006). Cortical abnormalities in BD investigated with MRI and voxel-based morphometry. *Neuroimage*, Vol.30, No.2, (April 2008), pp. 485–497, ISSN 1053-8119

Pavuluri, M.N., Yang, S., Kamineni, K., Passarotti, A.M., Srinivasan, G., Harral, E.M., Sweeney, J.A., & Zhou, X.J. (2009). Diffusion tensor imaging study of white matter fiber tracts in pediatric bipolar disorder and attention-deficit/hyperactivity disorder. *Biological Psychiatry*, Vol.65, No.7, (April 2009), pp. 586-93, ISSN 0006-3223

Pearlson, G.C., Garbacz, D.J., Tompkins, R.H., Ahn, H.S., Gutterman, D.F., Veroff, A.E., & DePaulo, J.R. (1984). Clinical correlates of lateral ventricular enlargement in bipolar affective disorder. *The American Journal of Psychiatry*, Vol.141, No.2, (February 1984), pp. 253-256, ISSN 0002-953X

Pearlson, G.D., & Veroff, A.E. (1981). Computerized tomographic scan changes in manic-depressive illness. *The Lancet*, Vol.2, No.8244, (August 1981), pp. 470, ISSN 0140-6736

Pearlson, G.D., Barta, P.E., Powers, R.E., Menon, R.R., Richards, S.S., Aylward, E.H., et al. (1997). Ziskind-Somerfeld Research Award 1996. Medial and superior temporal gyral volumes and cerebral asymmetry in schizophrenia versus bipolar disorder. *Biological Psychiatry*, Vol.41, No.1, (January 1997), pp. 1–14, ISSN 0006-3223

Person, C., Koessler, L., Louis-Dorr, V., Wolf, D., Maillard, L., & Marie, P.Y. (2010). Analysis of the relationship between interictal electrical source imaging and PET hypometabolism. *Engineering in Medicine and Biology Society (EMBC), 2010 Annual International Conference of the IEEE*, pp. 3723-6, ISBN 978-1-4244-4123-5, Buenos Aires, August 31-September 4, 2010.

Phelps M.E., Hoffman E.J., Mullani N.A., Ter-Pogossian M.M. (1975). Application of annihilation coincidence detection to transaxial reconstruction tomography. *Journal of Nuclear Medicine*, Vol.16, No.3, (March 1975), pp.210-224, ISSN 0161-5505

Phillips M.L., Vieta E. (2007). Identifying functional neuroimaging biomarkers of bipolar disorder: toward DSM-V. Schizophrenia bulletin. Vol. 33, No. 4, (Jul 2007), pp. 893-904, ISSN 0586-7614

Quigley, H., Colloby, S.J., & O'Brien, J.T. (2010). PET imaging of brain amyloid in dementia: a review. *International Journal of Geriatric Psychiatry*, (December 2010), epub ahead of print.

Regenold, W., Hisley, K., Phatak, P., Marano, C.M., Obuchowski, A., Lefkowitz, D.M., Sassan, A., Ohri, S., Phillips, T.L., Dosanjh, N., Conley, R.R., & Gullapalli, R. (2008). Relationship of cerebrospinal fluid glucose metabolites to MRI deep white matter hyperintensities and treatment resistance in bipolar disorder patients. *Bipolar Disorders*, Vol.10, No.7, (November 2008), pp. 753–764, ISSN 1398-5647

Rieder, R.O., Mann, L.S., Weinberger, D.R., van Kammen, D.P., Post, R.M. (1983). Computed tomographic scans in patients with schizophrenia, schizoaffective, and bipolar affective disorder. *Archives of General Psychiatry*, Vol.40, No.7, (July 1983), pp. 735–739, ISSN 0003-990X

Roncali E., Cherry S.R. (2011). Application of silicon photomultipliers to positron emission tomography. *Annals of Biomedical Engineering*, Vol.39, No.4, (April 2011), pp. 1358-77, ISSN 0090-6964

Salas-Gonzalez, D., Górriz, J.M., Ramírez, J., Illán, I.A., López, M., Segovia, F., Chaves, R., Padilla, P., & Puntonet, C.G. (2010). Feature selection using factor analysis for Alzheimer's diagnosis using 18F-FDG PET images. *Medical Physiology*, Vol.37, No.11, (November 2010), pp. 6084-95, ISSN 1985-4811

Savitz, J., & Drevets, W.C. (2009). Bipolar and major depressive disorder: neuroimaging the developmental-degenerative divide. *Neuroscience & Biobehavioral Reviews*, Vol.33, No.5, (May 2009), pp. 699-771, ISSN 0149-7634

Scherk, H., Kemmer, C., Usher, J., Reith, W., Falkai, P., & Gruber, O. (2008). No change to grey and white matter volumes in bipolar I disorder patients. *European Archives of Psychiatry and Clinical Neuroscience*, Vol.258, No.6, (September 2008), pp. 345–349, ISSN 0940-1334 (a)

Scherk H., Backens M., Schneider-Axmann T., Kemmer C., Usher J., Reith W., Falkai P., Gruber O. (2008). Neurochemical pathology in hippocampus in euthymic patients with bipolar I disorder. *Acta Psychiatrica Scandinavica*, Vol.117, No.4, (April 2008), pp. 283-288, 0001-690X (b)

Schlaepfer, T.E., Harris, G.J., Tien, A.Y., Peng, L.W., Lee, S., Federman, E.B., Chase, G.A., Barta, P.E., Pearlson, G.D. (1994). Decreased regional cortical gray matter volume in schizophrenia. *The American Journal of Psychiatry*, Vol.151, No.6, (June 1994), pp. 842–848, ISSN 0002-953X

Schlegel, S., & Kretzschmar, K. (1987). Computed tomography in affective disorders, part I. Ventricular and sulcal measurements. *Biological Psychiatry*, Vol.22, No.1, (January 1987), pp. 4-14, ISSN 0006-3223

Schulte T., Müller-Oehring E.M., Pfefferbaum A., Sullivan E.V. (2010). Neurocircuitry of emotion and cognition in alcoholism: contributions from white matter fiber tractography. *Dialogues in Clinical Neuroscience*, Vol.12, No.4, (2010), pp. 554-560, ISSN 1294-8322

Soares, J.C., & Mann, J.J. (1997). The anatomy of mood disorders – review of structural neuro-imaging studies. *Biological Psychiatry*, Vol.41, No.1, (January 1997), pp. 86–106, ISSN 0006-3223

Steffens, D.C., & Krishnan, K.R.R. (1998). Structural Neuroimaging and Mood Disorders: Recent Findings, Implications for Classification, and Future Directions. *Biological Psychiatry*, Vol.43, No.10, (May 15), pp. 705-712, ISSN 0006-3223

Stoll, A.L., Renshaw, P.F., Yurgelun-Todd, D.A., & Cohen, B.M. (2000). Neuroimaging in bipolar disorder: what have we learned? *Biological Psychiatry*, Vol.48, No.6, (September 2000), pp. 505–517, ISSN 0006-3223

Stork C., Renshae P.F. (2005). Mitochondrial dysfunction in bipolar disorder: evidence from magnetic resonance spectroscopy research. *Molecular Psychiatry*, Vol.10, No.10, (October 2005), pp. 900-19, ISSN 1359-4184

Strakowski, S.M., DelBello, M.P., Zimmerman, M.E., Getz, G.E., Mills, N.P., Ret, J., Shear, P., & Adler, C.M. (2002). Ventricular and periventricular structural volumes in first-versus multiple-episode bipolar disorder. *The American Journal of Psychiatry*, Vol.159, No.11, (November 2002), pp. 1841–1847, ISSN 0002-953X

Strakowski, S.M., Wilson, D.R., Tohen, M., Woods, B.T., Douglass, A.W., & Stoll, A.L. (1993). Structural brain abnormalities in first-episode mania. *Biological Psychiatry*, Vol.33, No.8-9, (April 15-May 1), pp. 602–609, ISSN 0006-3223

Suhara, T., Nakayama, K., Inoue, O., Fukuda, H., Shimizu, M., Mori, A., & Tateno, Y. (1992). D1 dopamine receptor binding in mood disorders measured by positron emission tomography. *Psychopharmacology*, Vol.106, No.1, (1992), pp. 14-18, ISSN 0033-3158

Sullivan, G.M., Ogden, R.T., Oquendo, M.A., Kumar, J.S., Simpson, N., Huang, Y.Y., Mann, J.J., & Parsey, R.V. (2009). Positron emission tomography quantification of serotonin-1A receptor binding in medication-free bipolar depression. *Biological Psychiatry*, Vol.66, No.3, (August 2009), pp. 223-230, ISSN 0006-3223

Supprian, T., Reiche, W., Schmitz, B., Grunwald, I., Backens, M., Hofmann, E., Georg, T., Falkai, P., & Reith, W. (2004). MRI of the brainstem in patients with major depression, bipolar affective disorder and normal controls. *Psychiatry Research*, Vol.131, No.3., (September 2004), pp. 269– 276, ISSN 0022-3956

Sussmann, J.E., Lymer, G.K., McKirdy, J., Moorhead, T.W., Muñoz Maniega, S., Job, D., Hall, J., Bastin, M.E., Johnstone, E.C:, Lawrie, S.M., & McIntosh, A.M. (2009). White matter abnormalities in bipolar disorder and schizophrenia detected using diffusion tensor magnetic resonance imaging. *Bipolar Disorders*, Vol.11, No.1, (February 2009), pp. 11-18, ISSN 1398-5647

Swayze, V.W., Andreasen, N.C., Alliger, R.J., Yuh, W.T.C., & Ehrhard, J.C. (1992). Subcortical and temporal structures in affective disorder and schizophrenia: A magnetic resonance imaging study. *Biological Psychiatry*, Vol.31, No.3, (February 1992), pp. 221–240, ISSN 0006-3223

Takahashi, T., Malhi, G.S., Wood, S.J., Yücel, M., Walterfang, M., Tanino, R., Suzuki, M., & Pantelis, C. (2010). Insular cortex volume in established bipolar affective disorder: A preliminary MRI study. *Psychiatry Research*, Vol.182, No.2, (May 2010), pp. 187–190, ISSN 0022-3956

Ter-Pogossian M.M., Phelps M.E., Hoffman E.J., Mullani N.A. (1975). A positron-emission transaxial tomograph for nuclear imaging (PETT). *Radiology*, Vol.114, No.1, (January 1975), pp. 89-98, ISSN 0033-8419

Townsend, J., Bookheimer, S.Y., Foland-Ross, L.C., Sugar, C.A., & Altshuler, L.L. (2010). fMRI abnormalities in dorsolateral prefrontal cortex during a working memory task in manic, euthymic and depressed bipolar subjects. *Psychiatry Research*, Vol.182, No.1, (April 2010), pp. 22-29, ISSN 0022-3956

Usher, J., Leucht, S., Falkai, P., & Scherk, H. (2010). Correlation between amygdala volume and age in bipolar disorder— A systematic review and meta-analysis of structural MRI studies. *Psychiatry Research*, Vol.182, No.1, (April 2010),pp. 1–8, ISSN 0022-3956

Van der Schot, A.C., Vonk, R., Brans, R.G., van Haren, N.E., Koolschijn, P.C., Nuboer, V., Schnack, H.G., van Baal, G.C., Boomsma, D.I., Nolen, W.A., Hulshoff Pol, H.E., & Kahn, R.S. (2009). Influence of Genes and Environment on Brain Volumes in Twin Pairs Concordant and Discordant for BD. *Archives of General Psychiatry*, Vol.66, No.2, (February 2009), pp. 142-151, ISSN 0003-990X

Van der Werf-Eldering, M.J., Burger, H., Holthausen, E.A., Aleman, A., & Nolen, W.A. (2010). Cognitive functioning in patients with bipolar disorder: association with depressive symptoms and alcohol use. *PLoS One*, Vol.5, No.9, (September 2010), pp. e13032, ISSN 1932-6203

Versace, A., Almeida, J.R., Hassel, S., Walsh, N.D., Novelli, M., Klein, C.R., Kupfer, D.J., & Phillips, M.L. (2008). Elevated left and reduced right orbitomedial prefrontal fractional anisotropy in adults with bipolar disorder revealed by tract-based spatial statistics. *Archives of General Psychiatry*, Vol.65, No.9, (September 2008), pp. 1041-1052, ISSN 0003-990X

Versace, A., Thompson, W.K., Zhou, D., Almeida, J.R., Hassel, S., Klein, C.R., Kupfer, D.J., & Phillips, M.L. (2010). Abnormal left and right amygdala-orbitofrontal cortical functional connectivity to emotional faces: state versus trait vulnerability markers of depression in bipolar disorder. *Biological Psychiatry*, Vol.67, No.5, (March 2010), pp. 422-431, ISSN 0006-3223

Videbech, P. (1997). MRI findings in patients with affective disorder: a meta-analysis. *Acta Psychiatrica Scandinavica*, Vol.96, No.3, (September 1997), pp. 157–168, ISSN 0001-690X

Vyas N.S., Patel N.H., Nijran K.S., Al-Nahhas A., Puri B.K. (2011). The use of PET imaging in studying cognition, genetics and pharmacotherapeutic interventions in schizophrenia. *Expert Review of Neurotherapeutics*, Vol.11, No.1, (January 2011), pp. 37-51, ISSN 1473-7175

Wang, F., Kalmar, J.H., He, Y., Jackowski, M., Chepenik, L.G., Edmiston, E.E., Tie, K., Gong, G., Shah, M.P., Jones, M., Uderman, J., Constable, R.T., & Blumberg, H.P. (2009). Functional and structural connectivity between the perigenual anterior cingulate and amygdala in bipolar disorder. *Biological Psychiatry,* Vol.66, No.5, (September 2009), pp. 516-21,ISSN 0006-3223

Wiesel, F.A. (1989). Positron emission tomography in psychiatry. *Psychiatric Developments,* Vol.7, No.1, (1989), pp. 19-47, 0262-9283.

Wingo, A., Wingo, T., Harvey, P., & Baldessarini, R. (2009). Effects of lithium on cognitive performance: a meta-analysis. *Journal of Clinical Psychiatry,* Vol.70, No.11, (November 2009), pp. 1588-1597, ISSN 0160-6689

Wolf, F., Brüne, M., & Assion, H.J. (2010). Theory of mind and neurocognitive functioning in patients with bipolar disorder. *Bipolar Disorders,* Vol.12, No.6, pp. 657-666, ISSN 1398-5647

Yates, D.B., Dittmann, S., Kapczinski, F., & Trentini, C.M. (2010). Cognitive abilities and clinical variables in bipolar I depressed and euthymic patients and controls. *Journal of Psychiatric Research,* Vol.45, No.4, (April 2011), pp. 495-504, ISSN 0022-3956

Yatham, L.N., Liddle P.F., Shiah, I.S., Lam, R.W., Ngan, E., Scarrow, G., Imperial, M., Stoessl, J., Sossi, V., & Ruth, T.J. (2002). PET study of [(18)F]6-fluoro-L-dopa uptake in neuroleptic- and mood-stabilizer-naive first-episode nonpsychotic mania: effects of treatment with divalproex sodium. *The American Journal of Psychiatry,* Vol.159, No.5, (May 2002), pp. 768-774, ISSN 0002-953X (a)

Yatham, L.N., Liddle, P.F., Lam, R.W., Shiah, I.S., Lane, C., Stoessl, A.J., Sossi, V., & Ruth, T.J. (2002). PET study of the effects of valproate on dopamine D(2) receptors in neuroleptic- and mood-stabilizer-naive patients with nonpsychotic mania. *The American Journal of Psychiatry,* Vol.159, No.10, (October 2002), pp. 1718-1723, ISSN 0002-953X (b)

Yatham, L.N., Liddle, P.F., Erez, J., Kauer-Sant'Anna, M., Lam, R.W., Imperial, M., Sossi, V., & Ruth, T.J. (2010). Brain serotonin-2 receptors in acute mania. *The British Journal of Psychiatry,* Vol.196, No.1, (January 2010), pp. 47-51, ISSN 0007-1250

Yildiz-Yesiloglu, A., & Ankerst, D.P. (2006). Neurochemical alterations of the brain in bipolar disorder and their implications for pathophysiology: a systematic review of the in vivo proton magnetic resonance spectroscopy findings. *Progress in Neuropsychopharmacology and Biological Psychiatry,* Vol.30, No.6, (August 2006), pp. 969-995, ISSN 0278-5846

Young, R.C., Nambudiri, D.E., Jain, H,. de Asis, J.M., & Alexopoulos, G.S. (1999). Brain computed tomography in geriatric manic disorder. *Biological Psychiatry,* Vol.45, No.8, (April 1999), pp.1063-1065, ISSN 0006-3223 (a)

Young, R.C., Patel, A., Meyers, B.S., Kakuma, T., & Alexopoulos, G.S. (1999). Alpha(1)-acid glycoprotein, age, and sex in mood disorders. *The American Journal of Geriatric Psychiatry,* Vol.7, No.4, (1999), pp. 331-334, ISSN 1064-7481 (b)

2

Human Oscillatory EEG Activities Representing Working Memory Capacity

Masahiro Kawasaki

Rhythm-based Brain Computation Unit, RIKEN, BSI-TOYOTA Collaboration Center,
Japan

1. Introduction

We can flexibly process and make decisions regarding multiple types of information in daily situations such as driving and cooking. However, human error is increased in complex or combined tasks (relative to simple tasks) because our information processing capacity is limited. This limited cognitive function is associated with working memory (WM), which is proposed to be a higher-level human ability to memorize, maintain, and manipulate mental representations in the mind for a short time (Baddeley, 1986). Most theorists think that WM function includes active manipulation as well as passive short-term maintenance. An often-used metaphor for working memory is "the blackboard of the mind." For example, imagine that you are rearranging the furniture in your room. You can move around the furniture in your mind, that is, transform the imagination any number of times. To guide behavior and make decisions about what to do next, WM temporarily selects and retains task-relevant information such as recently processed sensory input, retrieved information from long-term memory, or mentally manipulated images. Thus, WM is directly linked to any and all other brain functions, including perception, movement, emotion, and problem solving.

Baddeley & Hitch (1974) proposed a basic psychological model in which WM is divided into separate components, the "storage system" and the "central executive". The "storage system" consists of 2 temporary storage buffers for visual information (visuospatial sketch pad, i.e., visual working memory) and auditory-verbal information (phonological loop, i.e., verbal working memory) and an episodic buffer for long-term memory, whereas the "central executive" controls the allocations of attention, selects relevant information, and manipulates information held in the storage systems (Baddeley, 1986; Baddeley & Hitch, 1974; Phillips, 1974; Baddeley, 2000). Extensive experimental evidence from behavioral performance of normal subjects, lesion studies, and neuroimaging studies supports this view. For example, performance in dual tasks requiring 2 separate perceptual domains (i.e., a visual and a verbal task, or a mental processing task and a maintenance task) is nearly as efficient as performance of individual tasks (for a review, Cowan, 2001; Della Sala & Logie, 1993). These findings indicate that the visual and verbal WM are separated.

Both visual and verbal WM have 3 phases: encoding, which imports the relevant information in memory; maintenance, which stores the encoded information; and retrieval (or rehearsal), which briefly uses the information for a task. To investigate the neural substrate for WM, previous electrophysiological studies in nonhuman primates and human neuroimaging studies have shown sustained neural activity over the retention interval in distributed brain regions including frontal, parietal, occipital, and temporal areas during maintenance of relevant information (e.g., Chafee & Godman-Rakic, 1998). If these brain regions are actually involved in maintaining mental representations, their activities are thought to be correlated with WM capacity. In fact, brain activity has been reported to increase with increasing number of objects to be remembered and saturated below the limited WM capacity (Todd & Marois, 2004; Vogel & Machizawa, 2004). Frontal regions also represent the limitation of executive functions, since activity there is increased during engagement in dual tasks (Marois & Ivanoff, 2005). These results suggest that frontal regions are associated with executive functions and posterior regions are involved in maintenance of mental representations. Thus, although much is known concerning the brain areas involved in various WM functions, understanding how these brain areas temporally communicate is more difficult.

To address this issue, measuring electrophysiological (EEG) data during WM tasks and analyzing the synchronizations in local areas and between different areas has proved particularly useful (Varela et al., 2001). Our previous EEG studies used mental calculation as the auditory WM task and mental spatial manipulation as the visual WM task (Kawasaki et al., 2010). The EEG results clearly demonstrated that the frontal theta (4–6 Hz) activity increased during the manipulation periods on both WM tasks, and the parietal and temporal alpha activities were enhanced only during the maintenance periods on the auditory and visual WM task, respectively. Phase synchronization analysis revealed significant theta synchronizations between the frontal and parietal regions for visual WM and between the frontal and temporal regions for auditory WM. These results indicated that long-range theta synchronizations could connect the different brain regions to manipulate task-relevant representations. Interestingly, the concurrent theta and alpha phases were significantly synchronized in task-relevant storage areas, which suggests the presence of gating mechanisms to extract stored information. Theta and alpha activities thus play an important role in several WM functions; however little is known regarding how these oscillations represent WM limitations.

This chapter describes investigations into the neural dynamics of EEG oscillatory activities that underlie the capacity limitations for executive functions and storage buffers in WM, particularly for visual infomation. To advance understanding of the detailed brain networks involved, the use and interpretation of EEG time-frequency analyses such as wavelet analysis and the role of each EEG oscillatory activity in WM functions is discussed, and 2 experiments are described. Visual storage systems were investigated using delayed-matching-to-sample tasks with visual stimuli, and a dual WM task with visual and auditory representations was used to identify the bottleneck of the central executive function. These EEG findings may contribute to understanding the causes of human error.

2. Capacity limitations of working memory

To investigate the limitation of visual WM (VWM) storage capacity, previous behavioral and neuroimaging studies used a change detection paradigm, namely, delayed matching to sample (DMS) tasks with a visual stimulus. In this paradim, multiple visual items are presented (sample display) and participants are required to memorize and retain these items over retention intervals. The number of items within the sample display is manipulated. Following the retention interval, one probe item (test display) or multiple probe items (whole display) are presented at one location within the sample array, and participants are then required to judge whether a change has occurred or not. These 2 tests have shown different performance scores, since VWM storage capacity is vulnerable to visual interference created during the encoding period (Wheeler & Treisman, 2002). Therefore, many behavioral and neuroimaging studies have applied the single-probe test. To avoid the possibility of using verbal strategies, most studies involving the DMS task used very short exposure duration for the sample display (about 150 ms), and require participants to engage in phonological tasks simltaneously, e.g., repeating a word during the sample display and retention intervals (Baddeley, Lewis & Vallar, 1984).

Many previous studies have proposed a VWM capacity of 3 or 4 items (Luck & Vogel, 1997) because the accuracy rates for many DMS tasks systematically decrease as the number of items increases beyond 3 or 4. More recently, one study demonstrated that VWM capacity decreases as object complexity increases, and proposed that VWM capacity varies by the type of features (Alvarez & Cavanagh, 2004). The authors used complex items, Chinese characters, which are thought to be a combination of simple shapes. Although the issue retains some controversy, many studies have demonstrated consensus on the existence of large individual differences in VWM capacity.

To estimate the capacity of VWM in terms of objects stored in DMS tasks, Cowan (2001) has proposed a model that takes both hit rates (accurately detecting a change) and correct rejection rates (accurately reporting no change when none occurred) into account. The model estimates hit rates and correct rejection rates with the following equations:

$$H = \frac{K}{N} + \frac{(N-K)}{N} \times g \tag{1}$$

$$CR = \frac{K}{N} + \frac{(N-K)}{N} \times (1-g) \tag{2}$$

where K denotes the estimated number of items stored in VWM, N is the total number of items presented in the sample display, H is the probability of a hit rate, CR is the probability of a correct rejection rate, and g is the guessing rate for coincidentally giving a correct answer. The theory assumes that when one of the items within the VWM capacity (K/N; Fig. 1 purple area) changed, subjects could detect whether the change occurred. In contrast, they could not detect whether a change occurred in objects exceeding the capacity ($(N-K)/N$; Fig. 1 green area).

However, in some cases subjects happened to answer correctly on some portion of the trials (g) under an alternative forced-choice paradigm or, in another portion of the trials ($1-g$), coincidentally report correctly that no change occurred in the no-change trial, although they could not detect this. This guessing rate could not be estimated from the performance of the DMS tasks. Thus, given the hit rates and correct rejection rates for a particular set size, these equations (1) and (2) can be solved for the set size:

$$K = N \times (H + CR - 1) \tag{3}$$

The Cowan's K value is obtained from the set size of each sample display as each subject's VWM capacity for a given material.

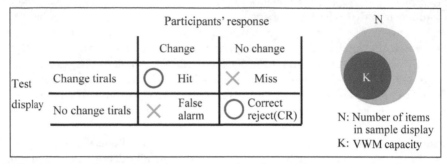

Fig. 1. Combination of participants' response and trial type (change or not) in change detection paradigm (left) and a model of Cowan's formula (right).

Unlike VWM, the WM capacity for executive functions has been evaluated using dual WM tasks. Although no interference exists between independent storage components such as visual and verbal storage, simultaneously processing more than 2 information sources that require mental manipulation and reactions is thought to be difficult. Previous studies have revealed a psychological refractory period, in which a second task elicits a longer reaction time when the interval between the first and second tasks (i.e., stimulus onset asynchrony; SOA) is short (Marois & Ivanoff, 2005). That is to say, if the 2 tasks seem to be processed simultaneously, the performance is degraded. This phenomenon is known to be a bottleneck of the central executive function.

3. Neural substrates for working memory

Over many years, numerous researchers have attempted to localize and characterize the neural implementation of VWM and dissociate its functions. Lesion studies have reported that damage to the prefrontal cortex (PFC) in monkeys impairs performance on DMS tasks with a short delay, but not on visual discrimination tasks that do not require maintenance of information (Goldman-Rakic, 1987). Likewise, electrophysiological recording studies of nonhuman primates have revealed sustained neuronal firing in the PFC during the retention interval of DMS tasks, and interpreted the activity as maintaining the previously presented representations (Fuster & Alexander, 1971; Kubota & Niki, 1971). Therefore, the PFC was believed to be the neural substrate for VWM over a longer period. Since then, numerous physiological studies have shown neurons specifically active during the delay period in a vast network of brain regions including the PFC (e.g., Funahashi, Bruce, & Goldman-Rakic, 1989), the posterior parietal cortex (e.g., Chafee & Godman-Rakic, 1998), and visual processing cortices (Bisley & Pasternak, 2000; Miyashita & Chang, 1988).

Consistent with this interpretation, human neuroimaging studies have also revealed that the blood flow in these regions continually increased during the retention interval (Courtney et al., 1997, 1998; Postle & D'Esposito, 1999). Although considerable evidence supports the sustained delay-period activity, DMS tasks include many requirements (e.g., preparation of actions) in addition to maintenance. Therefore, recent fMRI studies have assumed that the blood oxygen level-dependent (BOLD) signal captures a population of neuronal activity that may reflect the representation of multiple items to be maintained, and have indeed shown that a subset of the distributed network demonstrated delay-period activity sensitive to the number of items in the sample display (Diwadkar et al., 2000; Glahn et al., 2002; Jha & McCarthey 2000; Linden et al., 2003). The VWM load-sensitive network includes the frontal, parietal, and visual cortices. Notably, some studies have revealed that activity in the posterior parietal cortex is correlated with the number of items to be remembered (Cowan's K value) and indicated that this area actually stored the representations (Kawasaki et al., 2008; Todd & Marois, 2004, 2005; Vogel & Machizawa, 2004; Xu & Chun, 2006).

In contrast to the posterior parietal and visual cortices, anterior regions including the frontal cortex have also been associated with executive processes such as attentional selection and manipulation of information (Curtis & D'Esposito, 2003). For instance, in studies using a spatial WM task that requires participants to memorize the spatial locations of simultaneous or sequentially presented items and, after a delay, select one relevant location, the prefrontal cortex has been reported to show transient activity during the selection period and no sustained activity during the retention interval (Rowe et al., 2000). Furthermore, the frontal cortex is particularly sensitive to the number of listed items to be maintained in VWM in the n-back task, which requires participants to maintain a series of items and their order, select a relevant item from VWM, and compare it with the earlier item (Smith & Jonides, 1999). Moreover, the frontal cortex is proposed to serve in maintaining task-specific goals (Miller & Cohen, 2001; Passingham & Sakai, 2004) and assist in maintaining high loads and/or long retention intervals (Braver et al., 1997; Linden et al., 2003).

Although, thus far, many neuroimaging studies have identified the neural substrate for the storage systems and central executive of WM, they have not dealt with how these brain areas temporally communicate. To address this issue, some studies have investigated the dynamic relationships governing brain activity by focusing on electroencephalograph (EEG) oscillations, which are closely related to synchronization of a large number of neurons underlying a particular function (Varela et al., 2001). Previous human scalp-recorded EEG studies have revealed modulated theta (about 4–8 Hz) and alpha (about 9–12 Hz) rhythms in distributed brain regions and phase synchronization between them during various WM tasks (Jensen & Tesche, 2002; Kawasaki & Watanabe, 2007; Klimesch et al., 2008; Mizuhara et al., 2004; Sauseng et al., 2005). Frontal theta activity in particular has been associated with the mental manipulation of WM, because these oscillations were enhanced in tasks such as mental calculation and image transfomation (Kawasaki et al., 2010). In contrast, posterior alpha activities are thought to be involved in the WM storage systems, because these oscillations are mainly observed in the retention intervals of many WM tasks. However, whether these oscillatory activities are increased or decreased during each WM period remains controversial. Furthermore, little is known regarding how these oscillations represent WM limitations; therefore, their detailed mechanisms have not yet been identified. To clarify the functional role of the theta and alpha oscillations in WM, the study described in the following 2 sections used EEG data measured during DMS and dual WM tasks to demonstrate 2 types of EEG activity that were correlated with the WM capacities for visual storage and central executive systems.

4. EEG oscillations for visual storage capacity

This section describes the investigation of EEG oscillatory activity correlated with VWM capacity, which aimed to identify the roles of different oscillations in the VWM storage systems (e.g., maintenance of high or low VWM demands). EEG data was measured during the DMS task.

4.1 Delayed matching to sample task

Fourteen healthy, right-handed volunteers (10 male and 4 female; mean age = 25.6 ± 4.2 years, range 21–38 years) with normal or corrected-to-normal visual acuity, normal hearing acuity, and normal motor performance took part in the delayed matching to sample tasks. All participants gave written informed consent, which was approved by the Ethical Committee of the RIKEN (in accordance with the Declaration of Helsinki), before the experiments were performed.

Participants faced a computer screen and were asked to memorize the colors of 3 or 6 colored disks (size, 1° × 1°; color, white, red, green, blue, yellow, magenta, cyan, or orange) that were distributed at random locations within an invisible 3 × 3 cell matrix in a black rectangle (size, 10° × 10°) for 0.2 s (Fig. 2, sample display). After a 2-s retention interval, one disk was presented at one location within the sample array (test display), and participants were asked to judge whether its color matched the disk at the same location in the sample display via a button press while the fixation point was red for 2 s. In one trial, the color of the probe disk matched the sample disk, and in a second trial, the color of the probe disk did not match. After the judgment, a feedback stimulus indicating whether the answer was correct (O) or incorrect (X) was presented. The duration of the inter-trial interval (ITI) was 2 s. Each participant completed 4 separate sessions which consisted of 48 trials. A behavioral training session before the EEG-measurement sessions was provided for all participants.

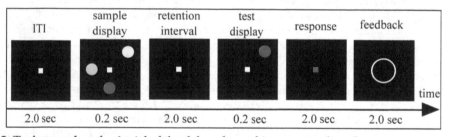

Fig. 2. Task procedure for 1 trial of the delayed-matching-to-sample task.

4.2 EEG measurements and analyses

An EEG was continuously recorded using 60 scalp electrodes embedded in an electrode cap in accordance with the extended version of the International 10/20 System of Electrode Placement. The sampling rate was 500 Hz. Reference electrodes were placed on the right and left earlobes. Artifacts due to eye blinks and movements were detected by electro-oculogram (EOG) electrodes placed above and below the left eye to monitor eye blinks and vertical eye movements, and electrodes placed 1 cm from the right and left eyes to monitor horizontal eye movements. Trials in which the amplitude of any electrode of an EEG epoch exceeded plus or minus 100 μV were rejected from the offline analysis. These EEG data were amplified using NeuroScan equipment (Compumedics NeuroScan Corp., Charlotte, NC) and filtered with a band-pass range from 0.1 Hz to 50 Hz.

We analyzed the EEG data for the correct trials. These epochs were subjected to infomax independent component analysis (ICA) with the use of EEGLAB (Delorme & Makeig, 2004;

Institute for Neural Computation, University of California, San Diego, CA) running under Matlab (Mathworks, Natick, MA). ICA components that were significantly correlated with vertical or horizontal EOGs were regarded as components related to eye movement or other artifacts and were reduced or eliminated from the data. The ICA-corrected data were recalculated using regressions on the remaining components.

To accurately evaluate cortical activity under the scalp EEG electrodes without error due to volume conduction, we used a current source density analysis at each electrode position. The spherical Laplace operator was applied to the voltage distribution on the surface of the scalp using the following parameters: the order of the spline, $m = 4$, and the maximum degree of the Legendre polynomial, $n = 50$, with a precision of 10^{-5} (Perrin et al., 1989).

Time-frequency (TF) amplitudes and phases were calculated by wavelet transforms based on Morlet's wavelets, having a Gaussian shape in the time domain (SD σ_t) and frequency domain (SD σ_f) around a center frequency (f) (Tallon-Baudry et al., 1997). The TF amplitude $E(t, f)$ for each time point of each trial was the squared norm of the result of the convolution of the original EEG signal $s(t)$ with the complex Morlet's wavelet function $w(t, f)$:

$$w(t, f) = (\sigma_t \sqrt{\pi})^{-1/2} \exp(-t^2 / 2\sigma_t^2) \exp(i2\pi ft) \tag{4}$$

$$E(t, f) = |w(t, f) \otimes s(t)|^2 \tag{5}$$

where $\sigma_f = 1/(2\pi\sigma_t)$. The wavelet used was characterized by a constant ratio ($f/\sigma_f = 7$), with f ranging from 1 Hz to 40 Hz in 0.5-Hz steps. The TF amplitude was averaged across single trials for events and conditions. The event-related TF amplitude was calculated by subtracting the baseline data measure in the ITI for each frequency band. For all statistical analyses, a nonparametric Wilcoxon signed-rank test was used across the events or conditions because the distributions of the TF amplitude populations were far from Gaussian.

4.3 Results

Accuracy rates (percent correct) for lower numbers of presented objects were higher than those for larger numbers of presented objects (3 objects: 90.2 ± 2.0%; 6 objects: 72.6 ± 2.8%). A one-factor analysis of variance (ANOVA) revealed a main effect of the number of objects ($F_{1, 26} = 24.3$, $P < 0.01$) and the accuracy rates demonstrated a significant difference (Wilcoxon signed-rank test; $Z = 3.71$, $P < 0.01$).

The VWM capacity was estimated by Cowan's K formula (see Section 2; 3 objects: $K = 2.41 \pm 0.12$; 6 objects: $K = 2.71 \pm 0.33$). A one-factor ANOVA revealed no main effect of the number of objects ($F_{1, 26} = 0.64$, $P = 0.43$), and no significant difference between K-values was detected between 3 and 6 objects ($Z = 1.18$, $P = 0.24$). These results suggested that the VWM capacity in our experiments was limited to approximately 2.7 objects.

Brain activity was evaluated using the averaged time-frequency amplitudes of the EEG data obtained during the DMS task. The EEG results demonstrated that parietal alpha amplitudes (about 12 Hz) sustainably and significantly increased during the retention intervals (POz electrode: $Z = 2.11$, $P < 0.04$), whereas enhancement of the frontal theta delay-period amplitudes (about 6 Hz) was not observed (Fz electrode: $Z = 0.18$, $P = 0.85$). Frontal theta activity during maintenance of 6 objects was significantly higher than that for maintenance of 3 obejcts (3 objects: -0.28 ± 0.21 μV; 6 objects: 0.55 ± 0.40 μV; $Z = 2.12$, $P < 0.04$). In contrast, parietal alpha activity demonstrated an opposing pattern (3 objects: 2.06 ±

0.66 µV; 6 objects: 0.45 ± 0.45 µV; $Z = 1.97$, $P < 0.05$). Interestingly, frontal theta activity was significantly and positively correlated with the VWM capacity of the individual (Fz electrode: $r(14) = 0.39$, $P < 0.05$), whereas the parietal alpha activity was negatively correlated with the VWM capacity (Poz electrode: $r(14) = -0.44$, $P < 0.05$).

4.4 Discussion
The observed VWM capacity was about 3 objects, which is consistent with many previous findings using simple visual features (Luck & Vogel, 1997). In relation to the behavioral results, the EEG results revealed that the frontal theta and parietal alpha amplitudes were sustainably enhanced during the retention interval of the DMS task. Interestingly, frontal theta activity demonstrated a positive correlation with individual WM capacity, whereas parietal alpha activity demonstrated a negative correlation.

In addition to confirming previous reports that these oscillations are involved in VWM (; Klimesch et al., 2008; Jensen & Tesch, 2002; Jensen et al., 2002), the present study was able to dissociate their functions. Frontal theta activities have been associated with central executive functions including mental manipulation and calculation tasks (Kawasaki et al., 2010) and in supporting VWM storage during high-VWM loads and demands (Curtis & D'Esposito, 2003; Kawasaki & Watanabe, 2007; Sakai et al., 2002). Parietal alpha activity has been proposed to reflect simple WM storage. Indeed, many neuroimaging studies using the DMS task with simple visual features (e.g., color) have shown that parietal activity was correlated with VWM capacity and decreased beyond the limit of VWM capacity, unlike increased frontal activity (Linden et al., 2003; Rypma et al., 2002). These results suggested that parietal alpha activity may be involved essentially only in the maintenance of limited visual information, whereas the frontal theta activity seems to assist in VWM storage under high VWM demand, as if instead of the suppressed alpha activity.

5. EEG oscillations for central executive

This section describes the investigation of EEG oscillatory activities that represent the WM limitations for executive functions by comparing dual and single WM tasks. The dual tasks required 2 separate perceptual domains: mental manipulation with visual stimuli and the mental calculations with auditory stimuli.

5.1 Dual WM task for visual and auditory representations
Fourteen healthy volunteers (10 male and 4 female; mean age = 27.92 ± 6.76 years, range 21–41 years; 13 right-handed) with normal or corrected-to-normal visual acuity, normal hearing acuity, and normal motor performance took part in the single visual and dual WM tasks. All participants gave written informed consent, which was approved by the Ethical Committee of the RIKEN (in accordance with the Declaration of Helsinki), before the experiments were performed.

For the single VWM task, at the beginning of each trial, 5 × 5 gridded squares and a red circle included within one of those squares were presented on the computer screen as the visual stimulus for 1 s (Fig. 3A). The participants were required to memorize and then maintain the position of the red circle for 2 s after the visual stimulus disappeared. A white arrow designating a direction (up, down, right, or left) to which the participants should move the red circle in their minds was then presented at the center of screen for 1 s. The participants manipulated the mental representations for 2 s. Like the auditory working memory condition, the participants were required to repeat the mental manipulation 4 times, and then determine whether the position of the red circle which they mentally moved matched a probe visual stimulus (test display). In half of the trials, the probe stimulus matched the mental representation. In the remaining trials, the wrong probe was presented by changing only the fourth direction of movement from the initial position. The participants were asked to indicate via button press whether the probe stimulus was correct or not while the fixation point was red for 2 s. The duration of the ITI was 2 s. The size of the red circle and gridded squares was $1° \times 1°$ and $5° \times 5°$ ($1° \times 1°$ per square), respectively.

For the dual WM task, the participants were asked to complete an auditory WM task simultaneously to the visual tast (Fig. 3B). When the visual stimuli described above were presented on the computer screen, a word indicating a one-digit number was simultaneously presented as the auditory stimulus through the headphones of both ears for 1 s (sample display). The auditory WM task requried the participants to memorize and maintain the presented number with rehearsal in their minds and, after a 2-s retention interval, to update the number by adding the another presented one-digit number for 2 s. After this a total of 4 incidences of auditory and visual manipulation, auditory and visual stimuli were simultaneously presented again, and participants were required to judge whether or not they were identical to the manipulated mental representation for both auditory and visual tasks (test display). In half of the trials, both the auditory and visual probe stimulus matched the mental representations. In the remaining trials, the incorrect probe for either the auditory or visual stimulus was presented, similar to the single VWM condition. The button press, duration of the inter-trial interval, and creation of the stimuli were identical to the single WM condition.

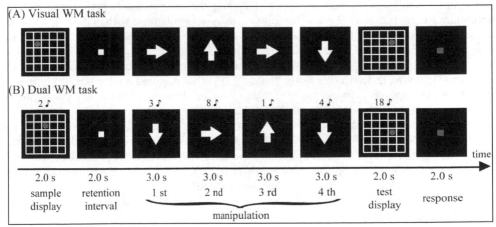

Fig. 3. Task procedure for one trial of the single visual WM (A) and dual WM (B) tasks.

5.2 EEG measurements and analyses
The same methods were used as described in Section 4.2.

5.3 Results
All participants performed all the WM tasks with high accuracy rates (mean accuracy rate (± s.d.), $97.3 \pm 4.7\%$ and $91.1 \pm 7.1\%$ for visual and dual WM conditions, respectively).

Significant differences in performance were detected between the single and dual WM conditons (Wilcoxon signed-rank test; $Z = 2.87$, $P < 0.01$), suggesting the presence of dual-task interference, that is, degraded performance of 2 simultaneous tasks relative to a single task (e.g., psychological refractory period) (Logan & Gordon, 2001; Pashler, 1994).

Time-frequency analyses of the recorded EEG data revealed enhanced theta amplitudes (4–6 Hz) of the 4 manipulation periods relative to those of the ITI in the frontal and parietal regions in both the single visual and dual WM conditions (single WM: AF3 electrode, $Z = 3.53$, $P < 0.01$; Pz electrode, $Z = 2.04$, $P < 0.05$; dual WM: AF3 electrode, $Z = 3.71$, $P < 0.01$; Pz electrode, $Z = 3.01$, $P < 0.01$). The increased frontal theta amplitudes during the dual WM conditions were significantly higher than those during the single VWM condition (AF3, $Z = 2.24$, $P < 0.03$), whereas this difference was not observed in the parietal theta activities (Pz, $Z = 0.68$, $P = 0.49$).

In addition to the theta amplitudes, alpha amplitudes (9–12 Hz) were increased only in the parietal regions during manipulation periods in the single visual WM condition (single WM: AF3, $Z = 1.15$, $P = 0.25$, Pz, $Z = 2.19$, $P < 0.05$; dual WM: AF3 electrode, $Z = 1.11$, $P < 0.27$; Pz electrode, $Z = 2.39$, $P < 0.02$). Parietal alpha amplitudes demonstrated no significant difference between the single and dual WM conditions (Pz, $Z = 1.78$, $P = 0.08$). Moreover, enhanced parietal alpha activity was observed during the retention intervals as well as the manipulation periods (Pz, $Z = 0.49$, $P = 0.62$).

5.4 Discussion

The EEG results concerning oscillatory amplitudes demonstrated the bottlenecks of central executive function in WM. In our recent study using single visual and auditory WM tasks, the frontal theta activity was mainly observed during the manipulation period and not the maintenance periods, whereas posterior alpha activity was enhanced both in the manipulation and maintenance periods (Kawasaki et al., 2010). Building upon those previous findings, the present study demonstrated that frontal theta activity further increased in the dual WM task in comparison to the single VWM task, whereas parietal alpha activity did not differ between the single and dual WM tasks. In this study, the dual WM task required a large amount of mental manipulation compared to the single WM task. However, the amount of visual representations to be remembered for the dual WM task was almost same that required for the single VWM task. Therefore, these results indicate that the bottlenecks for central executive function are represented by frontal theta activity, which is supported by the earlier evidence that the frontal cortex is associated with active manipulation, and the posterior regions are involved in simple maintenance (Curtis & D'Esposito, 2003; Postle et al., 1999; Rowe et al., 2000; Smith & Jonides, 1999; Wager & Smith, 2003). These results suggest that concurrent frontal theta and alpha activity is associated with the hierarchical control structures of the multiple operations involved in dual WM tasks.

6. Conclusion

Using data from 2 EEG experiments, this study has demonstrated the brain oscillations that are related to WM capacities for visual storage and central executive function. Frontal theta and parietal alpha activities represented the storage limitations under conditions of high and low WM demands, respectively. Moreover, frontal theta activity was also related to bottlenecks in central executive function, which is necessary to perform dual WM tasks. In addition to confirming previous findings concerning regional dissociations between WM functions, the present study further suggests important roles for these brain oscillations, which reflect different local synchronizations within specific cell assemblies, in the WM process: theta for manipulation and alpha for maintenance.

7. Acknowledgment

This research was supported by Grant-in-Aid for Scientific Research on Innovative Areas (21120005 & 22118510) and Grant-in-Aid for Young Scientists (B) (23700328). We would like to thank Yoko Yamaguchi for her help in discussions for this study, Eri Miyauchi for her support of our data analyses, and Yuta Kakimoto, Ken'ichi Sawai, and Saoko Ikuno for their support of our data acquisition.

8. References

Alvarez, G.A. & Cavanagh, P. (2004). The capacity of visual short-term memory is set both by visual information load and by number of objects. *Psychological Science*, Vol.15, No.2, (February 2004), pp. 106-111, ISSN 0956-7976.

Baddeley, A.D. & Hitch, G. (1974). Working memory, In: *Recent Advances in Learning and Motivation*, G.A. Bower GA (Ed), 47-90, Academic, New York.

Baddeley, A.D., Lewis, V.J., & Vallar, G. (1984). Exploring the articulatory loop. *Quarterly Journal of Experimental Psychology Section A: Human Experimental Psychology*, Vol.36, pp. 233-252.

Baddeley, A.D. (1986). *Working memory*. Clarendon Press, Oxford.

Baddeley, A.D. (2000). The episodic buffer: a new component of working memory? *Trends in Cognitive Sciences, Vol. 4, pp. 417-423.*

Bisley, J.W. & Pasternak, T. (2000). The multiple roles of visual cortical areas MT/MST in remembering the direction of visual motion. *Cerebral Cortex*, Vol.10, pp. 1053-1065.

Braver, T.S., Cohen, J.D., Nyström, L.E., Jonides, J., Smith, E.E., & Noll, D.C. (1997). A parametric study of prefrontal cortex involvement in human working memory. *Neuroimage*, Vol.5, pp. 49-62.

Chafee, M.V. & Goldman-Rakic, P.S. (1998). Matching patterns of activity in primate prefrontal area 8a and parietal area 7ip during a spatial working memory task. *Journal of Neurophysiology*, Vol.79, pp. 2919-2940.

Courtney, S.M., Ungerleider, L.G., Keil, K., & Haxby, J.V. (1997). Transient and sustained activity in a distributed neural system for human working memory. *Nature*, Vol.386, pp. 608-611.

Courtney, S.M., Petit, L., Maisog, J.M., Ungerleider, L.G., & Haxby, J.V. (1998). An area specialized for spatial working memory in human frontal cortex. *Science*, Vol.279, pp. 1347-1351.

Cowan, N. (2001). The magical number 4 in short-term memory: a consideration of mental storage capacity. *Behavioral Brain Science*, Vol.24, pp. 87-114.

Curtis, C.E. & D'Esposito, M. (2003). Persistent activity in the prefrontal cortex during working memory. *Trends in Neurosciences*, Vol.7, pp. 415-423.

Della Sala, S. & Logie, R. (1993). When working memory does not work. The role of working memory in neuropsychology, In: *Handbook of Neuropsychology*, F. Boller and H. Spinnler (Eds.), Vol.8, 1-63. Elsevier, Amsterdam, the Netherlands.

Delorme, A., & Makeig, S. (2004). EEGLAB: an open source toolbox for analysis of single-trial EEG dynamics. *Journal of Neuroscience Methods*, Vol.134, pp. 9-21.

Diwadkar, V.A., Carpenter, P.A. & Just, M.A. (2000). Collaborative activity between parietal and dorso-lateral prefrontal cortex in dynamic spatial working memory revealed by fMRI. *Neuroimage*, Vol.12, pp. 85-99.

Fuster, J.M. & Alexander, G.E. (1971). Neuron activity related to short-term memory. *Science*, Vol.173, pp. 652-654.

Funahashi, S., Bruce, C.J., and Goldman-Rakic, P.S. (1989). Mnemonic coding of visual space in the monkey's dorsolateral prefrontal cortex. *Journal of Neurophysiology*, Vol.61, pp. 331-349.

Glahn, D.C., Kim, J., Cohen, M.S., Poutanen, V.P., Therman, S., Bava, S., VanErp, T.G.M., Manninen, M., Huttunen, M., Lonnquvist, J., Standertskjold-Nordenstam, C.G., & Cannon, T.D. (2002). Maintenance and manipulation in spatial working memory: dissociations in the prefrontal cortex. *Neuroimage*, Vol.17, pp. 201-213.

Goldman-Rakic, P.S. (1987). Circuitry of primate prefrontal cortex and regulation of behavior by representational memory, In: *Handbook of Physiology*. F. Mountcastle & F. Plum (Eds.), 373-417, American Physiology Society, Washington DC, USA.

Jensen, O., & Tesche, C.D. (2002). Frontal theta activity in humans increases with memory load in a working memory task. *European Journal of Neuroscience*, Vol.15, pp. 1395-1399.

Jha, A.P. & McCarthy, G. (2000). The influence of memory load upon delay-interval activity in a working memory task: an event-related functional MRI study. *Journal of Cognitive Neuroscience*, Vol.12 (Suppl 2), pp. 90-105.

Kawasaki, M., & Watanabe, M. (2007). Oscillatory gamma and theta activity during repeated mental manipulations of a visual image. *Neuroscience Letters*, Vol.422, pp. 141-145.

Kawasaki, M., Watanabe, M., Okuda, J., Sakagami, M., & Aihara, K. (2008). Human posterior parietal cortex maintains color, shape and motion in visual short-term memory. *Brain Research*, Vol.1213, pp. 91-97.

Kawasaki, M., Kitajo, K., & Yamaguchi, Y. (2010). Dynamic links between theta executive functions and alpha storage buffers in auditory and visual working memory. *European Journal of Neuroscience*, Vol.31, pp. 1683-1689.

Klimesch, W., Freunberger, R., Sauseng, P., & Gruber, W. (2008). A short review of slow phase synchronization and memory: evidence for control processes in different memory systems? *Brain Research*, Vol.1235, pp. 31-44.

Kubota, K. & Niki, H. (1971). Prefrontal cortical unit activity and delayed alternation performance in monkeys. *Journal of Neurophysiology*, Vol.34, pp. 337-347.

Linden, D.E.J., Bittner, R.A., Muckli, L., Waltz, J.A., Kriegeskorte, N., Goebel, R., Singer, W., & Munk, M.H.J. (2003). Cortical capacity constraints of visual working memory: dissociation of fMRI load effects in a front-parietal network. *Neuroimage*, Vol.20, pp. 1518-1530.

Logan, G.D. & Gordon, R.D. (2001). Executive control of visual attention in dual-task situations. *Psychological Review*, Vol.108, pp. 393-434.

Luck, S.J. & Vogel, E.K. (1997). The capacity of visual working memory for features and conjunctions. *Nature*, Vol.390, pp. 279-281.

Marois, R. & Ivanoff, J. (2005). Capacity limits of information processing in the brain. *Trends in Cognitive Sciences*, Vol.9, pp. 296-305.

Miller, E.K. & Cohen, J.D. (2001). An integrative theory of prefrontal cortex function. *Annual Review of Neuroscience*, Vol.24, pp.167-202.

Miyashita, Y. & Chang, H.S. (1988). Neuronal correlate of pictorial short-term memory in the primate temporal cortex. *Nature*, Vol.331, pp. 68-70.

Mizuhara, H., Wang, L.Q., Kobayashi, K., & Yamaguchi, Y. (2004). A long-range cortical network emerging with theta oscillation in a mental task. *Neuroreport*, Vol.15, pp. 1233-1238.

Pashler, H. (1994). Dual-task interference in simple tasks: data and theory. *Psychological Bulletin*, Vol.116, pp. 220-244.

Passingham, R.E. & Sakai, K. (2004). Working memory: physiology and brain imaging. *Current Opinion in Neurobiology*, Vol.14, pp. 163-168.

Perrin, F., Pernier, J., Bertrand, O., & Echallier, J. F. (1989) Spherical splines for scalp potential and current density map reading. *Electroencephalography and Clinical Neurophysiology*, Vol.72, pp. 184-187.

Phillips W.A. (1974). On the distinction between sensory storage and short-term visual memory. *Perception & Psychophysics*, Vol.16, pp. 283-290.

Postle, B.R. & D'Esposito, M. (1999). Dissociation of human caudate nucleus activity in spatial and nonspatial working memory: An event-related fMRI study. *Cognitive Brain Research*, Vol.8, pp. 107-115.

Rowe, J.B., Toni, I., Josephs, O., Frackowiak, R.S., & Passingham, R.E. (2000). The prefrontal cortex: response selection or maintenance within working memory? *Science*, Vol.288, pp. 1656-1660.

Rypma, B., Berger, J.S., & D'Esposito, M. (2002) The influence of working-memory demand and subject performance on prefrontal cortical activity. *Journal of Cognitive Neuroscience*, Vol.14, pp. 721-731.

Sauseng, P., Klimesch, W., Schabus, M., & Doppelmayr, M. (2005). Fronto-parietal EEG coherence in theta and upper alpha reflect central executive functions of working memory. *International Journal of Psychophysiology*, Vol.57, pp. 97-103.

Smith, E.E. & Jonides, J. (1999). Storage and executive processes of the frontal lobes. *Science*, Vol.283, pp. 1657-1661.

Tallon-Baudry, C., Bertrand, O., Delpuech, C., & Pernier, J. (1997). Oscillatory gamma-band (30-70 Hz) activity induced by a visual search task in humans. *Journal of Neuroscience*, Vol.17, pp. 722-734.

Todd, J.J. & Marois, R. (2004). Capacity limit of visual short-term memory in human posterior parietal cortex. *Nature*, Vol.428, pp. 751-754.

Todd, J.J. & Marois, R. (2005) Posterior parietal cortex activity predicts individual differences in visual short-term memory capacity. *Cognitive, Affective, & Behavioral Neuroscience*, Vol.5, pp. 144-155.

Varela, F., Lachaux, J. P., Rodriguez, E., & Martinerie, J. (2001) The brainweb: phase synchronization and large-scale integration. *Nature Reviews Neuroscience*, Vol.2, pp. 229-239.

Vogel, E.K. & Machizawa, M.G. (2004). Neural activity predicts individual differences in visual working memory capacity. *Nature*, Vol.428, pp. 784-751.

Wager, T.D. & Smith, E.E. (2003) Neuroimaging studies of working memory: a meta-analysis. *Cognitive, Affective, & Behavioral Neuroscience*, Vol.3, pp.255-274.

Wheeler, M.E. & Treisman, A.M. (2002) Binding in short-term visual memory. *J Exp Psychol Gen*, Vol.131, pp. 65-72.

Xu, Y. & Chun, M.M. (2006). Dissociable neural mechanisms supporting visual short-term memory for objects. *Nature*, Vol.440, pp. 91-95.

3

Reinforcement Learning, High-Level Cognition, and the Human Brain

Massimo Silvetti and Tom Verguts
Ghent University
Belgium

1. Introduction

Reinforcement learning (RL) has a rich history tracing throughout the history of psychology. Already in the late 19th century Edward Thorndike proposed that if a stimulus is followed by a successful response, the stimulus-response bond will be strengthened. Consequently, the response will be emitted with greater likelihood upon later presentation of that same stimulus. This proposal already contains the two key principles of RL. The first principle concerns *associative learning*, the learning of associations between stimuli and responses. This theme was developed by John Watson. Building on the work of Ivan Pavlov, John Watson investigated the laws of classical conditioning, in particular, how a stimulus and a response become associated after repeated pairing. In the classical "Little Albert" experiment, Watson and Rayner (1920) repeatedly presented a rabbit together with a loud sound to the kid (little Albert); the rabbit initially evoked a neutral response, the loud sound initially evoked a fear response. After a while, also presentation of the rabbit alone evoked a fear response in the subject. In this same paper, the authors proposed that this principle of learning by association more generally is responsible for shaping (human) behavior. According to psychology handbooks John Watson hereby laid the foundation for behaviorism. The second principle is that *reinforcement* is key for human learning. Actions that are successful for the organism, will be strengthened and therefore repeated by the organism. This aspect was developed into a systematic research program by the second founder of behaviorism, Burrhus Skinner (e.g., Skinner, 1938).

The importance of RL for explaining human behavior started to be debated from the late 1940s. Scientific criticism toward RL arrived from two main fronts. The first was internal, deriving from experimental findings and theoretical considerations within psychology itself. The second derived from external developments, in particular, advancements in information theory and control theory. These criticisms led to a disinterest for RL lasting several decades. However, in recent years, RL has been revived, leading to a remarkable interdiscplinary confluence between computer science, neurophysiology, and cognitive neuroscience. In the current chapter, we describe the relevant mid-20th century criticisms and developments, and how these were considered and integrated in current versions of RL. In particular we focus on how RL can be used as a model for understanding high-level cognition. Finally, we link RL to the broader framework of neural Darwinism.

2. Internal criticisms to RL

During the 40s, more and more data were piling up demonstrating the insufficiency of behaviorism to account for human and animal behavior. For example, Tolman and colleagues showed that animals can and do learn even without obtaining reinforcement (Tolman, 1948). They performed a series of experiments on maze learning in rats. It was shown that animals left free to familiarize themselves with the maze before the reinforcement experimental session, were afterwards able to find the food in the maze much more efficiently than completely naive animals. To explain these findings Tolman introduced the concept of the "cognitive map", i.e. an internal representation of the maze that the rats used to find reinforcers more efficiently. Because of this and other demonstrations that animals hold some kind of internal representation of the environment (memory), Tolman formed part of what became known as "the cognitive revolution".

During the same period, but in the field of psychobiology, Donald Hebb wrote *The Organization of Behaviour* (1949), a seminal work in which for the first time a neurobiological theory of learning was proposed. Hebb suggested that the synaptic connection between two neurons improves its efficacy after repeated simultaneous activity of them. This law, properly called "Hebbian rule" and describing what was called "Hebbian Learning", provided the first neural hypothesis on the basis of memory, thus opening the "black box", which behaviorists considered not scientifically investigable. The depth of Hebb's intuition can be better understood if we consider that the Hebbian rule has been experimentally proven almost twenty years after its formulation, with the discover of synaptic long term potentiation (LTP) in the rabbit hippocampus (Lømo, 1966).

Another strong criticism came from psycholinguistics. In a famous review study, Noam Chomsky (1959) argued that the RL paradigm was not suitable to explain the generative feature of natural language (i.e. the possibility to express a quasi-infinite variety of verbal expressions). In the same work, Chomsky also provided a survey on research in animal behavior (e.g., imprinting) that seemed to be in striking contrast with key behaviorist tenets. Finally, and most importantly from the theoretical point of view, Chomsky showed that Skinner himself was obliged to introduce hypotheses about internal variables (e.g., internal self-reinforcements), in order to explain human verbal behavior.

3. External developments

An important role in the demise of RL derived from advances in information theory and control theory in engineering. This happened during the 1940-50s with the publication of several seminal works like those of Shannon (1948), Turing (1936) and Wiener (1948). Their importance consisted in showing that it was possible to formulate rigorous mathematical theories and models to study information processing. In control theory (Wiener, 1948), for instance, the term "control" referred to the auto-correction of internal parameters of a system based on a feedback signal indicating the error between the wished (or the expected) value of an internal parameter and its real value, typically provided by the environment. This general theory of control (called cybernetics) (literally from ancient Greek: "the art of piloting"), did not refer to a particular system: instead, it provided mathematical models to study control phenomena occurring *inside* any system, being animal or artificial or even social. A similar story holds for information theory (Shannon, 1948), which provided the concept of "information", a measure that did not refer to any directly measurable physical variable, but instead to the *internal* "surprise" of any system receiving an external signal.

These new disciplines showed that it was possible, and indeed a proficient and powerful approach, to investigate the internal functioning of systems (including biological organisms), by mathematical modelling of their hidden machinery that was not directly investigable. In this way, the philosophical-methodological assumption of behaviorism, according to which the scientific approach should be limited to strictly empirical investigation, was shown to be unnecessary for scientific progress.

4. Precursors to the return of RL

Because of these developments, behaviorism, and with it RL, was discredited for several decades. Instead an alternative paradigm became dominant, according to which the human mind could be construed as a computer that manipulates abstract symbols (e.g., Neisser, 1967; Atkinson and Shiffrin, 1968). However, in recent years the RL framework became influential again. At least two developments in the second part of the 20th century prepared a renewed interest for RL. The first originated in human learning theory; the second from a new discipline called connectionist psychology, which proposed itself as an alternative to the then canonical symbol-manipulation paradigm for the study of cognition.

4.1 Human learning theory and the Rescorla-Wagner model

Important phenomena observed in the behavioral lab could not be accounted for with the standard behaviorist conceptualization (Rescorla and Wagner, 1972). For example, blocking (Kamin, 1969) refers to the fact that an organism only learns about the contingency between two events to the extent that one of the events is unexpected. To account for blocking, Rescorla and Wagner added a crucial ingredient to an associative learning framework, namely prediction error. Prediction error refers to the difference between an external feedback signal indicating the correct response or stimulus on the one hand, and the response or stimulus predicted by the organism on the other. Here it is worth noting the influence (and indeed similarity) of the cybernetic concept of feedback on the formulation of the concept of prediction error. Rescorla and Wagner proposed a formal model which learned by updating associations between events (e.g., stimulus and response) using prediction error (Rescorla and Wagner, 1972). This model formed the basis for many human learning theories (e.g., Kruschke, 2008; Pearce and Hall, 1980; Van Hamme and Wasserman, 1994), and can be represented by the following equations:

$$\delta_t = \lambda_t - V_t \tag{1}$$

$$V_{t+1} = V_t + \alpha\delta_t \tag{2}$$

where δ is the prediction error, V is the prediction of the organism, and λ is the actual outcome from the environment. Equation 2 shows how the new expectations are updated by the prediction error from time point t to $t+1$; α is a learning rate parameter modulating the prediction error.

4.2 The connectionist approach

A second development preparing the cultural ground for reviving the field of RL was connectionist psychology. Here, the study of psychological phenomena was grounded on the construction of artificial neural networks, i.e. models simulating both the nervous system and cognitive processes, providing what was called a sub-symbolic explanation of cognition. This new field was inspired by the fast developing neurosciences; in particular, the scientists developing this new branch not only did not adhere to the dogma that theorizing should remain at the behavioral level, but they also attempted to bridge the explanatory gap between the biological level of neurons and synapses on the one hand, and the psychological level of language and other forms of high-level cognition on the other.

An important step was taken by McClelland, Rumelhart and colleagues (Rumelhart and McClelland, 1986). Models similar to theirs had been developed by other researchers before (Grossberg, 1973) but Rumelhart and McClelland developed a series of applications that made these connectionist models almost instantly influential. At the core of these models is again the Rescorla-Wagner idea that learning consists of updating associations based on prediction errors. However, the authors proposed a generalized learning rule (backpropagation), which allowed learning also for so-called "hidden units", that is, neurons that do not receive external feedback. In backpropagation, such neurons use as a prediction error a linear combination of prediction errors of other neurons that do receive external feedback. This development made the learning rule many orders more powerful than that of Rescorla and Wagner. With the more powerful learning rule, the connectionists were able to investigate linguistic phenomena such as past tense formation (Rumelhart and McClelland, 1987), naming aloud (Seidenberg and McClelland, 1989), and sentence comprehension (St. John and McClelland, 1990).

4.3 The new RL approach

With these important historical precedents, RL learning became influential again during the early 1990s partly because of its important contributions to Machine Learning, a branch of Artificial Intelligence. One of the main protagonists of this revival was Richard Sutton, who developed another generalization of the Rescorla-Wagner rule, called temporal-difference (TD) learning (Sutton, 1988). The original Rescorla-Wagner rule had a *spatial* limitation in the sense that not all neurons received feedback, and this problem was solved by backpropagation. Similarly, the Rescorla-Wagner rule also has a *temporal* limitation in the sense that feedback is not always available to the model – only when there is explicit supervisory feedback. The TD learning algorithm solved this latter problem, because it allowed learning by not only comparing a prediction with external feedback (which may or may not be available, depending on an appropriate teacher's availability), but additionally by comparing a prediction with an earlier prediction (which is always available). In this case the learning signal is the TD error (here denoted as δ^{TD}), in which both the comparisons between previous prediction and external feedback and previous prediction and current prediction play a role. The TD error signal can be written as follows:

$$\delta_{t+1}^{TD} = \lambda_{t+1} + \gamma V_{t+1} - V_t \tag{3}$$

where λ is the external feedback already defined in Equation (1) and γ is a discount factor. The symbol V was used before to denote the organism's prediction; in RL applications, it refers specifically to reward prediction. This rule is more powerful than the Rescorla-Wagner rule: For example, Tesauro (1989) demonstrated that a neural network equipped with TD learning can learn to play backgammon at a worldmaster level.

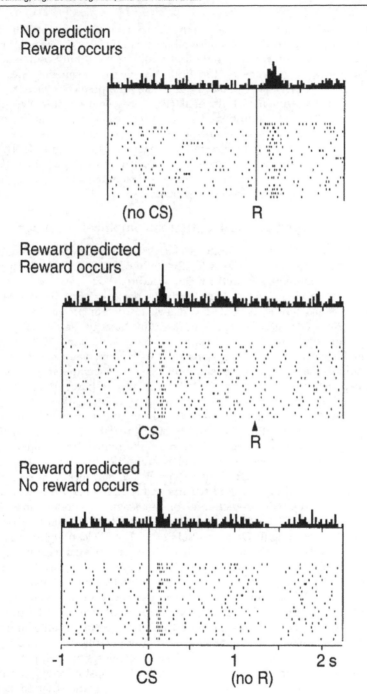

Fig. 1. Shifting of dopaminergic activity from reward to predictor of reward (CS). Reprinted with permission from Schultz et al. (1997).

A few years later, the RL paradigm received the decisive boost to come back to the attention of the broad scientific community. This derived from its official entrance into the domain of neurophysiology. In particular, with single-unit recording Wolfram Schulz and colleagues discovered dopaminergic neurons in the brainstem ventral tegmental area (VTA) and substantia nigra (SN) of macaque monkeys that exhibited a prediction error signature. In a classical conditioning experiment, Schultz et al. (1993) presented a conditioned stimulus (CS, e.g. a light), followed by an unconditioned stimulus (US, e.g. a drop of juice) some seconds later. Initially, dopaminergic neurons respond to the US only. After some trials, the dopaminergic neurons respond to the CS, but no longer to the US (Figure 1). This backward shift in time is exactly what was predicted by TD learning (Montague et al., 1996). Hence, this strongly suggested that the mammalian nervous system implements a RL (in particular, TD) algorithm to learn associations between stimuli.

5. RL in high-level cognition: Conceptual and empirical advances

Ever since the seminal findings of Schultz et al. (1993), the marriage between neuroscience and RL never stopped providing benefits for the study of learning and the nervous system. We here discuss a few highlights from the recent literature.

One conceptual development of RL consisted in the discovery that besides reward value, other value dimensions can be estimated and used to discount reward value (e.g., effort, Kennerley et al., 2006, or delay, Rudebeck et al., 2006). More generally, not only value but also upcoming states of the world can be estimated (Sutton and Barto, 1998). This allows the organism to make more far-sighted actions than with immediate values estimates only. Further, RL models have been proposed with the same computational power as the benchmark backpropagation algorithm (O'Reilly & Frank, 2004; Roelfsema and Van Ooyen, 2005), providing a biologically plausible alternative to backpropagation.

At the empirical level, clever experimental paradigms in combination with modern imaging technology allowed demonstrating the validity of RL models for human cognition. Using fMRI, Seymour et al. (2004) identified a TD signal in the human brain, similar to what was found by Schultz and colleagues in the monkey brain. Seymour et al. used a cued pain learning paradigm, in which a first CS (CS1) predicted (statistically) a second CS (CS2), which then (deterministically) predicted the upcoming pain level. In the striatum (ventral putamen), they observed a pain prediction error signal which responded to CS1 onset, and to CS2 if it differed from CS1 (i.e., was unpredicted based on CS1). Similar paradigms were used using appetitive learning (O'Doherty et al., 2003). The TD learning framework has also been applied extensively to EEG data, in particular the error-related negativity, for example in the work of Holroyd and Coles (2002). These authors successfully compared the performance of a TD learning-based computational model with the dynamics of the error-related negativity (ERN) from human volunteers. The model was aimed to clarify the roles of anterior cingulate cortex (ACC) and the ventral striatal structures in an instrumental conditioning paradigm. The authors proposed that the ventral striatum implements TD learning in order to estimate the value of external stimuli in terms of expected reward, while the ACC functions as a filter of several possible motor responses. In their proposal, the ACC would select the motor plans that are expected to be the most effective to achieve future rewards, based on the reward predictions computed by the ventral striatum. In this model, the ERN would be the result of ACC activity following the suppression of dopaminergic input from the ventral striatum. In a series of EEG experiments, Holroyd and Coles showed that their model was indeed able to predict several effects linked to the ERN, for example the fact that this EEG component appears only when there is a violation of the reward prediction.

Another example comes from the study of Parkinson's disease, a neurological disorder whose pathological basis consists of the degeneration of the dopaminergic neurons in the substantia nigra pars compacta, source of the main brainstem input to basal ganglia. Parkinson patients are impaired in learning from positive outcomes (reward), while performance is preserved for learning based on negative outcomes (punishment) (Frank et al., 2004). A neural model was proposed representing the interactions between basal ganglia, cortex and substantia nigra (Frank, 2005). In this model, the basal ganglia consists of two neural populations; "Go" neurons fire when an action planned in cortex is allowed to be implemented, whereas "No Go" neurons suppress the action planned in the cortex. Both Go and No Go populations learn by dopaminergic (i.e., reinforcement-related) bursts and dips coming from the substantia nigra. One of the advantages of the model consists in explaining several symptoms of Parkinson's disease. For instance, with reduced dopaminergic input (simulation of the substantia nigra degeneration), the basal ganglia are impaired at learning in Go neural populations, and hence impaired specifically in learning by rewards, just like human Parkinson patients. In addition, the model successfully predicts that this distinction between Go versus No Go learning holds true in high-level cognition as well (Frank et al., 2004).

Finally, it is worth describing briefly the work of Gläscher et al. (2010), which showed, by a combined computational and fMRI study, that the human brain also implements RL-like algorithms for creating abstract models of the environment. This study resembled the historical experiment of Tolman (1948). Volunteers were at first exposed to a simplified artificial environment, in which each single state was represented by an abstract figure (a fractal) (Figure 2). The subjects were asked to "navigate" inside this environment by performing binary choices (left or right). Each choice was followed by a transition to one of two possible states, each with some probability. In the first part of the experiment, subjects freely navigated in this environment, resembling Tolman's latent learning phase. In the second part, subjects received a monetary reward in some of the final states. In this way they had to exploit the latent learning acquired during the first part of the experiment to maximize reward, again as in Tolman's paradigm. Through a model-based analysis of the fMRI signal from both experimental phases, the authors localized the brain regions involved in both the latent learning (leading to a cognitive map or model of the environment) and the subsequent model-driven RL. While the RL-related areas were those typically found in the literature (ventral striatum and dopaminergic system), the areas involved in the formation of cognitive maps were the dorsolateral prefrontal cortex and intraparietal sulci.

The merit of this work consisted not only in the localization of two separate circuits for RL and environment-model (cognitive map) learning, but also in the demonstration that the two processes can be based on very similar computational mechanisms. One is the already described "prediction error" (Equation (1)), the other the "state prediction error". The latter is formally similar to the prediction error (comparison between predictions and real outcomes), but it deals with environmental state transitions. The mathematical form of the state prediction error (δ^{SPE}) is the following (note the similarity with Equation (1)):

$$\delta_t^{SPE} = 1 - T_t\left(s,a,s'\right) \tag{4}$$

where the value 1 corresponds to the probability of being in the current state (s'; with probability 1), and $T(s,a,s')$ is the expected probability of transition from previous state s (the previous state) to the current state given (chosen) action a. The expectation T is updated by means of the state prediction error:

$$T_{t+1}(s,a,s') = T_t(s,a,s') + \alpha\delta_t^{SPE}$$ (5)

In conclusion, this work showed that prediction error and state prediction error are similar computations but calculated in different brain circuits. This suggested a neurophysiological and computational basis of Tolman's discoveries sixty years before.

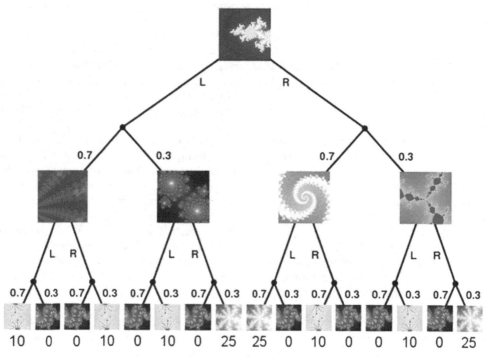

Fig. 2. Formal structure of state space in Gläscher et al.'s experiment. Reprinted with permission from Gläscher et al. (2010).

6. A case study: RL, cognitive control, and anterior cingulate cortex

One of the remaining mysteries of the human mind is executive functioning or cognitive control – the rapid modulation of behavior when called for by unexpected circumstances. In the symbol-manipulation paradigm, executive functioning was proposed to originate from a central executive endowed with two or more "slave systems" (typically the visuospatial sketch pad and the phonologic loop; Baddeley and Hitch, 1974). Detailed models have been developed of the slave systems (Burgess and Hitch, 1999), and in general great progress has been made in understanding them. However, the role of the central executive has remained poorly understood. To tackle this issue, researchers have tried recasting executive functioning in neural models. We will describe these models and demonstrate how the union of RL and connectionist models provides steps toward understanding the neural basis of cognitive control.

6.1 Associative models of cognitive control

Working within the connectionist framework, Cohen et al. (1990) proposed a model of the Stroop task, a widely used index of cognitive control. In this task, subjects are shown a color word in a given ink color, with the color and word either congruent (e.g., the word RED written in red), or incongruent (e.g., the word RED written in green). The subject's task is to name the ink color. Because word reading is automatic in literate adults, cognitive control is required to override the automatic tendency to read the word. Although subjects can do this, a congruency cost is typically observed, with incongruent trials slower than congruent ones. The Stroop task is widely used in clinical contexts to assess executive functioning, and differentiates between healthy subjects and various patient groups suffering from impairments in cognitive control (e.g., ADHD, Willcutt et al., 2005; Parkinson's disease, Bonnin et al., 2010). In the Cohen et al. model, a distinction is made between an input layer for the relevant dimension and an input layer for the irrelevant dimension, each projecting to a response layer. Crucially, Cohen et al. added task demand units which bias responding toward the relevant dimension (input layer). This brings top-down modulation in an associative model framework.

Botvinick et al. (2001) further developed the model of Cohen et al. They argued that the earlier model did not specify when cognitive control is required. In particular, cognitive control is required only on incongruent trials (e.g., RED written in green), not on congruent ones. For this purpose, they introduced the notion of response conflict, measuring the extent to which responses are simultaneously active. They proposed the conflict monitoring model, according to which response conflict is calculated in anterior cingulate cortex (ACC). Conceptually, this was an advance over the previous model, because not only top-down modulation but also the trial-by-trial cognitive control could be captured in an associative learning framework. In addition, it has been highly influential and allowed accounting for many data. For example, using fMRI Botvinick et al. (1999) demonstrated that human ACC was more active on incongruent trials following a congruent trial than on incongruent trials following an incongruent trial. This finding contradicted the popular notion that ACC activity reflects executive control itself (because the subject should be more "controlled" after an incongruent trial), but was in line with the conflict monitoring model because there should be more conflict after a congruent trial. Note that this model is also a control model in the cybernetic sense mentioned before: It detects when something goes wrong, and when so, it leads to adaptation in the system.

Verguts and Notebaert (2008, 2009) further developed this line of work. They started from the fact that the conflict monitoring model specifies when control should be exerted, but not where (see also Blais et al., 2007). To confront this issue, the authors proposed a neural model in which the implementation of cognitive control was based on an error signal modulating the Hebbian learning between active model neurons. This error signal was, like in Gläscher et al.'s work, borrowed from the RL domain. The new measure, which could be called "conflict prediction error", was computed by comparing the actual amount of conflict, evoked by a stimulus, with the expected mean amount of conflict. This model successfully predicted that cognitive control should not extend across different task input dimensions

(Notebaert and Verguts, 2008) or even across task effectors (Braem et al., in press). Consistent with the model, it was recently demonstrated that ACC responds to item-specific congruencies, not block-level congruencies (Blais and Bunge, 2011).

6.2 New evidence on ACC function: Insights from RL-based neural modelling

Besides conflict monitoring, several other functions have been attributed to the ACC. In humans, evidence using EEG and fMRI pointed toward a role in error processing (Gehring et al., 1993), error likelihood (Brown and Braver, 2005), or volatility (Behrens et al., 2007). Moreover, in the single-cell literature, no direct evidence has been found for conflict monitoring (Cole et al., 2009), while, on the other hand, there is strong evidence for reinforcement processing (Rushworth and Behrens, 2008). More specifically, single-cell recording studies revealed the presence in ACC of three different types of neural units. One population codes for reward expectation, discharging as a function of the expected reward following the presentation of an external cue or the planning of an action. A second population codes for positive prediction error (i.e. when the outcome was better than predicted). Finally, another population codes for negative prediction errors (i.e. when the outcome was worse than predicted). We recently attempted to integrate these different levels of data and theories from the point of view of the RL framework. The model we proposed (Silvetti et al., 2011), the Reward Value Prediction Model (RVPM) demonstrated that all these findings can be understood from the same computational machinery which calculates values and deviations between observed reinforcement and expected values in an RL framework. The global function of the ACC however, remained similar to that in the conflict monitoring model and later versions of it: it is to detect if something is unexpected, and if so, to take action and adapt the cognitive system.

The evolution sketched here, from abstract cybernetic control models to the RVPM, represents a general trend in RL, in which computational, cognitive, and neuroscience concepts are increasingly integrated. Despite this success, not all features of RL have received appropriate attention in the literature. In the final section, we look at an aspect of RL that has been underrepresented.

7. RL and neural Darwinism

Despite the variety in levels of abstraction and purpose of the different models that we described, most of them implement what is sometimes called a triple-factor learning rule (Ashby et al., 2007; Arbuthnott et al., 2000). This means that three factors are multiplied for the purpose of changes in model weights: the first two factors are activation of input and output neurons, constituting the Hebbian component. The third factor is a RL-like signal, which provides some evaluation of the current situation (is it rewarding, unexpected, etc; henceforth, value signal). The value signal indicates the valence of an environmental state or of an internal state of the individual. It can be both encoded by dopaminergic signals (Holroyd & Coles, 2001) or by noradrenergic signals (e.g., Gläscher et al., 2010; Verguts & Notebaert, 2009).

This general scheme of Hebbian learning modulated by value provides an instantiation of the theory of Neural Darwinism (ND; Edelman, 1978). ND is a large scale theory on brain processes with roots in evolutionary theory and immunology. The basic idea of ND consists in the analogy between the Darwinian process of natural selection of individual organisms, and the selection of the most appropriate neural connections between a large population of them. The general learning rule described above implements such a scheme. Because of the Hebbian component (input and output cells active together), individual synapses (which connect input and output neurons) are selected; and because of the value signal, the most appropriate synapses are chosen.

Just like in Darwinism applied to natural evolution, one key ingredient of ND is variation (called degeneracy by Edelman, 1978), or exploration when the unit of variation is not the individual synapse but rather responses (Aston-Jones & Cohen, 2001). From this variation, a selection can be made, based on an appropriate value signal. Computationally, Dehaene et al. (1987) demonstrated that temporal sequence learning can be achieved by such a variation-and-selection process. In neuroimaging, Daw et al. (2006) demonstrated that frontopolar cortex was used when subjects were in an exploration (rather than exploitation) phase of learning. Besides a few exceptions, however, variation and selection remain poorly studied. Given that it is a key component of RL, we suggest that its further exploration will learn us much more about high-level cognition and its implementation in the human brain.

8. Acknowledgements

MS and TV were supported by BOF/GOA Grant BOF08/GOA/011.

9. References

Arbuthnott, G. W., Ingham, C. A., & Wickens, J. R. (2000). Dopamine and synaptic plasticity in the neostriatum. *Journal of Anatomy, 196,* 587-596.

Ashby, F. G., Ennis, J. M., & Spiering, B. J. (2007). A neurobiological theory of automaticity in perceptual categorization. *Psychological Review, 114,* 632-656.

Aston-Jones, G., & Cohen, J. D. (2005). An integrative theory of locus coeruleus-norepinephrine function: Adaptive gain and optimal performance. *Annual Review of Neuroscience, 28,* 403-450.

Atkinson, R.C., and Shiffrin, R.M. (1968). "Human memory: A proposed system and its control processes," in *The psychology of learning and motivation.* (New York: Academic Press), 89-195.

Baddeley, A.D., and Hitch, G. (1974). "Working memory," in *The psychology of learning and motivation: Advances in research and theory,* ed. G.H. Bower. (New York: Academic Press).

Behrens, T.E., Woolrich, M.W., Walton, M.E., and Rushworth, M.F. (2007). Learning the value of information in an uncertain world. *Nat Neurosci* 10, 1214-1221.

Blais, C., and Bunge, S. (2011). Behavioral and neural evidence for item-specific performance monitoring. *J Cogn Neurosci* 22, 2758-2767.

Blais, C., Robidoux, S., Risko, E.F., and Besner, D. (2007). Item-specific adaptation and the conflict-monitoring hypothesis: a computational model. *Psychol Rev* 114, 1076-1086.

Bonnin, C.A., Houeto, J.L., Gil, R., and Bouquet, C.A. (2010). Adjustments of conflict monitoring in Parkinson's disease. *Neuropsychology* 24, 542-546.

Botvinick, M., Braver, T.S., Barch, D.M., Carter, C.S., and Cohen, J.D. (2001). Conflict monitoring and cognitive control. *Psychol Rev* 108, 624-652.

Botvinick, M., Nystrom, L.E., Fissell, K., Carter, C.S., and Cohen, J.D. (1999). Conflict monitoring versus selection-for-action in anterior cingulate cortex. *Nature* 402, 179-181.

Braem, S., Verguts, T., & Notebaert, W. (in press). Conflict adaptation by means of associative learning. *Journal of Experimental Psychology: Human Perception & Performance.*

Brown, J.W., and Braver, T.S. (2005). Learned predictions of error likelihood in the anterior cingulate cortex. *Science* 307, 1118-1121.

Burgess, N., and Hitch, G.J. (1999). Memory for Serial Order: A Network Model of the Phonological Loop and its Timing. *Psychological Review* 106, 551-581.

Chomsky, N. (1959). Review of Verbal Behavior by B.F. Skinner. *Language* 35, 26-58.

Cohen, J.D., Dunbar, K., and Mcclelland, J.L. (1990). On the control of automatic processes: a parallel distributed processing account of the Stroop effect. *Psychol Rev* 97, 332-361.

Cole, M.W., Yeung, N., Freiwald, W.A., and Botvinick, M. (2009). Cingulate cortex: diverging data from humans and monkeys. *Trends Neurosci* 32, 566-574.

Daw, N. D., O'Doherty, J. P., Dayan, P., Seymour, B., & Dolan, R. J. (2006). Cortical substrates for exploratory decisions in humans. *Nature, 441,* 876-879.

Dehaene, S., Changeux, J.-P., & Nadal, J.-P. (1987). Neural networks that learn temporal sequences by selection. *Proceedings of the National Academy of Sciences: USA, 84,* 2727-2731.

Edelman, G. (1978). *The Mindful Brain.* Cambridge, Ma: MIT press.

Frank, M.J., Seeberger, L.C., and O'reilly R, C. (2004). By carrot or by stick: cognitive reinforcement learning in parkinsonism. *Science* 306, 1940-1943.

Frank, M.J. (2005). Dynamic dopamine modulations in the basal ganglia: A neurocomputational account of cognitive deficits in medicated and nonmedicated Parkinsonism. *Journal of Cognitive Neuroscience, 17,* 51-72.

Gehring, W.J., Goss, B., Coles, M.G.H., Meyer, D.E., and Donchin, E. (1993). A Neural System for Error Detection and Compensation. *Psychological Science* 4, 385-390

Gläscher, J., Daw, N., Dayan, P., and O'doherty, J.P. (2010). States versus rewards: dissociable neural prediction error signals underlying model-based and model-free reinforcement learning. *Neuron* 66, 585-595.

Grossberg, S. (1973). Contour enhancement, short term memory, and constanciesin reverberating neural networks. *Studies in Applied Mathematics* 11, 213-257.

Hebb, D. (1949). *The organization of behavior; a neuropsychological theory.* New York Wiley-Interscience.

Holroyd, C.B., and Coles, M.G. (2002). The neural basis of human error processing: reinforcement learning, dopamine, and the error-related negativity. *Psychol Rev* 109, 679-709.

Kamin, L.J. (1969). "Predictability, surprise, attention, and conditioning.," in *Punishment and Aversive Behavior.,* eds. B.A. Campbell & R.M. Church. (New York: Appleton-Century-Crofts), 279-296.

Kennerley, S.W., Walton, M.E., Behrens, T.E., Buckley, M.J., and Rushworth, M.F. (2006). Optimal decision making and the anterior cingulate cortex. *Nat Neurosci* 9, 940-947.

Kruschke, J.K. (2008). Bayesian approaches to associative learning: from passive to active learning. *Learn Behav* 36, 210-226.

Lømo, T. (1966). Frequency potentiation of excitatory synaptic activity in the dentate area of the hippocampal formation. *Acta Physiologica Scandinavia* 68 Suppl. 277, 128.

Montague, P.R., Dayan, P., and Sejnowski, T.J. (1996). A framework for mesencephalic dopamine systems based on predictive Hebbian learning. *J Neurosci* 16, 1936-1947.

Neisser, U. (1967). *Cognitive psychology*. New York: Appleton-Century-Crofts.

Notebaert, W., and Verguts, T. (2008). Cognitive control acts locally. *Cognition* 106, 1071-1080.

O'doherty, J.P., Dayan, P., Friston, K., Critchley, H., and Dolan, R.J. (2003). Temporal difference models and reward-related learning in the human brain. *Neuron* 38, 329-337.

O'Reilly, R. C., & Frank, M. J. (2004). Making working memory work: A computational model of learning in the prefrontal cortex and basal ganglia. *Neural Computation, 18,* 283-328.

Pearce, J.M., and Hall, G. (1980). A model for Pavlovian learning: variations in the effectiveness of conditioned but not of unconditioned stimuli. *Psychol Rev* 87, 532-552.

Rescorla, R.A., and Wagner, A.R. (1972). "A theory of Pavlovian conditioning: variation in the effectiveness of reinforcement and nonreinforcement," in *Classical conditioning II: current research and theory,* eds. A.H. Black & W.F. Prokasy. (New York: Appleton-Century-Crofts), 64-99.

Roelfsema, P.R., and Van Ooyen, A. (2005). Attention-gated reinforcement learning of internal representations for classification. *Neural Computation* 17, 2176-2214.

Rudebeck, P.H., Walton, M.E., Smyth, A.N., Bannerman, D.M., and Rushworth, M.F. (2006). Separate neural pathways process different decision costs. *Nat Neurosci* 9, 1161-1168.

Rumelhart, D.E., and Mc Clelland, J.L. (1986). *Parallel Distributed Processing: Explorations in the Microstructure of Cognition*. Cambridge, MA: MIT Press.

Rumelhart, D.E., and Mcclelland, J.L. (1987). Learning the past tenses of english verbs: Implicit rules or parallel distributed processing, in *Mechanisms of Language Acquisition,* ed. B. Macwhinney. (Mahwah, NJ: Erlbaum), 194-248.

Rushworth, M.F., and Behrens, T.E. (2008). Choice, uncertainty and value in prefrontal and cingulate cortex. *Nat Neurosci* 11, 389-397.

Schultz, W., Apicella, P., and Ljungberg, T. (1993). Responses of monkey dopamine neurons to reward and conditioned stimuli during successive steps of learning a delayed response task. *J Neurosci* 13, 900-913.

Schultz, W., Dayan, P., & Montague, P. R. (1997). A neural substrate of prediction and reward. *Science, 275,* 1593-1599.

Seidenberg, M.S., and Mc Clelland, J.L. (1989). A Distributed, Developmental Model of Word Recognition and Naming. *Psychological Review* 96, 523-568.

Seymour, B., O'doherty, J.P., Dayan, P., Koltzenburg, M., Jones, A.K., Dolan, R.J., Friston, K.J., and Frackowiak, R.S. (2004). Temporal difference models describe higher-order learning in humans. *Nature* 429, 664-667.

Shannon, C.E. (1948). A Mathematical Theory of Communication. *The Bell System Technical Journal* 27, 379–423, 623–656.

Silvetti, M., Seurinck, R., and Verguts, T. (2011). Value and prediction error in the medial frontal cortex: integrating the single-unit and systems levels of analysis. *Frontiers in Human Neuroscience*, 5:75.

Skinner, B. F. (1938). *The behavior of organisms: An experimental analysis*. New York: Appleton-Century-Crofts.

St. John, M.F., and Mcclelland, J.L. (1990). Learning and applying contextual constraints in sentence comprehension. *Artificial Intelligence* 46, 217-257.

Sutton, R.S. (1988). Learning to Predict by the Method of Temporal Differences. *Machine Learning* 3, 9-44.

Sutton, R.S., and Barto, A.G. (1998). *Reinforcement learning : an introduction.* Cambridge (MA): MIT Press.

Tesauro, G. (1989). Neurogammon wins Computer Olympiad. *Neural Computation* 1, 321-323.

Tolman, E.C. (1948). Cognitive maps in rats and men. *Psychological Review* 55, 189-208.

Turing, A.M. (1936). On Computable Numbers, with an Application to the Entscheidungsproblem. *Proceedings of the London Mathematical Society* 2, 230–265.

Van Hamme, L.J., and Wasserman, E.A. (1994). Cue competition in causality judgements: The role of nonpresentation of compound stimulus elements. *Learning and Motivation* 25, 127–151.

Verguts, T., and Notebaert, W. (2008). Hebbian learning of cognitive control: dealing with specific and nonspecific adaptation. *Psychol Rev* 115, 518-525.

Verguts, T., and Notebaert, W. (2009). Adaptation by binding: a learning account of cognitive control. *Trends Cogn Sci* 13, 252-257.

Wiener, N. (1948). *Cybernetics or Control and Communication in the Animal and the Machine.* Paris: Hermann & Cie Editeurs.

Willcutt, E.G., Doyle, A.E., Nigg, J.T., Faraone, S.V., and Pennington, B.F. (2005). Validity of the executive function theory of attention-deficit/hyperactivity disorder: a meta-analytic review. *Biol Psychiatry* 57, 1336-1346.

4

What Does Cerebral Oxygenation Tell Us About Central Motor Output?

Nicolas Bourdillon and Stéphane Perrey

Movement To Health (M2H), Montpellier-1 University, Euromov
France

1. Introduction

Since the fifth Century Athens, when Hippocrates identified the brain as the source of thought and understanding, humanity has been preoccupied with its functions. Anatomical descriptions have been brought to modernity by Andreas Vesalius in the sixteenth century (Vesalius, 1543) while underlying mechanisms have awaited the discovery of "bio-electricity" by Luigi Galvani in the eighteenth century to emerge (Galvani, 1791). In the nineteenth century, famous physicians such as Paul Broca or Carl Wernicke have demonstrated the role of the brain in cognitive tasks, studying patients with neurological disorders (Broca, 2004; Wernicke, 1894). From the late twentieth century to present day, neuroimaging techniques have allowed explorations in healthy subjects providing very precise locations of brain regions involved in cognitive and motor functions.

For the advancement of theory it is essential to acknowledge the strengths and limitations of available neuroimaging techniques so that converging evidence on the basis of multiple modes of investigation can be brought to bear on current controversies in the literature. Electroencephalography (EEG) was chronologically the first technique to open the way to the study of brain functions in exercising subjects (Swartz and Goldensohn, 1998). While one of the most direct methods to non-invasively measure the electrical signal arising from the synchronous firing of neurons, spatial resolution and lack of information from areas deeper than the cortex are its main limitations. Magnetoencephalography (MEG) is also a direct measure of the electrical activity of neurons and has a better spatial resolution as compared with EEG. However, the lack of detection in deep brain structures and the threshold detection (at least 50,000 neurons active simultaneously are needed) make MEG main disadvantages (Shibasaki, 2008). Functional imaging such as positron emission tomography (PET), single photon emission computed tomography (SPECT) and functional magnetic resonance imaging (fMRI) overcome the EEG and MEG limitations as they can detect neuronal activity as deep in the brain as experimenters desire (Cui et al., 2011; Villringer, 1997). However, the measure is indirect as it relies on blood supply for fMRI or on radioactive tracers for PET and SPECT (Jantzen et al., 2008; Tashiro et al., 2008). Additionally, except for EEG, the experimental environments of the earlier described techniques are very restricting with regards to physical exercise. Subjects and experimenters are limited to sit or laid positions and to breathe, eye, wrist and ankle movements. Actually, *in vivo* determination of brain functions in humans requires flexible, accessible and rapid monitoring techniques (Kikukawa et al., 2008; Perrey, 2008;

Rasmussen et al., 2007). Near infrared spectroscopy (NIRS) is perhaps the technique which best gathers these qualities; which may account for the increasing popularity of NIRS among research teams in recent years.

2. Near infrared spectroscopy in humans

As suggested by its name, the NIRS technique relies on red and infrared light diffusion through the living tissues. Physically, NIRS systems consist of numerous probes designed to be attached directly on the skin, over the area(s) to explore. Either optical fibres or regular electrical wires link the probes to a dedicated hardware, which in turn feeds a computer with experimental data. Probes are made of light transmitters and light receivers; the light power emission, the receiver gain and the interoptode distance can be adapted to match with the characteristics and depth of the areas under investigation. However, those three parameters necessarily come as inputs for the NIRS dedicated software which drives the record session.

2.1 Principles of physics underlying the NIRS technique

Back in the eighteenth century, the brilliant French scientist Pierre Bouguer (1698-1758) is probably the true father of photometry (Bouguer, 1729). The goal of his publication entitled "Essais sur la gradation de la lumière" in 1729 was to quantify how much light is lost when travelling through a given atmospheric layer. To achieve his work, he empirically characterizes materials with an optical density (OD) as follows:

$$OD = \log\left(\frac{I_0}{I}\right) \tag{1}$$

where I_0 is the intensity of the incident light and I the intensity of the transmitted light. More than one hundred years later, the German scientist August Beer (1825-1863), based on Jean-Henri Lambert's (1728-1777) and Pierre Bouguer's works, published "Einleitung in die höhere Optik" (1853), where he defined transmittance of light rather than its loss when travelling through a tissue (Beer, 1853). What is now known as the Beer-Lambert's law is a different version of Bouguer's idea (eq.1). The Beer-Lambert's law (eq.2) states that there is a logarithmic dependence between the transmission of light (T) and the product of the absorption coefficient of the substance the light travelled through (α) and the distance travelled by the light (also called path length, l).

$$T = 10^{\alpha l} \tag{2}$$

In turn, the absorption coefficient α depends on the product of the extinction coefficients (ε) and the concentration (c) of the absorbers in the material. In liquids, the Beer-Lambert's law is often written as follows:

$$T = 10^{\varepsilon c l} \tag{3}$$

Equations 1 and 3 imply that there is a linear relationship between Bouguer's optical density and the concentration of species in the material explored:

$$OD = \varepsilon c l \tag{4}$$

From equation 4 (illustrated by fig.1), the main idea of NIRS is to compute the concentration of species (c) by measuring the OD according to Bouguer's definition (eq.1) and, inserting the a priori known extinction coefficients for species and the path length of light (eq. 4).

Panel A   Panel B

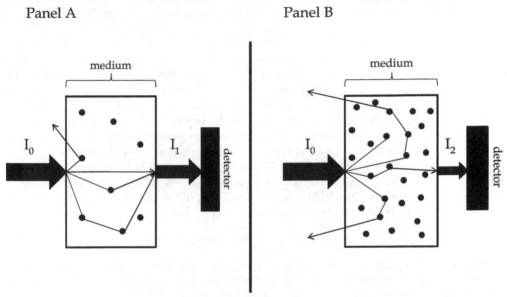

Fig. 1. Illustration of the Beer-Lambert's law. In panel A, the medium has a low OD (transmitted light I_1 is close to incident light I_0); the concentration of absorbing species is low. In panel B, OD is higher (larger difference between I_2 and I_0 than between I_1 and I_0), so is the concentration of absorbing species.

2.2 Application of NIRS to living tissues

At least six conditions have to be fulfilled in order for the Beer-Lambert's law to be valid:

- the absorbers must act independently from each others;
- the absorbing medium must be homogeneous in the interaction volume;
- the absorbing medium must not scatter the radiation;
- the incident radiation must consist of parallel rays, each travelling the same length in the medium;
- the incident radiation must be monochromatic;
- the incident radiation must not influence the atoms in the medium.

Living tissues, especially in humans, are doubtlessly among the most structured and complex in the universe. Their characteristics do not match with the Beer-Lambert's law prerequisites on numerous points. Therefore, the modified Beer-Lambert's law has to be applied in NIRS. As stated in the fifth point of the prerequisites, the incident light must be monochromatic (i.e. only one wavelength λ). In human tissues, lots of chemical species absorb light and account for its loss when travelling. However, there is a range of wavelengths at which light travel is much facilitated. Intuitively, when, in a dark environment, one looks at a flashlight through his finger or his hand, red is invariably the dominant colour. The physical explanation is that the red light travel through the human tissues is easier than for any other wavelengths. Implicitly, in the red portion of the visible light, there are a limited number of chemical species which are responsible for the majority of light absorption and diffusion. These species are known to give its colour to the tissue and have been judiciously named chromophores. In human tissues, it is well known that haemoglobin is responsible for the colour given to tissues; in physics, haemoglobin is the chromophore whose concentration can be measured using Bouguer's idea.

2.2.1 The chromophores
Haemoglobin is a metalloprotein which transports 98% of the oxygen in most vertebrates' blood. When oxygen binds to the iron complex, it causes the iron ion to move back, and changes the optical properties of the molecule. At the human scale the phenomenon is perceptible and results in the long standing view that the red blood is filled-up with oxygen while the blue one has lost the majority of its initial quantity of oxygen. In physics, it can be considered that there are two distinct chromophores: oxygenated haemoglobin (O_2Hb) and deoxygenated haemoglobin (HHb). Therefore, according to Bouguer's idea one can compute the concentration of oxy and deoxyhaemoglobin in a tissue by measuring the changes in OD (eq. 4). However, the OD in human tissues is not strictly dependant on haemoglobin. In an imaginary case where there would be no haemoglobin in the explored area, the tissue would still absorb light. Consequently, eq.4 should be rewritten as:

$$OD_{(\lambda)} = \varepsilon_{(\lambda)} \cdot c \cdot 1 + ODr_{(\lambda)} \tag{5}$$

where ODr is the y-intercept of the linear relation and denotes the OD of the living tissue when there is no haemoglobin. λ denotes the chosen wavelength for the monochromatic light.

2.2.2 Two wavelengths
The Beer-Lambert's law states that the measured optical density is the sum of the absorbance of the two chromophores. Eq. 5 becomes eq. 6 with the two chromophores appearing:

$$OD_{(\lambda)} = \varepsilon_{O2Hb(\lambda)} \cdot c_{O2Hb} \cdot 1 + \varepsilon_{HHb(\lambda)} \cdot c_{HHb} \cdot 1 + ODr_{(\lambda)} \tag{6}$$

There are two unknowns in eq. 6 (ie. c_{O2Hb} and c_{HHb}). Thus, two equations are needed to solve the system. The two equations are provided by firing at two different wavelengths λ_1 and λ_2.

$$\begin{cases} OD_{(\lambda1)} = \varepsilon_{O2Hb(\lambda1)} \cdot c_{O2Hb} \cdot 1 + \varepsilon_{HHb(\lambda1)} \cdot c_{HHb} \cdot 1 + ODr_{(\lambda1)} \\ OD_{(\lambda2)} = \varepsilon_{O2Hb(\lambda2)} \cdot c_{O2Hb} \cdot 1 + \varepsilon_{HHb(\lambda2)} \cdot c_{HHb} \cdot 1 + ODr_{(\lambda2)} \end{cases} \tag{7}$$

The main idea is that one needs as many wavelengths as there are chromophores in the investigated area. Only one equation is exposed further down this line for clarity purpose. Note that NIRS systems perform every computation to solve the systems of equations.

2.2.3 Application of the modified Beer-Lambert's law
Since physiologists use NIRS to compute the haemoglobin concentration, the modified Beer-Lambert's law is then written:

$$c = \frac{(OD_{(\lambda)} - ODr_{(\lambda)})}{\varepsilon_{(\lambda)} \cdot 1} \tag{8}$$

In eq. 8, OD is measured using Bouguer's idea (eq.1), ε is known from the physicists who are able to measure it (fig.2), ODr and l are unknown but necessary to the computation of c.

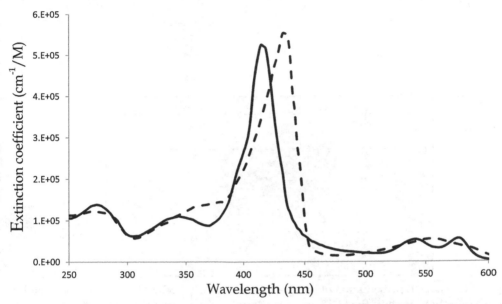

Fig. 2. Molar extinction coefficient for haemoglobin in water. O_2Hb: plain line; HHb: dashed line; x axis: wavelength (λ) in nm; y axis: extinction coefficient (ε) in cm-1/M. Data compiled by Scott Prahl (Prahl, 2008).

ODr is not expected to change radically in a short lap of time. In other words, it is considered constant between two light impulsions a few tenths of seconds away. Therefore, considering two light impulsions at t_0 and t_1, it is possible to write:

$$c_{t0} - c_{t1} = \frac{(OD_{(\lambda)t0} - ODr_{(\lambda)})}{\varepsilon_{(\lambda)} \cdot l} - \frac{(OD_{(\lambda)t1} - ODr_{(\lambda)})}{\varepsilon_{(\lambda)} \cdot l} \qquad (9)$$

which simplifies into

$$c_{t0} - c_{t1} = \frac{(OD_{(\lambda)t0} - OD_{(\lambda)t1})}{\varepsilon_{(\lambda)} \cdot l} \qquad (10)$$

Eq. 10 states that the concentration variations depend on the measured OD variations. The advantage of the subtraction in eq. 9 is to get rid of the unknown ODr. However, the absolute concentration of the chromophore becomes unknown as only a concentration difference (or variation) can be computed.

The last unknown parameter missing to compute the concentration variation is l, the path length of light between the transmitter and the receptor (fig. 3). Its measure is almost impossible due to the numerous interactions between the matter and the light in living tissues (Ijichi et al., 2005). Three methods are available to approach the path length:

- the differential path length factor (DPF)
- the time of flight
- the Monte Carlo simulation

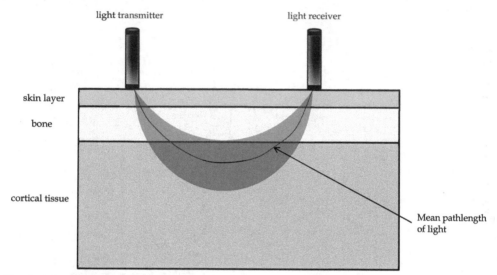

Fig. 3. Schematic representation of NIRS applied to human cerebral tissues. The mean path length of light represents the l.DPF in eq.11. Roughly, the maximum depth of the mean path length of light is believed to be half of the emitter to receiver distance.

The DPF method is doubtlessly the easiest to use but also the less precise and less satisfactory. Regrettably it is the most common method nowadays. In this method, l is considered the most direct way between the light transmitter and receptor, DPF is multiplied to l to lengthen the global path length, eq. 10 is then written:

$$\Delta c = \frac{\Delta OD_{(\lambda)}}{\varepsilon_{(\lambda)} \cdot l \cdot DPF} \tag{11}$$

DPF is arbitrarily set from abacus found in the literature. Only a few studies give the DPF, often as a function of age (Duncan et al., 1995; Essenpreis et al., 1993a; Essenpreis et al., 1993b; Firbank et al., 1993; Ijichi et al., 2005; Kohl et al., 1998a; Kohl et al., 1998b; Nolte et al., 1998; Pringle et al., 1999; Ultman and Piantadosi, 1991; van der Zee et al., 1992; Zhao et al., 2002). Another way to approach the path length of light is to measure the time of flight between the light transmitter and the receptor. The speed of light in the vacuum is used to compute the path length. This method is more precise than the DPF method but costly financially and in terms of load of computation. Billion of photons are detected by the receptor at each light impulsion. One of the advantages is the possibility to select the photons to study; the first detected photons have a priori a shorter path length, which means that they did not go deep into the tissues (Ferrante et al., 2009). The latest photons, which have a longer path length, went a priori deeper into the tissues and carry more information. Finally, the Monte Carlo simulation is a statistical method representing the distribution of energy in the explored volume. It is a way to assume the random path length of photons between the light transmitter and the receptor (Hiraoka et al., 1993; Simpson et al., 1998; Zhang et al., 2007a, b). This is the most precise method nowadays, usable with regular measurement devices but costly in terms of computation. The Monte Carlo method might be performed after the monitoring session as computers may not be powerful enough to ensure simultaneously proper recording of the data and Monte Carlo analysis (Avrillier et al., 1998a; Avrillier et al., 1998b). Roughly, for all methods the maximum depth of the mean path length of light is believed to be half of the emitter to receiver distance.

3. Signal characteristics and interpretations

NIRS data consist of oxy and deoxyhaemoglobin time series (Fig. 4 and Fig. 5), with sampling rate usually ranging from 2 to 20Hz, and occasionally above. Usual measurement sites exclude locations where large arteries or veins would be reachable by the NIRS light as experimenters are rather interested in tissue data. In the tissues, the light crosses three types of blood vessels:
-    arterioles (diameter below 100μm, average 20-30μm)
-    capillaries (average diameter 5-10μm)
-    venules (average diameter 8-30μm)

NIRS signal is believed to originate in its major part from the venous compartment (approx. 70%); however, vasomotion makes the part of each segment variable (Bourdillon et al., 2009; Peltonen et al., 2009). Briefly, capillaries form an extensive network which connects the arterial and venous sides of the vascular system. The blood flow through a given capillary bed strongly depends on the vascular tone of the parent arteriole and the pre-capillary sphincters. Both adjust the local blood flow to meet the physiological demands. Despite the smooth muscles of the arterioles and sphincters are connected to the sympathetic nervous system, the vascular tone is largely dependent on the local factors (Segal, 2005). Concerning the motor areas of the brain, it is generally assumed that, when activated, the neurons increase their firing rates to generate the motor command and thus increase their metabolic demands (Villringer, 1997). One of the consequences is to increase the local blood flow; this

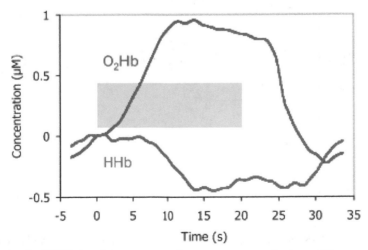

Fig. 4. Example of a NIRS signal pattern over the motor cortex during a 20 seconds lasting handgrip task (Wolf et al., 2007).

phenomenon can be detected by NIRS. It is obvious that the NIRS measurements are indirect with regards to neuronal activity and rely on the assumption that the latter is coupled to blood supply. Moreover, NIRS measures the concentrations of oxy and deoxyhaemoglobin (the sum of both, Hbtot, giving a proxy of local blood volume), not the blood flow nor the oxygen consumption. Fig. 4 shows a typical NIRS record during a simple motor task (handgrip).

3.1 Patterns

Empirically, activation pattern in the motor cortex is identified as an increase in oxyhaemoglobin concomitant to a decrease in deoxyhaemoglobin (Fig. 4). The reasons which give the activation pattern such a shape are not fully elucidated (Dai et al., 2001; Harada et al., 2006; Matsuura et al., 2011). However, it is commonly thought that the vasodilation caused by the increase in metabolic demand from the firing neurons overcomes the needs in oxygen; which results in an apparent increase in tissue oxygenation as measured by NIRS (Franceschini and Boas, 2004; Gervain et al., 2011; Leff et al., 2011; Rooks et al., 2010; Shibasaki, 2008; Shibuya and Tachi, 2006). The amplitudes of changes in oxy and deoxyhaemoglobin within the motor cortex areas have been shown to be dependent on the force production: the stronger the push, the higher the oxyhaemoglobin (Shibuya and Tachi, 2006; Smith et al., 2003). However, at low levels of force, there might be no detection by the NIRS systems (at least 10% of maximal voluntary contraction needed); while at high levels (about 50% of maximal voluntary contraction and above) there might be no plateau but only a peak in oxyhaemoglobin (Ekkekakis, 2009). This type of activation pattern is valid only for steady systemic variables (ie. globally non moving body). The NIRS signal, as it comes from the circulatory system, is strongly dependent on the cardio-respiratory parameters. Modifications in cardiac output, autonomic nervous system balance, hormonal response,

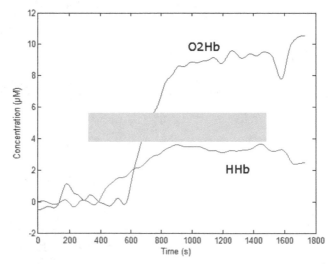

Fig. 5. Example of a NIRS signal pattern over the motor cortex during a high intensity whole body cycling exercise at a constant work rate from baseline level (warm up) at 600 s. Personal data.

blood concentration in oxygen or carbon dioxide, baroreflexes and neural feedbacks from metabo and mecano receptors in the skeletal muscle potentially affect the vascular tone and thus the NIRS signal. Consequently, in subjects exercising at high metabolic rates (elevated oxygen consumption), with hyperventilation, hyper/hypocapnia and high cardiac output, the NIRS signal is rather dependant on systemic variables than on motor command (Pereira et al., 2007; Rasmussen et al., 2007). Fig. 5 shows a typical NIRS response from the motor cortex of a subject exercising on a cycloergometer above the ventilatory threshold for 20 minutes (Rooks et al., 2010; Rupp and Perrey, 2008). The amplitudes of the variations are way larger as compared with fig. 4 and the "activation pattern" is altered as there is no apparent decrease in deoxyhaemoglobin. In any case, the interpretation of the NIRS signals has to be modulated following the experimental design and the systemic conditions (Gervain et al., 2011; Rooks et al., 2010).

3.2 Delay
As shown in fig. 4 or fig. 5, there is a delay between the stimulus, the neural responses and the hemodynamic modifications as detected by the NIRS systems (Cui et al., 2010b; Yasui et al., 2010). If the NIRS signal depends on the motor command, the delay has been shown to range between 2 and 5 seconds (Fig. 4). In the case of fig. 5 the NIRS signal is rather dependant on systemic parameters (i.e. ventilation) and the delay ranges between 1 and 4 minutes. Such variations in delays are due to the facts that the NIRS records of cerebral hemodynamic parameters depend whether on the motor command or on systemic parameters, following the experimental design. To date, the time course analysis of NIRS signals has yet to be established, notably with regards to the transition periods and the experimental designs.

3.3 NIRS computed indicators
The only parameters measured by NIRS are the optical densities at two (or more) wavelengths as stated in the part 2.2.2 of this article. O_2Hb and HHb are directly computed variables; the computer usually performs calculations during data acquisition. Afterwards, experimenters are using to computing other parameters from O_2Hb and HHb to present NIRS data. Among the most often found parameters in the literature there are: the difference between O_2Hb and HHb (usually abbreviated $O_2Hbdiff$ or Hbdiff); the tissue or capillary saturation (usually abbreviated StO_2 or ScO_2) and the tissue oxygenation index (TOI). TOI, StO_2 and ScO_2 are given by the simple formula:

$$TOI = \frac{O_2Hb}{O_2Hb + HHb} \tag{12}$$

These indicators are thought to summarize O_2Hb and HHb signals and reflect tissue oxygenation. However, physical exercise results in a large heterogeneous increase in cerebral oxygenation (Rooks et al., 2010). It seems that the primary factor influencing this increase is the intensity of exercise, followed by the training status of the subjects, age, health status (i.e., patients vs. healthy subjects) and methodology.

3.4 Pre-processing
In most studies, NIRS data is pre-processed in order to improve the signal quality (Boas et al., 2004). The first step typically aims at removing noise (Gervain et al., 2011). The noise

comes from the devices as well as from physiological parameters not a priori linked to the stimulation (eg. Exercise) and are thus undesirable (Nolte et al., 1998). This kind of noise is considered high frequency with regards to the frequencies of interest (Cui et al., 2010a). Low-pass filters are used to remove heart rate, blood pressure variations, breath, swallowing etc. Usually, the cut-off frequency ranges between 0.1 and 1Hz. Detrending is performed using a high-pass filter when NIRS signals slowly drift throughout the experimental session. High-pass filters usually range between 0.01 and 0.05Hz. However experimenters must care as the frequencies of interest could be part of this range. Finally, experimenters have several tools to choose from to remove movement artefacts. If possible set a marker during the experimental session when the subject moved his head is a good start. Retrospectively, the eye of the physiologist is the first tool which can be used. However, its somehow objective behaviour and its inability to treat large amounts of data make its main limits. Abrupt changes in the signals can be detected and corrected by algorithms (Lloyd-Fox et al., 2010; Wilcox et al., 2008). However, the thresholds must be defined carefully in order to preserve the changes that supposedly belong to the awaited hemodynamic response (Gervain et al., 2011).

3.5 Data analysis
Since NIRS is a relatively new technique for brain investigations, there is no standardised method to analyse data. Up to date, the only invariant is that different experimental designs require different analysis techniques.

In block-designed studies, experimenters are used to analysing time series by averaging multiple trials of the same condition. Mean variations and mean time courses are then obtained for each condition. The critical points of such techniques are the determination of the relevant windows of the time series and the baseline which it is compared to. Once determined, student t-test and analyses of variance are the most often used statistical methods.

More complex, three main freeware packages are downloadable and provide analysis methods derived from the BOLD signal of fMRI: HomER (Huppert et al., 2009), fOSA (Koh et al., 2007) and NIRS-SPM (Ye et al., 2009). The general linear model (GLM) and the statistical parametric mapping (SPM) offer the possibility to create three dimensional pictures of the brain, where activated/inhibited cortex areas are colour encoded (Friston et al., 1999; Plichta et al., 2007; Schroeter et al., 2004; Zarahn et al., 1997). In most studies, the NIRS records are performed off the MRI scan. Then, the input of the three dimensional coordinates of the optodes/channels is crucial for the reconstitution of the pictures. In the case of a co-record of NIRS and fMRI techniques, the coordinates of the NIRS optodes can be precisely assigned; else, skull measurements and probe placement are made either by reference to the 10-20 EEG system or by kinematic acquisition using such devices as optotrack or fastrack.

3.6 Dos and don'ts
Doubtlessly, the toughest part of the NIRS based studies, is to draw physiological and cognitive conclusions from the data. Multi-channel setups cover wide cortical zones and result in several time series and three dimensional coloured images in which probability to give statistically significant results is high. The question experimenters inevitably face is "What do those results mean?". A typical NIRS channel includes a great number of capillary

beds, corresponding to a greater number of neurons (estimated around 300,000 to 500,000) from various depths in the cortex (Gervain et al., 2011). The pool of capillary beds enlighten by a channel is believed to belong to a given cortex area, which supposedly has a single function. This makes a huge simplification if compared to the brain complexity and its capacity of integration, not to mention the neuro-vascular coupling assumption (see part 4.1.)! Moreover, probe placement is based on the skull anatomy as no direct access to the brain is allowed by NIRS (except in the case of fMRI co-recording) giving a probability to fire over multiple cortex areas or even over a wrong area. Additionally, the proportion of excitatory and inhibitory neurons in the volume aimed by NIRS is unknown yet potentially affects the results.

3.7 Confounding factors

At this stage of the article, the most impeding factors have been brought to discussion. However, some factors, not directly linked to the NIRS concepts nor to brain characteristics must be debated. Before entering the tissue of interest, light travels through the skin and the fat layers (as well as the hair and skull layers in case of brain investigations, Fig. 3). The skin colour (and hair colour) has been shown to influence light absorption (Pringle et al., 1999). Intuitively, human eyes perceive various skin colours because skin absorbs and reflects light depending on its properties. The same (or the opposite) happens in the near infrared portion of the spectrum. Light skins are believed to absorb light more than dark skins, while Asian originated skins are the less absorbent. NIRS gain or laser power must then be modulated to fit with the skin properties of a given subject; which can be performed automatically by the NIRS hardware before starting the data acquisition.

Skin blood flow is one of the main confounding factors as the haemoglobin molecules present in the capillary beds located in the skin are the first (and last) exposed to NIRS light (Tew et al., 2010). In exercising subjects, blood flow is increasing in proportion to the intensity of exercise, for well-known thermoregulation reasons. However, skin is not believed to consume more oxygen at high intensity as compared with low intensity exercises. This means that skin blood flow overcomes by far the local metabolic demands; which necessarily biases the NIRS measurements.

The fat and bone layers are probably easier to take into account as they can be integrated in the automatic gain setup which occurs in most modern NIRS devices, before data acquisition.

Finally, gender has been shown to influence NIRS responses to various stimuli, notably motor, cognitive tasks and emotions (Marumo et al., 2009; Yang et al., 2009).

4. Measuring the brain activities related to the motor stimulation using NIRS

4.1 Physiological processes associated with brain activity

Physiological events associated with brain activity can be subdivided into intracellular events, events occurring at the cell membranes and those that are mediated by neurovascular coupling and occur within the vascular space. Increased brain activity is correlated not only with oxygen consumption but also with glucose consumption. The brain has only negligible stores of glucose and therefore relies both on the circulating glucose and on the active transport system which moves glucose across the blood-brain barrier. Increased activity in brain cells is associated with an increase in glucose consumption and thus the intracellular glucose concentration might fall in the early activation period (Villringer and Dirnagl, 1995). This transient drop in glucose is accompanied by a transient rise in local lactate concentration (Villringer and Dirnagl, 1995). Magistretti and Pellerin (Magistretti and Pellerin, 1999a, b) have provided new insights on the role of astrocytes in coupling neuronal activity with energy metabolism. They propose an initial glycolytic processing which occurs in astrocytes during activation, resulting in a transient lactate overproduction; followed by a recoupling phase during which lactate is oxidised by neurons. In addition to the events taking place intracellularly, local brain activity induces a local arteriolar vasodilation (Villringer and Dirnagl, 1995). Although small arteries and arterioles probably contain less than 5% of the blood volume in the brain parenchyma, they control most of the resistance and therefore blood flow at a local level. As a consequence of local vasodilation the local cerebral blood volume as well as the blood flow increase. This relationship between neuronal activity and vascular response is termed "neurovascular coupling". In other words, the changes in Hbtot most probably reflect the match between oxygen supply and oxygen demand, whereas changes in O_2Hb reflect the alterations in cerebral blood flow, an overshoot in cerebral oxygenation during brain activation. Several NIRS studies conducted in the past fifteen years have demonstrated that activation- induced changes in brain activity can be assessed non-invasively during the performance of various whole-body motor activities (Maki et al., 1995; Obrig et al., 1996).

4.2 Brain activity and motor performance

The NIRS is applicable under a variety of conditions ranging from bedside monitoring in intensive care to documenting the effects of maximal whole body exercise in the physiology laboratory. To date, several studies have used NIRS to examine alterations in cerebral oxygenation during dynamic exercise, and have found an increase in cerebral oxygenation with medium and high-intensity exercise (Bhambhani et al., 2007; Shibuya et al., 2004a; Subudhi et al., 2007; Suzuki et al., 2004).

While a rather detailed understanding of brain activity during hand movement has been developed (Dettmers et al., 1995), less is known about the functional anatomy of motor control for leg or foot movements. Due to its advantages compared to other neuroimaging techniques, NIRS technique allows recording of cerebral activity during ordinary gait (Fig. 6). For instance, Miyai et al. (2001) were able to compare cerebral activities evoked during gait, alternating foot movements, arm swing and motor imagery of gait. Gait-related responses along the central sulcus were medial and caudal to activity associated with arm swing, in agreement with the known somatotopic organisation of the motor cortex (Perec, 1974). Crucially, these authors showed that walking increased cerebral activity bilaterally in the medial primary sensori-motor cortices and the supplementary motor area, and to a greater extent than the alternation of foot movements. Unfortunately, the spatial distribution and intensity of these responses were not statistically compared. In a different NIRS study, Suzuki et al. (2004) examined the effect of various walking speeds on cerebral activity. They demonstrated that cerebral activity in the prefrontal cortex and premotor cortex tended to increase as the locomotion speed increased, whereas cerebral activity in the medial sensori-motor cortex was not influenced by the locomotion speed. In summary, NIRS is particularly useful for studying the cortical bases of locomotion control. Unfortunately, given the limited depth penetration of the infrared light (a few centimetres from the skull surface), the NIRS technique can only assess the responses of the most superficial portions of the cerebral cortex.

Neuroimaging studies have reported a proportional relationship between cortical signals and exerted joint force in humans, indicating that brain signals are positively correlated to voluntary efforts, as a high level of effort is required for exerting greater muscle force (Liu et al., 2007; Liu et al., 2003). Recently several authors have proposed combining neuroimaging techniques with the classical twitch interpolation to investigate the central aspects of fatigue after and during ongoing exercise. Most studies on central fatigue have investigated isometric contractions of isolated muscle groups. Post et al. (2009) showed, during a sustained high force contraction, that the hemodynamic response (BOLD signal) in the most important motor (output) areas increased (primary sensorimotor cortex, supplementary motor area, premotor area), whereas the voluntary activation (accessed via the twitch-interpolation technique) of the index finger muscle during a unilateral task decreased with time. This finding suggests that although the central nervous system (CNS) increased its input to the motor areas, these increases did not overcome fatigue-related changes in the voluntary drive to the motor units. During a progressive maximal cycling exercise, Rupp and Perrey (2008) showed a decrease in prefrontal cortical oxygenation before motor performance failure, which may be compatible with the notion of a role for the prefrontal cortex in the reduction of motor output by the cessation of exercise. However, this finding was not associated with a decrease in voluntary activation, but measured 6 min post-exercise. Support for the role of a failure of the CNS to excite the motor neurons adequately (i.e., central fatigue) in fatigue during challenging exercises has been provided by the finding that voluntary activation of skeletal muscles is reduced after fatiguing exercise.

This suboptimal muscle activation has also been functionally observed via lowered surface electromyographic (EMG) activity on several occasions during fatiguing exercises (Mendez-Villanueva et al., 2007). However, what triggers these acute changes in the CNS behaviour remains to be determined. Central fatigue may be elicited by low brain oxygenation, i.e., by insufficient O_2 delivery and/or low pressure gradient to drive the diffusion of O_2 from the capillaries to the mitochondria. Direct and indirect evidences support the contention that inadequate cerebral oxygenation depresses cortical neuron excitability, although the mechanisms remain debated (for review see Nybo and Rasmussen, 2007). The non-invasive technique of NIRS offers real-time measurement of oxygenation and hemodynamic responses in tissues, and thus, constitutes a relevant tool to enhance our current knowledge of central (CNS) and peripheral (muscle) determinants of whole-body exercise performance. Some studies have reported that muscle deoxygenation occurs during repeated cycling tests (Racinais et al., 2007). However, exercises of this nature appear to induce a fairly constant level of deoxygenation in prime mover muscles across repetitions, and therefore authors have suggested that muscle O_2 uptake was well preserved and was not likely to represent a limiting factor. Data on cerebral oxygenation changes during fatiguing tests are currently presented in the literature. Based on studies conducted during constant workload exercise, incremental test to maximal effort (Rupp and Perrey, 2008), and supramaximal exercise (Shibuya et al., 2004b), the deoxygenation of the cerebral cortex has, in general, been incriminated in the cessation of exercise, or at least in the reduction of exercise intensity. This finding, however, is confounded by the availability of O_2 (Subudhi et al., 2007). Although an association exists between cerebral oxygenation and performance in various exercises, no studies have yet determined if a critical level of cerebral deoxygenation impairs whole body exercise. Shibuya and colleagues Shibuya et al. (2004a) reported a progressive cerebral deoxygenation during intermittent exercises. Specifically, these authors observed a reduction in $\Delta[O_2Hb]$ and $\Delta[Hbtot]$, while $\Delta[HHb]$ increased, over the course of seven, 30s cycling exercises performed at an intensity corresponding to 150% $\dot{V}O_2$max and interspersed with 15s of rest. It was concluded that fatigue, resulting from such intermittent supramaximal exercises, was related to a decrease in the cerebral oxygenation level.

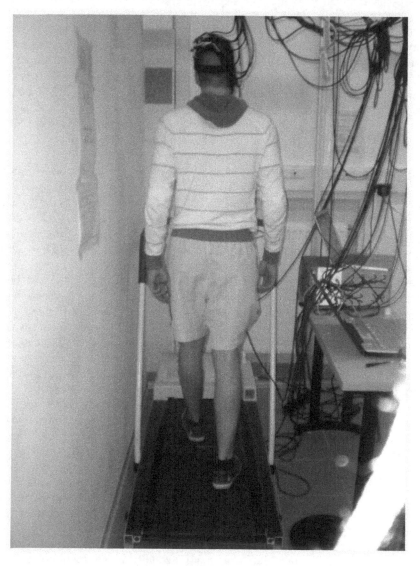

Fig. 6. Example of a NIRS setting while the subject is walking on a treadmill.

To date based on recent evidences; we may propose that reductions in cerebral oxygenation during exhaustive intensities are caused by decreased cerebral blood flow coupled with increased cerebral oxygen uptake (Gonzalez-Alonso et al., 2004). It has also been proposed that this change in flow and metabolism at high intensities is sensed or controlled by a 'central governor' so that during oxygen availability reduction, peak exercise performance is reduced to prevent the development of ischemia in vital organs including the brain (Noakes et al., 2005). In this way, an increase in Hbtot and a decrease in cerebral oxygenation represent potential metabolic indicators, signalling either directly or indirectly to sub-cortical and cortical motor areas of the brain to reduce muscle unit recruitment and thus protect the brain and peripheral organs.

5. Conclusion

NIRS utilises light to measure cortical haemoglobin concentration changes associated with neural activity. This technique is more tolerant compared with other comparable techniques, regarding the subjects' movements, thus allowing a wider range of experimental tasks in the range of dynamic exercises. However, it has some shortcomings that need to be addressed. In this chapter, we showed how technical obstacles could be overcome, how NIRS contributes to the mapping of exercise-related brain functions, and further promotes the understanding of human movement and motor performance. In this context, we propose NIRS as a potential mediator between physiology and neuroscience. Beside these advances in technique and analysis of the data, we believe that users should consider the methodology's strengths and weakness when designing a NIRS study.

6. References

Avrillier, S., Tinet, E., Tualle, J.M., (1998a). Real time inversion using Monte Carlo results for the determination of absorption coefficients in multi-layered tissues: application to non invasive muscle oxymetry (Part 1), Munich.

Avrillier, S., Tinet, E., Tualle, J.M., Costes, F., Revel, F., Ollivier, J.P., (1998b). Real time inversion using Monte Carlo results for the determination of absorption coefficients in multi-layered tissues: application to non invasive muscle oxymetry (Part 2), Munich.

Beer, A., (1853). Einleitung in die höhere Optik. Druck und Verlag von Friedrich Vieweg und Sohn.

Bhambhani, Y., Malik, R., Mookerjee, S., (2007). Cerebral oxygenation declines at exercise intensities above the respiratory compensation threshold. Respir Physiol Neurobiol 156, 2, (May 14), pp. (196-202), ISSN 1569-9048 (Print) 1569-9048 (Linking).

Boas, D.A., Dale, A.M., Franceschini, M.A., (2004). Diffuse optical imaging of brain activation: approaches to optimizing image sensitivity, resolution, and accuracy. Neuroimage 23 Suppl 1, pp. (S275-288), ISSN 1053-8119.

Bouguer, P., (1729). Essais la gradation de la lumière. Claude Jombert, Paris, France.

Bourdillon, N., Mollard, P., Letournel, M., Beaudry, M., Richalet, J.P., (2009). Interaction between hypoxia and training on NIRS signal during exercise: contribution of a mathematical model. Respir Physiol Neurobiol 169, 1, (Oct 31), pp. (50-61).

Broca, P., (2004). Ecrits sur l'aphasie (1861 - 1869). L'Harmattan, ISBN 2-7475-5925-4, Paris, France.

Cui, X., Bray, S., Bryant, D.M., Glover, G.H., Reiss, A.L., (2011). A quantitative comparison of NIRS and fMRI across multiple cognitive tasks. *Neuroimage* 54, 4, (Feb 14), pp. (2808-2821), ISSN 1095-9572 (Electronic) 1053-8119 (Linking).

Cui, X., Bray, S., Reiss, A.L., (2010a). Functional near infrared spectroscopy (NIRS) signal improvement based on negative correlation between oxygenated and deoxygenated hemoglobin dynamics. *Neuroimage* 49, 4, (Feb 15), pp. (3039-3046), ISSN 1095-9572 (Electronic) 1053-8119 (Linking).

Cui, X., Bray, S., Reiss, A.L., (2010b). Speeded near infrared spectroscopy (NIRS) response detection. *PLoS One* 5, 11, pp. (e15474), ISSN 1932-6203.

Dai, T.H., Liu, J.Z., Sahgal, V., Brown, R.W., Yue, G.H., (2001). Relationship between muscle output and functional MRI-measured brain activation. *Exp Brain Res* 140, 3, (Oct), pp. (290-300), ISSN 0014-4819.

Dettmers, C., Fink, G.R., Lemon, R.N., Stephan, K.M., Passingham, R.E., Silbersweig, D., Holmes, A., Ridding, M.C., Brooks, D.J., Frackowiak, R.S., (1995). Relation between cerebral activity and force in the motor areas of the human brain. *J Neurophysiol* 74, 2, (Aug), pp. (802-815), ISSN 0022-3077.

Duncan, A., Meek, J.H., Clemence, M., Elwell, C.E., Tyszczuk, L., Cope, M., Delpy, D.T., (1995). Optical pathlength measurements on adult head, calf and forearm and the head of the newborn infant using phase resolved optical spectroscopy. *Phys Med Biol* 40, 2, (Feb), pp. (295-304), ISSN 0031-9155.

Ekkekakis, P., (2009). Illuminating the black box: investigating prefrontal cortical hemodynamics during exercise with near-infrared spectroscopy. *J Sport Exerc Psychol* 31, 4, (Aug), pp. (505-553), ISSN 0895-2779.

Essenpreis, M., Cope, M., Elwell, C.E., Arridge, S.R., van der Zee, P., Delpy, D.T., (1993a). Wavelength dependence of the differential pathlength factor and the log slope in time-resolved tissue spectroscopy. *Adv Exp Med Biol* 333, pp. (9-20), ISSN 0065-2598.

Essenpreis, M., Elwell, C.E., Cope, M., van der Zee, P., Arridge, S.R., Delpy, D.T., (1993b). Spectral dependence of temporal point spread functions in human tissues. *Appl Opt* 32, 4, (Feb 1), pp. (418-425), ISSN 0003-6935.

Ferrante, S., Contini, D., Spinelli, L., Pedrocchi, A., Torricelli, A., Molteni, F., Ferrigno, G., Cubeddu, R., (2009). Monitoring muscle metabolic indexes by time-domain near-infrared spectroscopy during knee flex-extension induced by functional electrical stimulation. *J Biomed Opt* 14, 4, (Jul-Aug), pp. (044011), ISSN 1560-2281 (Electronic) 1083-3668 (Linking).

Firbank, M., Hiraoka, M., Essenpreis, M., Delpy, D.T., (1993). Measurement of the optical properties of the skull in the wavelength range 650-950 nm. *Phys Med Biol* 38, 4, (Apr), pp. (503-510), ISSN 0031-9155.

Franceschini, M.A., Boas, D.A., (2004). Noninvasive measurement of neuronal activity with near-infrared optical imaging. *Neuroimage* 21, 1, (Jan), pp. (372-386), ISSN 1053-8119.

Friston, K.J., Holmes, A.P., Price, C.J., Buchel, C., Worsley, K.J., (1999). Multisubject fMRI studies and conjunction analyses. *Neuroimage* 10, 4, (Oct), pp. (385-396), ISSN 1053-8119.

Galvani, L., (1791). De viribus electricitatis in motu musculari commentarius. Bologna, Italy.

Gervain, J., Mehler, J., Werker, J.F., Nelson, C.A., Csibra, G., Lloyd-Fox, S., Shukla, M., Aslin, R.N., (2011). Near-infrared spectroscopy: A report from the McDonnell infant methodology consortium. *Developmental Cognitive Neuroscience* 1, 1, pp. (22-46).

Gonzalez-Alonso, J., Dalsgaard, M.K., Osada, T., Volianitis, S., Dawson, E.A., Yoshiga, C.C., Secher, N.H., (2004). Brain and central haemodynamics and oxygenation during maximal exercise in humans. *J Physiol* 557, Pt 1, (May 15), pp. (331-342), ISSN 0022-3751 (Print) 0022-3751 (Linking).

Harada, H., Tanaka, M., Kato, T., (2006). Brain olfactory activation measured by near-infrared spectroscopy in humans. *J Laryngol Otol* 120, 8, (Aug), pp. (638-643), ISSN 1748-5460 (Electronic) 0022-2151 (Linking).

Hiraoka, M., Firbank, M., Essenpreis, M., Cope, M., Arridge, S.R., van der Zee, P., Delpy, D.T., (1993). A Monte Carlo investigation of optical pathlength in inhomogeneous tissue and its application to near-infrared spectroscopy. *Phys Med Biol* 38, 12, (Dec), pp. (1859-1876), ISSN 0031-9155.

Huppert, T.J., Diamond, S.G., Franceschini, M.A., Boas, D.A., (2009). HomER: a review of time-series analysis methods for near-infrared spectroscopy of the brain. *Appl Opt* 48, 10, (Apr 1), pp. (D280-298), ISSN 1539-4522 (Electronic) 0003-6935 (Linking).

Ijichi, S., Kusaka, T., Isobe, K., Okubo, K., Kawada, K., Namba, M., Okada, H., Nishida, T., Imai, T., Itoh, S., (2005). Developmental changes of optical properties in neonates determined by near-infrared time-resolved spectroscopy. *Pediatr Res* 58, 3, (Sep), pp. (568-573), ISSN 0031-3998.

Jantzen, K.J., Oullier, O., Scott Kelso, J.A., (2008). Neuroimaging coordination dynamics in the sport sciences. *Methods* 45, 4, (Aug), pp. (325-335), ISSN 1095-9130 (Electronic) 1046-2023 (Linking).

Kikukawa, A., Kobayashi, A., Miyamoto, Y., (2008). Monitoring of pre-frontal oxygen status in helicopter pilots using near-infrared spectrophotometers. *Dyn Med* 7, pp. (10), ISSN 1476-5918.

Koh, P.H., Glaser, D.E., Flandin, G., Kiebel, S., Butterworth, B., Maki, A., Delpy, D.T., Elwell, C.E., (2007). Functional optical signal analysis: a software tool for near-infrared spectroscopy data processing incorporating statistical parametric mapping. *J Biomed Opt* 12, 6, (Nov-Dec), pp. (064010), ISSN 1083-3668.

Kohl, M., Lindauer, U., Dirnagl, U., Villringer, A., (1998a). Separation of changes in light scattering and chromophore concentrations during cortical spreading depression in rats. *Opt Lett* 23, 7, (Apr 1), pp. (555-557), ISSN 0146-9592.

Kohl, M., Nolte, C., Heekeren, H.R., Horst, S., Scholz, U., Obrig, H., Villringer, A., (1998b). Determination of the wavelength dependence of the differential pathlength factor from near-infrared pulse signals. *Phys Med Biol* 43, 6, (Jun), pp. (1771-1782), ISSN 0031-9155.

Leff, D.R., Orihuela-Espina, F., Elwell, C.E., Athanasiou, T., Delpy, D.T., Darzi, A.W., Yang, G.Z., (2011). Assessment of the cerebral cortex during motor task behaviours in adults: a systematic review of functional near infrared spectroscopy (fNIRS) studies. *Neuroimage* 54, 4, (Feb 14), pp. (2922-2936), ISSN 1095-9572 (Electronic) 1053-8119 (Linking).

Liu, J.Z., Lewandowski, B., Karakasis, C., Yao, B., Siemionow, V., Sahgal, V., Yue, G.H., (2007). Shifting of activation center in the brain during muscle fatigue: an explanation of minimal central fatigue? *Neuroimage* 35, 1, (Mar), pp. (299-307), ISSN 1053-8119.

Liu, J.Z., Shan, Z.Y., Zhang, L.D., Sahgal, V., Brown, R.W., Yue, G.H., (2003). Human brain activation during sustained and intermittent submaximal fatigue muscle contractions: an FMRI study. *J Neurophysiol* 90, 1, (Jul), pp. (300-312), ISSN 0022-3077 (Print) 0022-3077 (Linking).

Lloyd-Fox, S., Blasi, A., Everdell, N., Elwell, C.E., Johnson, M.H., (2010). Selective Cortical Mapping of Biological Motion Processing in Young Infants. *J Cogn Neurosci*, (Oct 18), ISSN 1530-8898 (Electronic) 0898-929X (Linking).

Magistretti, P.J., Pellerin, L., (1999a). Astrocytes Couple Synaptic Activity to Glucose Utilization in the Brain. *News Physiol Sci* 14, (Oct), pp. (177-182), ISSN 0886-1714.

Magistretti, P.J., Pellerin, L., (1999b). Cellular mechanisms of brain energy metabolism and their relevance to functional brain imaging. *Philos Trans R Soc Lond B Biol Sci* 354, 1387, (Jul 29), pp. (1155-1163), ISSN 0962-8436.

Maki, A., Yamashita, Y., Ito, Y., Watanabe, E., Mayanagi, Y., Koizumi, H., (1995). Spatial and temporal analysis of human motor activity using noninvasive NIR topography. *Med Phys* 22, 12, (Dec), pp. (1997-2005), ISSN 0094-2405.

Marumo, K., Takizawa, R., Kawakubo, Y., Onitsuka, T., Kasai, K., (2009). Gender difference in right lateral prefrontal hemodynamic response while viewing fearful faces: a multi-channel near-infrared spectroscopy study. *Neurosci Res* 63, 2, (Feb), pp. (89-94), ISSN 0168-0102.

Matsuura, C., Gomes, P.S., Haykowsky, M., Bhambhani, Y., (2011). Cerebral and muscle oxygenation changes during static and dynamic knee extensions to voluntary fatigue in healthy men and women: a near infrared spectroscopy study. *Clin Physiol Funct Imaging* 31, 2, (Mar), pp. (114-123), ISSN 1475-097X (Electronic) 1475-0961 (Linking).

Mendez-Villanueva, A., Hamer, P., Bishop, D., (2007). Physical fitness and performance. Fatigue responses during repeated sprints matched for initial mechanical output. *Med Sci Sports Exerc* 39, 12, (Dec), pp. (2219-2225), ISSN 0195-9131.

Miyai, I., Tanabe, H.C., Sase, I., Eda, H., Oda, I., Konishi, I., Tsunazawa, Y., Suzuki, T., Yanagida, T., Kubota, K., (2001). Cortical mapping of gait in humans: a near-infrared spectroscopic topography study. *Neuroimage* 14, 5, (Nov), pp. (1186-1192), ISSN 1053-8119.

Noakes, T.D., St Clair Gibson, A., Lambert, E.V., (2005). From catastrophe to complexity: a novel model of integrative central neural regulation of effort and fatigue during exercise in humans: summary and conclusions. *Br J Sports Med* 39, 2, (Feb), pp. (120-124), ISSN 1473-0480 (Electronic) 0306-3674 (Linking).

Nolte, C., Kohl, M., Scholz, U., Weih, M., Villringer, A., (1998). Characterization of the pulse signal over the human head by near infrared spectroscopy. *Adv Exp Med Biol* 454, pp. (115-123), ISSN 0065-2598.

Nybo, L., Rasmussen, P., (2007). Inadequate cerebral oxygen delivery and central fatigue during strenuous exercise. *Exerc Sport Sci Rev* 35, 3, (Jul), pp. (110-118), ISSN 0091-6331.

Obrig, H., Hirth, C., Junge-Hulsing, J.G., Doge, C., Wolf, T., Dirnagl, U., Villringer, A., (1996). Cerebral oxygenation changes in response to motor stimulation. *J Appl Physiol* 81, 3, (Sep), pp. (1174-1183), ISSN 8750-7587 (Print) 0161-7567 (Linking).

Peltonen, J.E., Paterson, D.H., Shoemaker, J.K., Delorey, D.S., Dumanoir, G.R., Petrella, R.J., Kowalchuk, J.M., (2009). Cerebral and muscle deoxygenation, hypoxic ventilatory chemosensitivity and cerebrovascular responsiveness during incremental exercise. *Respir Physiol Neurobiol* 169, 1, (Oct 31), pp. (24-35), ISSN 1878-1519 (Electronic) 1569-9048 (Linking).

Perec, G., (1974). Experimental demonstration of the tomatotopic organization in the Soprano (Cantatrix sopranica L.).

Pereira, M.I., Gomes, P.S., Bhambhani, Y.N., (2007). A brief review of the use of near infrared spectroscopy with particular interest in resistance exercise. *Sports Med* 37, 7, pp. (615-624), ISSN 0112-1642.

Perrey, S., (2008). Non-invasive NIR spectroscopy of human brain function during exercise. *Methods* 45, 4, (Aug), pp. (289-299), ISSN 1095-9130 (Electronic) 1046-2023 (Linking).

Plichta, M.M., Heinzel, S., Ehlis, A.C., Pauli, P., Fallgatter, A.J., (2007). Model-based analysis of rapid event-related functional near-infrared spectroscopy (NIRS) data: a parametric validation study. *Neuroimage* 35, 2, (Apr 1), pp. (625-634), ISSN 1053-8119.

Post, M., Steens, A., Renken, R., Maurits, N.M., Zijdewind, I., (2009). Voluntary activation and cortical activity during a sustained maximal contraction: an fMRI study. *Hum Brain Mapp* 30, 3, (Mar), pp. (1014-1027), ISSN 1097-0193 (Electronic) 1065-9471 (Linking).

Prahl, S., (2008). Tabulated molar extinction coefficient for hemoglobin in water. Values compiled using data provided by Gratzer WB, Medical Research Council Labs, Holly Hill London and Kollias N, Wellman laboratories, Harvard Medical School, Boston. *http://omlc.ogi.edu/spectra/hemoglobin/summary.html*.

Pringle, J., Roberts, C., Kohl, M., Lekeux, P., (1999). Near infrared spectroscopy in large animals: optical pathlength and influence of hair covering and epidermal pigmentation. *Vet J* 158, 1, (Jul), pp. (48-52), ISSN 1090-0233.

Racinais, S., Bishop, D., Denis, R., Lattier, G., Mendez-Villaneuva, A., Perrey, S., (2007). Muscle deoxygenation and neural drive to the muscle during repeated sprint cycling. *Med Sci Sports Exerc* 39, 2, (Feb), pp. (268-274), ISSN 0195-9131.

Rasmussen, P., Dawson, E.A., Nybo, L., van Lieshout, J.J., Secher, N.H., Gjedde, A., (2007). Capillary-oxygenation-level-dependent near-infrared spectrometry in frontal lobe of humans. *J Cereb Blood Flow Metab* 27, 5, (May), pp. (1082-1093), ISSN 0271-678X.

Rooks, C.R., Thom, N.J., McCully, K.K., Dishman, R.K., (2010). Effects of incremental exercise on cerebral oxygenation measured by near-infrared spectroscopy: a systematic review. *Prog Neurobiol* 92, 2, (Oct), pp. (134-150), ISSN 1873-5118 (Electronic) 0301-0082 (Linking).

Rupp, T., Perrey, S., (2008). Prefrontal cortex oxygenation and neuromuscular responses to exhaustive exercise. *Eur J Appl Physiol* 102, 2, (Jan), pp. (153-163), ISSN 1439-6327 (Electronic) 1439-6319 (Linking).

Schroeter, M.L., Bucheler, M.M., Muller, K., Uludag, K., Obrig, H., Lohmann, G., Tittgemeyer, M., Villringer, A., von Cramon, D.Y., (2004). Towards a standard analysis for functional near-infrared imaging. *Neuroimage* 21, 1, (Jan), pp. (283-290), ISSN 1053-8119.

Segal, S.S., (2005). Regulation of blood flow in the microcirculation. *Microcirculation* 12, 1, (Jan-Feb), pp. (33-45), ISSN 1073-9688.

Shibasaki, H., (2008). Human brain mapping: hemodynamic response and electrophysiology. *Clin Neurophysiol* 119, 4, (Apr), pp. (731-743), ISSN 1388-2457.

Shibuya, K., Tachi, M., (2006). Oxygenation in the motor cortex during exhaustive pinching exercise. *Respir Physiol Neurobiol* 153, 3, (Oct 27), pp. (261-266), ISSN 1569-9048.

Shibuya, K., Tanaka, J., Kuboyama, N., Murai, S., Ogaki, T., (2004a). Cerebral cortex activity during supramaximal exhaustive exercise. *J Sports Med Phys Fitness* 44, 2, (Jun), pp. (215-219), ISSN 0022-4707.

Shibuya, K., Tanaka, J., Kuboyama, N., Ogaki, T., (2004b). Cerebral oxygenation during intermittent supramaximal exercise. *Respir Physiol Neurobiol* 140, 2, (May 20), pp. (165-172), ISSN 1569-9048.

Simpson, C.R., Kohl, M., Essenpreis, M., Cope, M., (1998). Near-infrared optical properties of ex vivo human skin and subcutaneous tissues measured using the Monte Carlo inversion technique. *Phys Med Biol* 43, 9, (Sep), pp. (2465-2478), ISSN 0031-9155.

Smith, G.V., Alon, G., Roys, S.R., Gullapalli, R.P., (2003). Functional MRI determination of a dose-response relationship to lower extremity neuromuscular electrical stimulation in healthy subjects. *Exp Brain Res* 150, 1, (May), pp. (33-39), ISSN 0014-4819.

Subudhi, A.W., Dimmen, A.C., Roach, R.C., (2007). Effects of acute hypoxia on cerebral and muscle oxygenation during incremental exercise. *J Appl Physiol* 103, 1, (Jul), pp. (177-183), ISSN 8750-7587 (Print) 0161-7567 (Linking).

Suzuki, M., Miyai, I., Ono, T., Oda, I., Konishi, I., Kochiyama, T., Kubota, K., (2004). Prefrontal and premotor cortices are involved in adapting walking and running speed on the treadmill: an optical imaging study. *Neuroimage* 23, 3, (Nov), pp. (1020-1026), ISSN 1053-8119.

Swartz, B.E., Goldensohn, E.S., (1998). Timeline of the history of EEG and associated fields. *Electroencephalogr Clin Neurophysiol* 106, 2, (Feb), pp. (173-176), ISSN 0013-4694.

Tashiro, M., Itoh, M., Fujimoto, T., Masud, M.M., Watanuki, S., Yanai, K., (2008). Application of positron emission tomography to neuroimaging in sports sciences. *Methods* 45, 4, (Aug), pp. (300-306), ISSN 1095-9130 (Electronic) 1046-2023 (Linking).

Tew, G.A., Ruddock, A.D., Saxton, J.M., (2010). Skin blood flow differentially affects near-infrared spectroscopy-derived measures of muscle oxygen saturation and blood volume at rest and during dynamic leg exercise. *Eur J Appl Physiol* 110, 5, (Nov), pp. (1083-1089), ISSN 1439-6327 (Electronic) 1439-6319 (Linking).

Ultman, J.S., Piantadosi, C.A., (1991). Differential pathlength factor for diffuse photon scattering through tissue by a pulse-response method. *Math Biosci* 107, 1, (Nov), pp. (73-82), ISSN 0025-5564.

van der Zee, P., Cope, M., Arridge, S.R., Essenpreis, M., Potter, L.A., Edwards, A.D., Wyatt, J.S., McCormick, D.C., Roth, S.C., Reynolds, E.O., et al., (1992). Experimentally measured optical pathlengths for the adult head, calf and forearm and the head of the newborn infant as a function of inter optode spacing. *Adv Exp Med Biol* 316, pp. (143-153), ISSN 0065-2598.

Vesalius, A., (1543). De humani corporis fabrica. Brown University, Providence, Rhodes Island.

Villringer, A., (1997). Understanding functional neuroimaging methods based on neurovascular coupling. *Adv Exp Med Biol* 413, pp. (177-193), ISSN 0065-2598.

Villringer, A., Dirnagl, U., (1995). Coupling of brain activity and cerebral blood flow: basis of functional neuroimaging. *Cerebrovasc Brain Metab Rev* 7, 3, (Fall), pp. (240-276), ISSN 1040-8827.

Wernicke, C., (1894). Grundriss der Psychiatrie in klinischen Vorlesungen. Wrocław, Poland.

Wilcox, T., Bortfeld, H., Woods, R., Wruck, E., Boas, D.A., (2008). Hemodynamic response to featural changes in the occipital and inferior temporal cortex in infants: a preliminary methodological exploration. *Dev Sci* 11, 3, (May), pp. (361-370), ISSN 1467-7687 (Electronic) 1363-755X (Linking).

Wolf, M., Ferrari, M., Quaresima, V., (2007). Progress of near-infrared spectroscopy and topography for brain and muscle clinical applications. *J Biomed Opt* 12, 6, (Nov-Dec), pp. (062104), ISSN 1083-3668.

Yang, H., Wang, Y., Zhou, Z., Gong, H., Luo, Q., Lu, Z., (2009). Sex differences in prefrontal hemodynamic response to mental arithmetic as assessed by near-infrared spectroscopy. *Gend Med* 6, 4, (Dec), pp. (565-574), ISSN 1878-7398 (Electronic) 1550-8579 (Linking).

Yasui, H., Takamoto, K., Hori, E., Urakawa, S., Nagashima, Y., Yada, Y., Ono, T., Nishijo, H., (2010). Significant correlation between autonomic nervous activity and cerebral hemodynamics during thermotherapy on the neck. *Auton Neurosci* 156, 1-2, (Aug 25), pp. (96-103), ISSN 1872-7484 (Electronic) 1566-0702 (Linking).

Ye, J.C., Tak, S., Jang, K.E., Jung, J., Jang, J., (2009). NIRS-SPM: statistical parametric mapping for near-infrared spectroscopy. *Neuroimage* 44, 2, (Jan 15), pp. (428-447), ISSN 1095-9572 (Electronic) 1053-8119 (Linking).

Zarahn, E., Aguirre, G.K., D'Esposito, M., (1997). Empirical analyses of BOLD fMRI statistics. I. Spatially unsmoothed data collected under null-hypothesis conditions. *Neuroimage* 5, 3, (Apr), pp. (179-197), ISSN 1053-8119.

Zhang, Q., Brown, E.N., Strangman, G.E., (2007a). Adaptive filtering for global interference cancellation and real-time recovery of evoked brain activity: a Monte Carlo simulation study. *J Biomed Opt* 12, 4, (Jul-Aug), pp. (044014), ISSN 1083-3668.

Zhang, Q., Brown, E.N., Strangman, G.E., (2007b). Adaptive filtering to reduce global interference in evoked brain activity detection: a human subject case study. *J Biomed Opt* 12, 6, (Nov-Dec), pp. (064009), ISSN 1083-3668.

Zhao, H., Tanikawa, Y., Gao, F., Onodera, Y., Sassaroli, A., Tanaka, K., Yamada, Y., (2002). Maps of optical differential pathlength factor of human adult forehead, somatosensory motor and occipital regions at multi-wavelengths in NIR. *Phys Med Biol* 47, 12, (Jun 21), pp. (2075-2093), ISSN 0031-9155.

5

Intermanual and Intermodal Transfer in Human Newborns: Neonatal Behavioral Evidence and Neurocognitive Approach

Arlette Streri[1] and Edouard Gentaz[2]
[1]Paris Descartes University/LPP UMR 8158 CNRS, Paris
[2]Pierre Mendès-France University/LPNC UMR 5105 CNRS, Grenoble
France

1. Introduction

Until recently, newborns had typically been described as displaying mainly involuntary reactions and clumsy arm movements. However, in recent years investigation of exploratory perception of objects has emerged as key area research. Newborns' hands have often been described as closed or exhibiting either grasping or avoidance reactions which are inappropriate behaviors for holding an object and gathering and processing information (Katz, 1925; Roland and Mortensen 1987; Twitchell, 1965). However, besides possessing manual brief reactions (reflex), newborns are also able to handle small objects and to perceive their properties. To reveal this tactile ability, researchers have applied a habituation-dishabituation procedure to the tactile modality, just as in the visual modality (Streri & Pêcheux, 1986a). This procedure, which is controlled by the infant, is effective in revealing the early perceptual capacities of young babies (cf. Streri, 1993). It unfolds in two phases. The first phase, habituation, includes a series of trials in which the infants receive a small object in one hand. A trial begins when the infant holds the object and ends when the infant drops it or after a maximum duration defined by the experimenter. This process is repeated several times. As a consequence, the habituation process entails several grasps of determined duration (usually between 1 sec to 60 sec of holding). Trials continue until the habituation criterion is met. The newborn is judged to have been habituated when the duration of holding on any two consecutive trials, from the third onwards, totals a third (or a quarter, depending on age) or less of the total duration of the first two trials. Total holding time is taken as an indicator of the duration of familiarization. The mean number of trials taken to reach habituation ranges from four to twelve, and often varies with shape complexity. The decrease in holding times is considered to reveal the infants' ability to perceive and form a memory of the shape and subsequently recognize it. Then, in the dishabituation phase, a novel object is put in the infant's hand. If an increase in holding time of the novel object is observed, it is inferred that the baby is reacting to novelty, having noticed the difference between novel and familiar objects. That these processes reveal a form of mental representation of stimuli is now well established (cf. Pascalis & De Haan, 2003; Rovee-Collier & Barr, 2001).

Using this experimental procedure, Streri, Lhote, and Dutilleul (2000) showed that full-term newborns (the youngest was 16 hours old) were able to detect differences in the contours of two small objects (a smoothly curved cylinder versus a sharply angled prism) with both right and left hands. After habituation with one of the two objects placed in the right or left hand, the newborns reacted to novelty when a new object (the prism or cylinder) was put in their hand. This was the first evidence of habituation and reaction to novelty observed with the left as well as the right hand in human newborns. Thus, newborns are able to discriminate between curvilinear and rectilinear contours in small objects. However, this behavior does not show that babies have a clear representation of what they are holding in their hand. Because young infants are unable to perform the integration and synthesis of information in working memory required for haptic exploration, their shape perception is probably partial or limited to the detection of clues such as points, curves, presence or absence of a hole, etc. The information gathered is provided by the enclosure of the object (cf. Lederman & Klatzky, 1987), which seems to be an effective exploratory procedure for these limited purposes. To understand the emergence of these manual abilities in full-term newborns, it is important to recall the early maturation of touch (first among the senses to begin functioning) in the foetal period (from a cephalo-caudal point of view). Tactile receptors can be found in the epithelium of the mouth and the dermis of the peri-oral area as early as 8-9 gestational weeks. Meissner and Pacini corpuscles develop soon after. Tactile receptors are found on the face, the palms and the soles of the feet by 11 weeks. By the 15th week they are found on the trunk and proximal zones of arms and legs, and on the whole skin by the 20th week (Humphrey, 1964). Taken together, these data suggest that this ability to perceive various shapes with both hands observed in full-term newborns may be a "core ability" already present in the foetus. To investigate this hypothesis, the study of this manual ability in preterm babies is relevant and may reveal continuity in sensory functioning between foetal and neonatal periods, by determining whether preterm babies are able to extract information with their hands.

The current World Health Organization definition of premature is a baby born before 37 weeks of gestation, counting from the first day of the last menstrual period, where 40 weeks of gestation is the normal term. Moreover, the viability of foetuses is between 22 and 24 weeks of gestation, depending on the country. Studies about preterm babies and touch have generally focused on pain and developmental concerns (Sizun & Browne, 2005). They have shown that neonates' pain responses are influenced by the number of painful procedures previously experienced by the infant (Johnston & Stevens, 1996). Bartocci, Bergqvist, Lagercrantz and Anand (2006) showed that tactile and painful stimuli specifically activate somatosensory cortical areas. This result indicates that central integration of tactile information occurs in preterm newborns at 28-36 weeks of gestation. A link between hand movements and somatosensory cortical activation has also been shown in preterm newborns at 29-31 weeks of gestation (Milh et al., 2007). Recently, Lejeune, Audéoud, Marcus, Streri, Debillon and Gentaz (2010) investigated the ability of preterm babies' hands to discriminate between various shapes. Twenty-four preterm babies underwent a habituation phase followed by a test phase. The entire observation is performed in such a way the newborns cannot see their hands and the held object. In the test phase, twelve babies (experimental group) were tested with a novel object whereas twelve babies (control group) were tested with a familiar object (the one presented during the habituation phase). The shapes used were similar to those used by Streri et al (2000): a cylinder and a prism with identical object/hand surface ratio. These objects were smaller than those used by Streri et al. (2000) because preterm babies' hands are smaller than those of full term babies. The results revealed that when an object is placed in a preterm newborn's hand, holding time decreases trial by trial until the habituation criterion is reached. In the test phase, the experimental group held the novel object significantly longer compared to the preceding two habituation trials, in contrast to the control group in which this was not the case. These results suggest that preterm babies react differentially to a novel shape. These findings are in accordance with the early maturation of touch.

Taken together, these results show that preterm and full-term babies are able to memorize the shape of an object with each hand. These abilities reflect the very early existence of some internal representation of a stimulus. However, what is the nature of this internal representation? If it has some level of abstraction, newborns should be able to transfer object information from one hand to the other (low level of abstraction) or from one hand to the visual modality (high level of abstraction). Thus, the first goal of this chapter was to show that full-term and preterm newborns are capable of transferring shape and texture information from one hand to the other. The second goal was to show that full-term newborns are capable of transferring information between touch and vision in some, but not all, conditions. These limits or failures may be explained by neuroimaging evidence in adults.

2. Intermanual perception of object shape in human newborns

One reason for interest in intermanual transfer is its potential value in assessing communication between the two hemispheres and cerebral plasticity during cognitive development. Sann and Streri (2008a) investigated the inter-manual transfer of shape in twenty-four 2-day-old full-term newborns. After tactual habituation to a shape (prism or cylinder) in one hand, full-term newborns held the familiar shape longer in the opposite hand, and not the novel shape as usually expected in such procedure (Soroka, Corter, & Abramovitch, 1979). But in the same study, infants also exhibited inter-manual transfer of texture (smooth or granular), with a preference for the novel texture in the opposite hand. According to Sann and Streri (2008a), these discrepancies in performance between object properties indicate that the property of shape requires a more abstract and elaborate representation relative to texture. However, given the design of the study, it is not possible to draw definite conclusions about the type of shape information that was transferred: the entire shape of the object, edge information (round vs. angled), or other contrasts or differences. Regardless, these results provided evidence of intermanual transfer of shape in full-term newborns, confirming the hypothesis that the development of the corpus callosum at this stage is sufficient to permit some transfer of shape information between the two hands. Indeed, an fMRI study has demonstrated the essential contribution of posterior corpus callosum to the inter-hemispheric transfer of tactile information (Fabri et al., 2001, 2005).

Considering that the corpus callosum is less mature in preterm infants than full-term infants (Anderson, Laurent, Woodward, & Inder, 2006) and that very preterm birth (before 33 GW) may be associated with perinatal brain injury including the corpus callosum (Kontis et al., 2009), Lejeune et al. (in press) explored whether preterm infants are capable of inter-manual transfer of shape after the age of 33 GW. Using a classic tactile habituation-dishabituation procedure the authors predicted that after successive presentations of the same object, each preterm infant would show a decrease in holding time regardless of the hand tested or object shape. Second, the hypothesis of discrimination in intermanual transfer would be confirmed by differential treatment of novel and familiar objects in the opposite hand, as demonstrated previously in full-term newborns (Sann & Streri, 2008a). Thus, discrimination would be considered to have occurred when mean holding time for novel and familiar objects in the opposite hand differed significantly. Firstly, the results confirmed the occurrence of haptic manual habituation for each hand and for each shape in preterm infants between 33 and 34+6 GW. The second and main result was that, after habituation to the shape of an object in one hand, preterm infants held the novel object longer in the opposite hand. These results revealed intermanual transfer of shape in preterm infants between 33 and 34+6 GW for the first time. Fabri et al. (2005) showed the essential contribution of posterior corpus callosum to the inter-hemispheric transfer of tactile information: its development thus seems to be sufficient to permit the transfer of some shape information between hands in preterm infants between 33 and 34+6 GW. However, preterm infants' holding time in the opposite hand increased with both novel and familiar objects, although this increase was significantly greater for the novel object than for the familiar one. While the increase in holding time was expected for the novel object, confirming the presence of discrimination, the increase in holding time for the familiar object was more surprising. This second result relates to the influence of changing hands on manual discrimination. This pattern of results could be due to two factors, one peripheral and one central. At a peripheral level, the tactile receptors were not the same as those stimulated during habituation and the information collected by the opposite hand had to be sent to the central nervous system by another pathway. In addition, given that the infant participants had underdeveloped muscle tone, the increase in holding time could also be caused by muscle fatigue in the habituated hand, compared to the unfatigued contralateral hand. Any form of tactile stimulation of the contralateral hand would induce some degree of recovery from habituation. At a central level, comparing objects information collected from the two hands may require more time than during an intramanual discrimination. This increase in holding time could reflect the time required to transfer information between the two hemispheres via the corpus callosum.

Finally, the direction of preference (preference for novelty) differed from that observed in 2-day-old full-term newborns with a similar procedure. Lejeune et al. (in press) propose two interpretations for this difference. First, because it is impossible to determine what type of shape information was transferred (entire shape, edge information or other contrasts or differences), one possible interpretation could be that full-term and preterm infants extract different types of shape information, leading to this discrepancy of preference. A second interpretation could be that experience prevails over maturation. Preterm infants were tested at a lower post-conceptional age (34+3 GW) than full-term newborns (40+2 GW) but at a higher postnatal age (30 days *vs.* 2 days). Consequently, the results could be explained by a greater tactile experience *ex utero* than for the full-term newborns. However, 2-month-old full-term infants have also been found to demonstrate a familiar preference (Streri, Lemoine, & Devouche, 2008) even though their postnatal age was higher than that of our preterm infants. A second factor that could explain this second discrepancy is the type of tactile experience which, combined with the length of experience, might influence the direction of preference. Preterm infants in their incubators receive a great deal of repetitive and stereotyped tactile stimulations (daily care, feeding, medical examinations, etc.). Hospitalized infants experience up to 14 painful procedures per day and up to 53 different procedures during their first 15 days of life (Simons et al., 2003). Furthermore, Gimenez et al. (2008) showed that the maturation of brain tissue may be accelerated by factors associated with preterm birth, perhaps through the direct effects of the extrauterine environment. These particular tactile experiences could enhance the development of the intermanual transfer of information in preterm infants, even among younger infants who are at least 9 days old. In this case, according to the hypothesis proposed by Sann and Streri (2008a), preterm infants could have a more elaborate representation of shape than full-term newborns, leading to a preference for the novel shape in the opposite hand. However, these interpretations remain entirely speculative and post-hoc and require further investigation. More generally, the explanation of direction of preference is still debated in the infant studies literature, and seems to depend on several factors (e.g., Kerzerho, Streri, Gentaz, 2009; cf. Pascalis & De Haan, 2003). A preference indicates the presence of discrimination, whatever its direction, and suggests that the development of the corpus callosum is sufficient to permit some transfer of shape information between the two hands in preterm infants from 33 GW.

In conclusion, these results show that intermanual transfer of shape information is present at 33 GW in preterm infants. The occurrence of these intermanual abilities in full-term and preterm newborns suggests that some internal representation of a stimulus already has some level of abstraction. A second set of findings in favor of the existence of a higher-level internal representation stems from cross-modal studies on vision and touch in newborns.

3. Cross-modal transfer between touch and vision

In cognitive psychology, amodal perception is usually considered to be present at birth (see Streri, in press; Streri & Gentaz, 2009) as suggested by E. J. Gibson (1969). Beyond the details provided by individual sensory modalities, newborns are able to perceive a multimodal object as unified. However, the links between the haptic and the visual modalities are not fully established and will not be it until about the age of 15 years. Because newborns cannot engage in bimodal visual-haptic exploration of an object, a cross-modal transfer paradigm can be used to uncover the nature of these links and thereby evaluate young infants' ability to match the same object property captured by two modalities. However, cross-modal transfer tasks involve two successive phases (familiarization with an object in one modality and recognition test in a second modality). These tasks require cognitive processes (manual and visual information-processing capacities, memory load, etc.) that can weaken the links between sensory modalities and reveal failures in the establishment of amodal perception. Here we present a series of studies that illustrate these constraints.

3.1 Initial evidence in newborns

Newborns' visual abilities are weak. Nevertheless, numerous studies have revealed that babies can perceive speaking faces, photographs, objects, pictures, discriminate between large numbers, etc. (Coulon, Guellai and Streri, 2011; Féron, Gentaz, and Streri 2006; Guellai and Streri, 2011; Izard, Sann, Spelke and Streri, 2009; Meary, Kitromilides, Mazens, Graff and Gentaz, 2007; cf. Kellman and Arteberry, 1988, for a review). As discussed above, various studies have provided evidence that newborns are able to detect differences between shapes and textures with their hands (Streri et al. 2000; Molina and Jouen, 1998). All of these findings show that the prerequisites in both modalities are present to obtain cross-modal transfer between these senses.

Streri and Gentaz (2003; see also Streri and Gentaz, 2004) conducted an experiment on crossmodal transfer of shape information from the right hand to the eyes in 24 human newborns (mean age: 62 hours). They used an intersensory paired-preference procedure that included two phases: a haptic familiarization phase in which newborns were given an object to explore manually without seeing it, followed by a visual test phase in which infants were shown the familiar object paired with a novel one. Tactile objects were a small cylinder (10 mm in diameter) and a small prism (10 mm triangle base). Because the vision of newborns is immature and their visual acuity is weak, visual objects were the same 3D shapes, but much larger (45mm triangle base and 100mm in length for the prism and 30mm in diameter and 100mm in length for the cylinder). An experimental group (12 newborns) underwent the two phases successively (haptic then visual) whereas a baseline group (12 newborns) underwent only the visual test phase with the same objects as the experimental group but without haptic familiarization. Comparison of looking times between the two groups provided evidence of crossmodal recognition, with shapes explored by the hands of the experimental group recognized by the eyes. The newborns in the experimental group looked at the novel object for longer than the familiar one. In contrast, the newborns in the baseline group looked equally at both objects. Moreover, infants in the experimental group made more gaze shifts toward the novel object than the familiar object. In the baseline group this was not the case. Thus, this recognition in the experimental group stems from the haptic habituation phase. These results suggest that newborns recognized the familiar object through a visual comparison process as well as a comparison between the haptic and visual modalities. Moreover, the discrepancy between the sizes of the visual and tactile objects was apparently not relevant for crossmodal recognition. Shape alone seems to have been considered by newborns.

3.2 Limits of cross-modal shape transfer

Sann and Streri (2007) tested transfer from eyes to hand and from hand to eyes in order to ascertain whether this would demonstrate a complete primitive 'unity of the senses.' After haptic habituation to an object (cylinder or prism), the infants were shown the familiar and the novel shape in alternation. After visual habituation with either the cylinder or the prism, the familiar and the novel shape were put in the infant's right hand. The tactile objects were presented sequentially in an alternating manner. Again, visual recognition was observed following haptic habituation, but the reverse was not the case: no haptic recognition was found following visual habituation. Evidence of a visual recognition of shape also depended on the hand stimulated during the familiarization phase. No evidence of crossmodal recognition was found when the left hand was stimulated (Streri and Gentaz, 2004). Thus, cross-modal transfer seems not to be a general property of the newborn human; instead it is specific to certain parts of the body.

To understand this lack of bi-directional crossmodal transfer we must examine the differences between the ways that the two modalities process object shape. Vision processes shapes in a global manner, whereas touch processes information sequentially. Moreover, infants do not use efficient tactile exploratory procedures such as *"contour following"* to establish good representations of shapes (Lederman and Klatzky,, 1987). Earlier research performed on 2-month-old infants and using a bi-directional crossmodal shape transfer task (Streri 1987) revealed that two-month-old infants visually recognize an object that they have previously held, but do not manifest tactile recognition of an already-seen object. A plausible explanation of these results on lack of bi-directional crossmodal transfer is that, as in newborns, the levels of representation attained through each modality are not sufficiently equivalent to exchange information between sensory modalities. This hypothesis seems to be validated by the fact that if a two-month-old baby is presented with degraded visual stimulation (a bi-dimensional sketch of an 3D object) in which volumetric and textural aspects are missing, leading to a blurred percept, tactile recognition is possible, which is not the case with a visual volumetric object (Streri and Molina 1993). This result means that the infant's hand cannot sufficiently explore the held object to obtain a clear representation of this object.

A number of studies have also revealed that over the course of development, the links between the haptic and the visual modalities are fragile, often not bi-directional, and representation of objects is never complete: this holds not only in infancy (Rose and Orlian 1991; Streri 2007; Streri and Pêcheux 1986), but in children (Gori *et al.* 2008) and adults (Kawashima *et al.* 2002). For example, in a behavioral and PET study on human adults, Kawashima *et al.* found that the human brain mechanisms underlying crossmodal discrimination of object size follow two different pathways depending on the temporal order in which the stimuli are presented. They found crossmodal information transfer to be less accurate with VT transfer than with TV transfer. In addition, more brain areas were activated during VT than during TV. Crossmodal transfer of information is rarely reversible, and is generally asymmetrical even when it is bi-directional. However, in adults, these asymmetries can be due to experience, learning and maturation and the characteristics of these asymmetries cannot be used directly to explain the brains of newborns. To better understand results from newborns and two-month-olds, a comparison with another property (texture) in bi-directional cross-modal transfer tasks was carried out.

3.3 Shape vs. texture

The comparison between shape and texture, amodal properties, should allow testing the hypothesis of amodal perception in newborns and to shed light on the processes involved in information-gathering by both sensory modalities. However, shape is best processed by vision, whereas texture is thought to be best detected by touch (see Bushnell and Boudreau 1998; Klatzky *et al.* 1987). According to Guest and Spence (2003), texture is "more ecologically suited" to touch than to vision. In many studies on shape (a macrogeometric property), transfer from haptics to vision has been found to be easier than transfer from vision to haptics in both children and adults (Connolly and Jones 1970; Jones and Connoly 1970; Juurmaa and Lehtinen-Railo 1988; Newham and MacKenzie 1993; cf. Hatwell 1994). In contrast, when the transfer concerns texture (a microgeometric property), for which touch is as efficient as (if not better than) vision, this asymmetry does not appear.

Sann and Streri (2007) undertook a comparison between shape and texture in bi-directional crossmodal transfer tasks. They sought to examine how information is gathered and processed by the visual and tactile modalities and, as a consequence, to shed light on the perceptual mechanisms of newborns. If the perceptual mechanisms involved in gathering information on object properties are equivalent in both modalities at birth, then reverse crossmodal transfer would be expected. In contrast, if the perceptual mechanisms differ in the two modalities, then non-reversible transfer should be found. Thirty-two newborns participated in two experiments (16 in crossmodal transfer from vision to touch, and 16 in the reverse transfer). The stimuli were one smooth cylinder and one granular cylinder (a cylinder with pearls stuck on it). The results revealed crossmodal recognition of texture in both directions.

The findings suggest that for the property of texture, exchanges between the sensory modalities are bi-directional. Complete cross-modal transfer occurs with texture but not shape. However, this is true if only the object is volumetric and not flat, because newborns do not use the *"lateral motion"* exploratory procedure to detect differences between the textures of flat objects (Sann and Streri, 2008b). Cross-modal transfer between hands also reveals differences between shape and texture properties, and suggests that establishing representations of object shape is difficult for newborns. How should these results be explained? Human infants are particularly immature at birth, and brain maturation is protracted until adulthood. Almost no neuroimaging data is available because non-invasive techniques are difficult to apply in healthy infants. For example, newborns and young infants are often asleep (however, see Fransson et al., 2010 for a review on the functional architecture of the infant brain). Adult neuroimaging data, in contrast, offer some insights on how the brain processes cross-modal tasks.

3.4 Neuroimaging data

On the basis of these findings, two main questions emerge: First, why is bi-directional intermodal transfer observed for texture and not for shape? Second, how is haptic input translated into a visual format in newborns, i.e. by an organism that has never both seen and felt a 3D object?

On the basis of animal and human studies, Hsiao (2008) claimed that 3D shape processing involves the integration of both proprioceptive and cutaneous inputs from the hand. As the hand explores objects, different combinations of neurons are activated, and object recognition occurs as these 3D spatial views of the object are integrated. Cutaneous inputs related to 2D stimulus form and texture properties do not need such integration and may be processed differently than 3D shape in cortex. Cutaneous inputs stemming from the form and texture of 2D stimuli are processed in area 3b of SI cortex, whereas the sensitivity of neurons in area 2 to cutaneous inputs depends on hand conformation and its changes. Moreover, according to Hsiao (1998), the mechanisms underlying the early stages of 2D form processing are similar for vision and touch. Newborns' exploration of objects is very weak, and they may not be able to establish the 3D representations needed to perform tactile recognition after visual exploration of the object. Since texture and 2D form are similar in vision and touch, this data could explain why in 2-month-olds intermodal transfer from visual 2D object to haptic 3D objects is found, but not transfer from visual 3D objects to haptic 3D objects. Similarly, this data could explain the bi-directional transfer of texture between touch and vision observed in newborns.

Moreover, neuroimaging data from human adults suggests a functional separation in the cortical processing of micro- and macrogeometric cues (Roland et al. 1988). In this study, adults had to discriminate the length, shape, and roughness of objects with their right hand. Discrimination of object roughness activated lateral parietal opercular cortex significantly more than length or shape discrimination. Shape and length discrimination activated the anterior part of the intraparietal sulcus (IPA) more than roughness discrimination. More recently, Merabet *et al.* (2004) confirmed the existence of this functional separation and suggested that occipital (visual) cortex is functionally involved in tactile tasks requiring fine spatial judgments in normally sighted individuals. More specifically, a transient disruption of visual cortical areas using rTMS (repetitive Transcranial Magnetic Stimulation) did not hinder texture judgments, but impaired subjects' ability to judge the distance between dots in a raised dot pattern. Conversely, transient disruption of somatosensory cortex impaired texture judgments, while interdot distance judgments remained intact. In short, detection of shape and texture properties requires different exploratory procedures, and takes place in two different pathways in adult brains.

A second important question is that of how haptic input is translated into a visual format given that the sensory impressions are so different and that newborns have no experience with tactile and visual object inputs. To date, there is substantial neuroimaging evidence from adults showing that vision and touch are intimately connected, although views on this interconnectedness vary (see Amedi *et al.*, 2001; Sathian, 2005 for reviews). Cerebral cortical areas that were previously considered as exclusively visual, notably lateral occipital complex (LOC), are activated during haptic perception of shape (Lacey *et al.*, 2007). Crucially, LOC is activated in tactile recognition without mediation by visual recognition. Allen and Humphreys (2009) tested a patient with visual agnosia due to bilateral lesions of the ventral occipito-temporal cortex that had spared dorsal LOC. This patient's visual object recognition was impaired, but his tactile recognition was preserved. As a consequence, activation of dorsal LOC by tactile input can work directly through tactile inputs, and visual experience is unnecessary for LOC regions to be active in tactile object recognition. It seems plausible that visual imagery does not exist in newborns because they have little or no experience of the visual world of objects. It is possible that the LOC is activated in newborns brains when they explore an object haptically, and that the visual recognition of felt shape in cross-modal transfer tasks is not due to any visual imagery.

4. Conclusions

We recognize, understand, and interact with objects through both vision and touch (cf. Hatwell, Streri and Gentaz, 2003; Gentaz, 2009). In infancy, despite the various discrepancies between the haptic and visual modalities—such as asynchrony in the maturation and development of the different senses, distal vs. proximal inputs, and the contrast between the parallel character of vision and the sequential nature of the haptic modality—both systems detect regularities and irregularities when they are in contact with different objects, from birth onward. Conceivably, these two sensory systems may encode object properties such as shape and texture in similar ways. Behavioral evidence in newborns has revealed the involvement of different levels of abstraction in different types of transfer. Intermanual transfer of shape and texture seems to be bi-directional from birth. When newborns hold an object in one hand, left or right, its shape and texture are recognized by the other hand despite the immaturity of the corpus callosum. The maturity of the haptic sense is sufficient for gathering and processing information in a way that makes symmetrical correspondences between hands possible. This intermanual transfer may involve a low level of abstraction, because it does not require a change of representational format, since the steps involved, habituation and recognition, occur entirely within one modality—despite the fact that the transmission runs through the corpus callosum, which is immature at birth. Cross-modal transfers between vision and touch require a change of format and seem to be more difficult for newborns because of the higher level of abstraction involved.

Studies on crossmodal transfer tasks have revealed some links between the haptic and visual modalities at birth. Newborns are able to visually recognize a held object (Streri and

Gentaz 2003). This neonatal ability is independent of learning or the influence of the environment. However, by means of bi-directional crossmodal transfer tasks, Streri and colleagues have provided evidence on the perceptual mechanisms present at birth that constrain or limit the exchange of information between the sensory modalities. Newborns visually recognize the shape of a felt object, but are unable to recognize the shape of a seen object with their hands (Sann and Streri 2007). The link is obtained from the simplest information gathered, i.e. tactile information. Moreover, it is observed only with the newborn's right hand and not with the left (Streri and Gentaz 2004). A third striking result is that crossmodal transfer depends on object properties, being bidirectional with texture but not with shape (Sann and Streri 2007) — although this finding holds if, and only if, the felt textured object is volumetric, and not flat (Sann and Streri 2008b). For shape, just as for texture, the newborn's exploratory procedures are limited to the grasping reflex, which makes effective exploration of object properties impossible. All of these findings suggest that at birth, the links between the senses are specific to individual modalities and are not yet or entirely a general property of the brain.

Asymmetries in cross-modal transfer tasks continue to be found throughout the course of development. Several studies have also revealed that the links between the haptic and visual modalities are fragile, often not bi-directional, and representation of objects is never complete: this holds not only in infancy (Rose and Orlian 1991; Streri 2007; Streri and Pêcheux 1986b), but in children (Gori et al. 2008) and adults (Kawashima et al. 2002). Crossmodal transfer of information is rarely reversible, and is generally asymmetrical even when it is bi-directional (see Hatwell, Gentaz and Streri, 2003 for a review). The links between sensory modalities for object shape over the course of development appear to be flexible rather than immutable.

Why does cross-modal integration of spatial information develop in an asymmetrical manner? Several explanations may be offered. Sensory systems are not mature at birth, but become increasingly refined as children develop. Sometimes seen objects are observed to be well-recognized by touch, and more often, felt objects are well-recognized by vision. One possibility is that the sensory systems involved in spatial perception need to be continuously recalibrated during development, to take into account physical growth, such as changes in digit length (which affect haptic judgments), interocular separation, and eyeball length (affecting visual judgments). However, from birth, the links between the senses are more often effective when they begin with the hands rather than the eyes. Animal and adult neuroimaging studies also highlight asymmetries in cross-modal transfer tasks. Another suggestion would be that the links from eyes to hands are more effective for reaching and grasping objects than for cross-modal recognition. When we see an object, usually we take in information for some other purpose: e.g., transporting it to the mouth or somewhere else. In infancy, the hands are used as instruments to transport objects to the eyes or mouth, and the acquisition of this new ability develops to the detriment of the hands' perceptual function. Sensorimotor coordination triggered by the sight of an object is present from birth even though this ability mainly starts to be effective at about 4/5 months, at the beginning of prehension-vision. This ability may be better understood as the counterpart of cross-modal transfer from touch to vision. In both cases, perception and action are strongly linked. It is therefore important to note that sensory integration problems have often been observed in developmental disorders such as autism, dyslexia, and attention deficit disorder: understanding how incoming sensory information is transformed into outgoing motor commands is crucial for the diagnosis of such disorders (see Stein et al., 2009).

5. Acknowledgement

This work was supported by CNRS and by grants from the Agence Nationale de la Recherche (A.N.R.) and from the Institut Universitaire de France (I.U.F.).

6. References

Allen, H.A., & Humphreys, G.W. (2009). Direct tactile stimulation of dorsal occipito-temporal cortex in a visual agnostic. *Current Biology, 19*, 1044-1049.

Amedi, A., Kriegstein, K. von, Atteveldt, N. M. van, Beauchamp, M. S., Naumer, M.J. (2005). Functional imaging of human crossmodal identification and object recognition. *Experimental Brain Research, 166*, 559-571.

Anderson, N. G., Laurent, I., Woodward, L. J., & Inder T. E. (2006). Detection of impaired growth of the corpus callosum in premature infants. *Pediatrics, 118*, 951-960.

Bushnell, E.W. and Boudreau, J. P. (1998). Exploring and exploiting objects with the hands during infancy. In K. J. Connolly (Ed), *The psychobiology of the hand* (pp. 144-161). London: Mac Keith Press.

Connolly, K. and Jones, B. (1970). A developmental study of afferent-reafferent integration. *British Journal of Psychology, 61*, 259-266.

Coulon, M., Guellai, B., & Streri, A. (2011). Recognition of unfamiliar talking faces at birth. *International Journal of Behavioral Development, 35*, 282-287.

Bartocci M, Bergqvist LL, Lagercrantz H, Anand KJS (2006) Pain activates cortical areas in the preterm newborn brain. *Pain, 122*, 109-117.

Fabri, M., Del Pesce, M., Paggi, A., Polonara, G., Bartolini, M., Salvolini, U. and Manzoni, T. (2005). Contribution of posterior corpus callosum to the interhemispheric transfer of tactile information. *Cognitive Brain Research, 24*, 73-80.

Fabri, M., Polonara, G., Del Pesce, M., Quattrini, A., Salvolini, U., & Manzoni, T. (2001). Posterior corpus callosum and interhemispheric transfer of somatosensory information: An fRMI and neuropsychological study of partially callosotomized patient. *Journal of Cognitive Neuroscience, 13*, 1071-1079.

Féron, J., Gentaz, E. and Streri, A. (2006). Evidence of amodal representation of small numbers across visuo-tactile modalities in 5-month-old infants. *Cognitive Development, 21*, 81-92.

Fransson, P., Aden, Ulrika, Blennow, Mats, & Lagercrantz, H. (2010). The functional architecture of the infant brain as revealed by resting-state fMRI. *Cerebral Cortex*, doi:10.1093/cercir/bhq071.

Gentaz, E. (2009). *La main, le cerveau et le toucher (Hand, brain and touch)*. Paris: Dunod.

Gibson, E.J. (1969). *Principles of perceptual learning and development*. New York: Academic Press.

Gimenez, M., Miranda, M. J., Born, A. P., Nagy, Z., Rostrup, E., & Jernigan, T. L.(2008). Accelerated cerebral white matter development in preterm infants: a voxel-based morphometry study with diffusion tensor MR imaging. *Neuroimage, 41*, 728-734.

Gori, M., Del Viva, M., Sandini, G. and Burr, D. C. (2008). Young children do not integrate visual and haptic form information. *Current Biology, 18*, 1-5.

Guest, S. and Spence, C. (2003). Tactile dominance in speeded discrimination of textures. *Experimental Brain Research, 150*, 201-207.

Guellai, B., & Streri, A. (2011). Cues for early social skills: direct gaze modulates newborns' recognition of talking faces. *Plos One.* PONE-D-11-00014R1.

Hatwell, Y. (1994). Transferts intermodaux et intégration intermodale (crossmodal transfers and intersensory integration). In M. Richelle, J. Requin and M. Robert (Eds.), *Traité de psychologie expérimentale* (Vol 1, pp. 543-584). Paris: PUF.

Hatwell, Y., Gentaz, E., & Streri, A. (2003). *Touching for knowing. Cognitive psychology of tactile manual perception.* Johns Benjamins Publishing Compagny.

Humphrey, T. (1964). Some correlations between the appearance of human fetal reflexes and the development of the nervous system. *Progress in Brain Research, 4,* 93-135.

Hsiao, SS. (2008). Central mechanisms of tactile shape perception. *Current Opinion in Biology, 18,* 418-424.

Hsiao, SS. (1998). Similarities between touch and vision. In JW. Morley (ed.) *Neural aspects of tactile sensation* (pp 131-165). Amsterdam: Elsevier.

Izard, V., Sann, C., Spelke, E., and Streri, A. (2009). Newborn infants perceive abstract numbers. *Proceedings of the National Academy of Sciences USA, 106,* 10382-10385.

Johnston, C. C., & Stevens, B. J. (1996). Experience in a neonatal intensive care unit affects pain response. *Pediatrics, 98,* 925-930.

Jones, B., and Connolly, K. (1970). Memory effects in crossmodal matching. *British Journal of Psychology, 61,* 267-270.

Juurmaa, J., and Lehtinen-Railo, S. (1988). Visual experience and access to spatial knowledge. *Journal of Visual Impairment and Blindness, 88,* 157-170.

Katz, D. (1925/1989). *The world of touch* (translated by L.E. Krueger. 1989). Hillsdale, NJ: Erlbaum.

Kawashima, R., Watanabe, J. Kato, Takashi, Nakamura, A., Hatano, K., Schormann, T., Sato, K., Fukuda, H., Ito, K. and Zilles, K. (2002). Direction of crossmodal information transfer affects human brain activation: A PET study. *European Journal of Neuroscience, 16,* 137-144.

Kellman, P. J. and Arterberry, M. E. (1988). *The cradle of knowledge.* Cambridge MA: MIT Press.

Kerzerho, S., Streri, A., and Gentaz, E (2009). Factors influencing the manual discriminations of orientations in 5-month-old infants. *Perception, 38,* 44-51.

Klatzky, R. L., Lederman, S. J., and Reed, C. (1987). There's more to touch than meets the eye: The salience of object attributes for haptic with and without vision. *Journal of Experimental Psychology: General, 116,* 356-369.

Kontis, D., Catani, M., Cuddy, M., Walshe, M., Nosarti, C., Jones, D., et al. (2009). Diffusion tensor MRI of the corpus callosum and cognitive function in adults born preterm. *NeuroReport, 20,* 424-428.

Lacey, S., Campbell, C., and Sathian, K. (2007). Vision and touch: Multiple or multisensory representations of objects? *Perception, 36,* 1513-1521.

Lederman, S. J., and Klatzky, R. L. (1987). Hand movements: A window into haptic object recognition. *Cognitive Psychology, 19,* 342-368.

Lejeune, F., Audeoud, F., Marcus, L., Streri, A., Debillon, T. and Gentaz, E. (in press). Intermanual transfer of shapes in preterm human infants from 33 to 34+6weeks post-conceptional age. *Child Development.*

Lejeune, F., Audeoud, F., Marcus, L., Streri, A., Debillon, T., & Gentaz, E. (2010). The manual habituation and discrimination of shapes in preterm human infants from 33 to 34+6 post-conceptional age. *PLoS ONE, 5*: e9108. doi:10.1371/journal.pone.0009108.

Meary, D., Kitromilides, E., Mazens, K., Christian Graff & Edouard Gentaz (2007). Four-Day-Old Human Neonates Look Longer at Non-Biological Motions of a Single Point-of-Light. *PLoS ONE 2(1): e186*.

Merabet, L., Thut, G., Murray, B., Andrews, J., Hsiao, S. and Pascual-Leone, A. (2004). Feeling by sight or seeing by touch? *Neuron, 42*, 173-179.

Milh M, Kaminska A, Huon C, Lapillonne A, Ben-Ari Y, et al. (2007) Rapid oscillations and early motor activity in premature human neonate. *Cerebral Cortex, 17*, 1582-1594.

Molina, M., & Jouen, F. (1998). Modulation of the palmar grasp behavior in neonates according to texture property. *Infant Behavior and Development, 21*, 659-666.

Newham, C. and McKenzie, B. E. (1993). Crossmodal transfer of sequential and haptic information by clumsy children. *Perception, 22*, 1061-1073.

Pascalis, O., & De Haan, M. (2003). Recognition memory and novelty preference: what model? In H. Hayne & J. Fagen (Eds.), *Progress in infancy research* (Vol. 3, pp 95-120). New Jersey: Lawrence Erlbaum Associates.

Roland, P. E. and Mortensen, E. (1987). Somatosensory detection of microgeometry, macrogeometry and kinaesthesia in man. *Brain Research Review, 12*, 1-42.

Roland, P. E., O'Sullivan, B. and Kawashima, R. (1998). Shape and roughness activate different somatosensory areas in the human brain. *Proceedings of the National Academy of Sciences USA, 95*, 3295-3300.

Rose, S. A. and Orlian, E. K. (1991). Asymmetries in infant crossmodal transfer. *Child Development, 62*, 706-718.

Rovee-Collier, C., and Barr, R. (2001). Infant learning and memory. In G. Bremner and A. Fogel (Eds.), *Handbook of infant development* (pp. 139-168). Malden, MA: Blackwell Publishing.

Sann, C., & Streri, A. (2008a). Intermanual transfer of object texture and shape in human neonates. *Neuropsychologia, 46*, 698-703.

Sann, C., & Streri, A. (2008b). The limits of newborn's grasping to detect texture in a crossmodal transfer task. *Infant Behavior and Development, 31*, 523-531.

Sann, C., and Streri, A. (2007). Perception of object shape and texture in human newborns: evidence from crossmodal transfer tasks. *Developmental Science, 10*, 398-409.

Sathian, K. (2005). Visual cortical activity during tactile perception in the sighted and the visually deprived. *Development Psychobiology, 46*, 279-286.

Simons, S. H., van Dijk, M., Anand, K. S., Roofthooft, D., van Lingen, R. A., & Tibboel, D. (2003). Do we still hurt newborn babies? A prospective study of procedural pain and analgesia in neonates. *Archives of Pediatrics & Adolescent Medicine, 157*, 1058-1064.

Sizun. J, & Browne, J.V. (2005). *Research on early developmental care for preterm neonates.* Paris: John Libbey Eurotext.

Soroka, S. M., Corter, C. M., & Abramovitch, R. (1979). Infants' tactual discrimination of novel and familiar tactual stimuli. *Child Development, 50*, 1251-1253.

Stein, B.E., Perrault Jr, T.J., Stanford, T.R., and Rowland, B.A. (2009). Postnatal experiences influence how the brain integrates information from different senses. *Frontiers in integrative neuroscience.* Do:10.3389/neuro.07.021.2009.

Streri, A. (1987). Tactile discrimination of shape and intermodal transfer in 2- to 3- month-old infants. *British Journal of Developmental Psychology, 5,* 213-220.

Streri, A. (1993). *Seeing, reaching, touching. The relations between vision and touch in infancy.* London: Halverster Wheatsheaf.

Streri, A., and Gentaz, E. (2003). Crossmodal recognition of shape from hand to eyes in human newborns. *Somatosensory and Motor Research, 20,* 11-16.

Streri, A., and Gentaz, E. (2004). Crossmodal recognition of shape from hand to eyes and handedness in human newborns. *Neuropsychologia, 42,* 1365-1369.

Streri, A. and Gentaz, E. (2009). The haptic abilities of the human newborn: a review. *Zeitschrift fur Entwicklungspychologogie und Padagogishe Psychologie, 41,* 173-180.

Streri, A. and Molina, M. (1993). Visual-tactual and tactual-visual transfer between objects and pictures in 2-month-old infants. *Perception, 22,* 1299-1318.

Streri, A., and Pêcheux, M. G. (1986a). Tactual habituation and discrimination of form in infancy: A comparison with vision. *Child Development, 57,* 100-104.

Streri, A., and Pêcheux, M. G. (1986b). Vision to touch and touch to vision transfer of form in 5-month-old infants. *British Journal of Developmental Psychology, 4,* 161-167.

Streri, A., Lemoine, C., and Devouche, E. (2008). Development of intermanual transfer information in infancy. *Developmental Psychobiology, 50,* 70-76.

Streri, A., Lhote, M., and Dutilleul, S. (2000). Haptic perception in newborns. *Developmental Science, 3,* 319-327.

Streri, A. (in press). Crossmodal interactions in the human newborn: New answers to Molyneux's question. In A.J. Bremner, D.J. Lewkowicz, and C. Spence (Eds). *Multisensory Development.* Oxford: Oxford University Press.

Twitchell, T. E. (1965). The automatic grasping responses of infants. *Neuropsychologia, 3,* 247-259.

6

Somatosensory Stimulation in Functional Neuroimaging: A Review

S.M. Golaszewski et al.[*]
[1]Department of Neurology and Neuroscience Institute,
Paracelsus Medical University Salzburg,
[2]Karl Landsteiner Institute for Neurorehabilitation and Space Neurology Vienna
Austria

1. Introduction

Functional brain imaging of the somatosensory system has evolved over the past two decades and it has become an important tool in the preoperative planning in neurosurgery, in the monitoring in neurorehabilitation and for the understanding of motor recovery after brain damage for the planning and optimization of neurorehabilitation strategies.

Mapping of movement related cortical areas and areas that are related to body sensation was initially performed during neurosurgical procedures using direct cortical stimulation (Penfield, 1937). Several functional brain mapping techniques have subsequently evolved (Toga and Mazziotta, 2002). The era of functional brain imaging began in the 1980s with the implementation of the Positron Emission Tomography (PET) which provided a measure of the regional cerebral blood flow. Since the 1990s functional brain imaging is dominated by the rise of functional magnetic resonance imaging (fMRI) based on the blood oxygenation level dependant (BOLD) effect that was discovered 1990 by Ogawa et al. (Ogawa et al., 1990;Ogawa et al., 1992). Subsequently continuous evolution and progress of fMRI as well as its increasing popularity and spreading clinical use as a highly sensitive diagnostic neuroimaging instrument suitable for the assessment of a large variety of neurological and neurosurgical indications made fMRI to the leading functional neuroimaging modality. In this chapter we review somatosensory stimulation in PET and fMRI during the past decades, their advantages and disadvantages, optimal stimulation protocols as well as corresponding brain maps of different approaches of somatosensory stimulation in functional brain imaging and their clinical and neurophysilogical applications.

2. Positron Emission Tomography

In the 1980s, Positron Emission Tomography (PET) was used for the first time to detect focal neuronal activation within the primary somatosensory cortex of humans induced by

[*] M. Seidl[1], M. Christova[2], E. Gallasch[2], A.B. Kunz[1,5], R. Nardone[1,3], E. Trinka[1] and F. Gerstenbrand[4,5]
[1]Department of Neurology and Neuroscience Institute, Paracelsus Medical University Salzburg, Austria
[2]Institute of Physiology, Medical University Graz, Austria
[3]Department of Neurology, F. Tappeiner Hospital Meran, Italy
[4]Department of Neurology, Medical University Innsbruck, Austria
[5]Karl Landsteiner Institute for Neurorehabilitation and Space Neurology Vienna, Austria

cutaneous vibratory stimulation with a vibration frequency of 50 Hz and an amplitude of 1 mm (Fox et al., 1987). $H_2^{15}O$ labeled water was used as a blood flow tracer. The cutaneous surfaces of lips, fingers, and toes were tested. Intense and highly focal distinct responses within the primary somatosensory cortex with a medial-to-lateral homunculus were seen in each subject. The study demonstrated that eliciting regional cerebral blood flow responses within the somatosensory cortex by cutaneous vibration provides a safe, rapid, and reproducible tool for locating and assessing its functional status and for the localization of the central sulcus that is crucial in preoperative neurosurgical planning. The study has established normative values for future applications of the vibration paradigm in functional brain imaging.

In 1990, Tempel and Perlmutter compared the regional cerebral blood flow responses to vibrotactile stimulation in patients with predominantly unilateral idiopathic focal dystonia and normal subjects using $H_2^{15}O$ PET (Tempel and Perlmutter, 1990). The somatosensory stimulation led to consistently localized and robust peak response in the primary sensorimotor cortex, contralateral to hand vibration in normal subjects. The sensorimotor response in dystonic patients was also consistently localized to the same area, but significantly reduced in magnitude when vibrating the affected as well as the unaffected hand. Furthermore, vibration induced a dystonic cramp in the stimulated arm and hand in some patients, but in no normal subjects. This abnormal sensorimotor response had important implications for the understanding of the pathophysiology of idiopathic dystonia. Two years later, Tempel and Perlmutter performed another significant $H_2^{15}O$ PET study with vibration-induced regional cerebral blood flow responses in healthy young and elder subjects in order to investigate whether vibration-induced regional cerebral blood flow responses change with increasing age (Tempel and Perlmutter, 1992). Left and right hand vibration led to consistent responses within the contralateral primary sensorimotor cortex and the supplementary motor area with no changes in the physiologically aging brain.

In the same year, Seitz and Roland were able to demonstrate with a vibratory stimulus to the right hand palm of healthy volunteers and $H_2^{15}O$ PET that activation of some cerebral structures is accompanied by deactivations of corresponding other structures elsewhere in the brain (Seitz and Roland, 1992). Increases in the regional cerebral blood flow were localized in the left primary somatosensory area, the left secondary somatosensory area, the left retroinsular field, the left anterior parietal cortex, the left primary motor area, and the left supplementary motor area. The decreases occurred bilaterally within the superior parietal cortex, paralimbic association areas, and the left globus pallidus. The mean global cerebral blood flow did not change compared with rest. The decreases in cerebral oxidative metabolism were interpreted as regional depressions of synaptic activity.

In an $H_2^{15}O$ PET study by Drevets et al., changes in the human primary and secondary somatosensory cortices during the period when somatosensory stimuli were expected were investigated (Drevets et al., 1995): In anticipation of either focal or innocuous touching, or localized, painful shocks, the blood flow decreased in the parts of the primary somatosensory cortex located outside the representation of the skin locus of the expected stimulus. Specifically, attending to an impending stimulus to the fingers produced a significant decrease in blood flow in the somatosensory zones for the face, whereas attending to stimulation of the toe produced decreases in the zones for the fingers and face. Decreases were more prominent in the side ipsilateral to the location of the expected stimulus. No significant changes in the blood flow occurred in the region of the cortex representing the skin locus of the expected stimulation. These results were concurrent with a model of spatial attention in which potential signal enhancement may rely on generalized suppression of background activity.

In the same year, Ibanez et al. demonstrated in a PET study that there is no evidence that the primary motor and supplementary motor area are involved in the generation of the P22 and N30 components of somatosensory evoked potentials (SSEPs) caused by electrical stimulation of the median nerve at the wrist (Ibanez et al., 1995). PET was performed in normal subjects to study the cerebral areas activated by median nerve electrical stimulation at frequencies of up to 20 Hz. Stimulation evoked a single focus of activation in the primary somatosensory area. An increase of the regional cerebral blood flow in this area was linearly correlated with stimulus frequencies of up to 4 Hz and then reached a plateau. The supplementary motor area was not significantly activated by stimulation at any of the frequencies tested. In contrast to the primary somatosensory area, the supplementary motor area showed no trend toward a correlation between the regional cerebral blood flow changes and the stimulus repetition rate. These results suggested that a contribution of the primary motor cortex and the supplementary motor area to the generation of the P22 and N30 components of SSEPs is unlikely.

$H_2^{15}O$ PET studies with different application forms and intensities of innocuous and noxious thermal stimuli were performed by Casey et al (Casey et al., 1994;Casey et al., 1996) to identify the forebrain and brain stem structures that are active during the perception of acute heat pain in humans. Healthy subjects received repetitive noxious (50°C) and innocuous (40°C) heat pulses with duration of five seconds to the forearm and each subject rated the subjective intensity of each stimulation series. Significant regional cerebral blood flow with a maximum at 50°C stimuli was found in the thalamus, the cingulate cortex, the secondary and primary somatosensory cortex, the insula, the medial dorsal midbrain and the cerebellar vermis. In the second study noxious and innocuous heat and cold thermal stimuli to the non-dominant arm of healthy subjects were applied.

A detailed analysis of somatosensory representations within the parietal postcentral gyral and the lateral sulcal-opercular cortex in a $H_2^{15}O$ PET study was performed by Burton et al. (Burton et al., 1997). To investigate the issue of possible multiple activation foci in these regions and possible differences due to stimulating skin directly or through an imposed tool, changes in the regional cerebral blood flow during passive tactile stimulation of one or two fingertips were studied. Restrained fingers were rubbed with embossed gratings using a rotating drum stimulator. For different scans, gratings touched the skin directly for optimal stimulation of cutaneous receptors (skin mode stimulation) or indirectly by using an imposed guitar plectrum snugly fitted to the same fingers (tool mode stimulation). The latter was expected to better stimulate deep receptors better. The subjects were asked to estimate the roughness after each scan. Direct skin contact activated statistically validated foci in both hemispheres, on the contralateral side these foci occurred in the anterior and posterior limbs of the postcentral gyrus and on the ipsilateral side only in the posterior limb. Tool mode stimulation activated one contralateral focus that was in the posterior limb of the postcentral gyrus. These results suggested at least two maps for distal fingertips in the primary somatosensory area with the anterior and posterior foci corresponding, respectively, to activations in the Brodmann area 3b and the junction between the Brodmann areas 1 and 2. In the contralateral secondary somatosensory area, skin mode stimulation activated a peak that was anterior and medial to a focus associated with tool mode stimulation. The magnitude of the PET counts contralateral to stimulation was higher in the anterior primary and secondary somatosensory regions during initial scans, but reversed to more activation in the posterior primary somatosensory region during later scans. These short-term practice effects suggested changes in neural activity with stimulus novelty.

Another method for selectively activating the cortical projections of deep receptors for proprioceptive perception in a study with $H_2^{15}O$ PET was presented by Mima et al. (Mima et al., 1999). Functional brain maps during active and passive finger movements driven by a servo-motor were compared. The authors were able to selectively activate proprioception with a minimal contribution from the epicritic sensation with a newly developed device. Proprioception was represented only within the contralateral primary and secondary somatosensory areas, whereas active movements were cortically represented within the contralateral primary sensorimotor cortex, the premotor cortex, the supplementary motor area, the bilateral secondary somatosensory areas, the basal ganglia and the ipsilateral cerebellum. In this study, differential brain maps for cortical representations of different components of the sensorimotor system were displayed for the first time in the field of functional neuroimaging.

Xu et al. elucidated the functional localization and somatotopic organization of pain perception in the human cerebral cortex with PET during selective painful stimulation. Response to painful stimuli to the hand and foot were elicited using a special CO_2 laser, which selectively activates nociceptive receptors (Xu et al., 1997). Multiple brain areas, including the bilateral secondary somatosensory areas and both insulas, the frontal lobe, and thalamus contralateral to the stimulus side were found to be involved in the response to painful stimulation. While the data indicate that the bilateral secondary somatosensory area plays an important role in pain perception, they also indicate that there is no pain-related somatotopic organization in the human secondary somatosensory cortex or insula. Pain processing during three levels of noxious stimulation that produced differential patterns of central activity was investigated by Derbyshire et al. (Derbyshire et al., 1997).

Bittar et al. investigated presurgical mapping of the primary somatosensory cortex compared with intraoperative cortical stimulation with $H_2^{15}O$ PET (Bittar et al., 1999a;Bittar et al., 1999b). PET scanning with vibrotactile stimulation of the face, the hands or the feet to localize the primary somatosensory area before surgical resection of the mass lesions or epileptogenic foci affecting the central area was performed in patients with brain tumor. With the aid of image-guided surgical systems, the location of significant activation foci on the PET scanning were compared with those of positive intraoperative cortical stimulation performed at craniotomy. In 95%, the PET activation foci were spatially concordant with the intraoperative cortical stimulation. Intraoperative cortical stimulation was positive in 40% of the stimulation sites where the PET did not result in statistically significant activation. According to these results, it was concluded that PET is an accurate method for mapping the primary somatosensory area prior to surgery.

Boecker et al. investigated the functional anatomy of somatosensory processing in two clinical conditions characterized by basal ganglia dysfunction in Parkinson's and Huntington's disease (Boecker et al., 1999) in a $H_2^{15}O$ PET study. Continuous unilateral high-frequency vibratory stimulation was applied to the immobilized metacarpal joint of the index finger. In the control subjects, the activation pattern was lateralized to the side opposite to the stimulus presentation, including the primary and secondary somatosensory areas, as well as subcortical (globus pallidus, ventrolateral thalamus) regions. Inter-group comparisons of the vibration-induced changes of the regional cerebral blood flow between patients and control subjects revealed differences in central somatosensory processing. In Parkinson's disease, decreased activation was found in the contralateral sensorimotor cortex, the lateral premotor cortex, the contralateral secondary somatosensory area, the contralateral posterior cingulate cortex, the bilateral prefrontal cortex (Brodmann area 10) and in the contralateral basal ganglia. In Huntington's disease, decreased activation was detected contralateral in the secondary somatosensory area, the parietal Brodmann areas 39 and 40, the lingual gyrus, the bilateral prefrontal cortex (Brodmann areas 8, 9, 10 and 44), the primary somatosensory area, and the contralateral basal ganglia. In both clinical diseases, relative enhanced activation of the ipsilateral somatosensory cortical areas, notably the caudal primary and secondary somatosensory regions as well as the insular cortex, could also be detected. The data show that Parkinson's and Huntington's disease, beyond well-established deficits in the central motor control, are characterized by abnormal cortical and subcortical activation on passive somatosensory stimulation. Furthermore, the finding that the activation increases in the ipsilateral somatosensory cortical areas may be interpreted as an indication of either altered central focusing and gating of the somatosensory impulses, or enhanced compensatory recruitment of the somatosensory areas.

A ^{18}F-fluorodeoxyglucose PET study with somatosensory stimulation in patients suffering from spinal cord injuries was performed by Roelcke et al. (Roelcke et al., 1997a) to assess the effect of a transverse spinal cord lesion on cerebral energy metabolism in view of sensorimotor reorganisation. PET was used to study resting cerebral glucose metabolism in patients with complete paraplegia or tetraplegia after spinal cord injury compared with healthy subjects. The global absolute glucose metabolism rate was lower in the spinal cord injury patients than in the healthy subjects. A relatively increased glucose metabolism was discovered particularly in the supplementary motor area, the anterior cingulate, and the putamen. A relatively reduced glucose metabolism was found in patients with spinal cord injury was found in the midbrain, the cerebellar hemispheres, and the temporal cortex. It was concluded that cerebral deafferentation due to reduction or loss of sensorimotor function results in the low level of an absolute global glucose metabolism rate found in patients with spinal cord injury. Relatively increased glucose metabolism in brain regions involved in attention and initiation of movement may be related to secondary disinhibition of these regions.

PET studies using noxious electrical stimuli to the median nerve were also performed on patients in persistent vegetative state (actually referred to as unresponsive wakefulness syndrome) to assess cortical pain processing (Kassubek et al., 2003;Laureys et al., 2002). Even though cortical metabolism (in FDG-PET) was decreased up to 40% of normal values, both studies showed reliable activations in residual parts of the pain processing networks in H_2[15]O PET. Compared to age-matched controls, noxious stimuli activated the primary somatosensory cortex, contralateral thalamus and midbrain, but failed to activate higher-order associative cortices (secondary somatosensory, bilateral posterior parietal, premotor, polysensory superior temporal and prefrontal cortices). These findings help to understand cortical processing after severe brain injury, however, but they can neither prove nor disprove awareness of pain or any other stimulus in this patient group.

3. Functional Magnetic Resonance Imaging

Somatosensory stimuli were applied in many functional magnetic resonance imaging (fMRI) studies. Especially light stimulation using air puffs (Stippich et al., 1999b) or other tactile stimuli (Hodge et al., 1998;Moore et al., 2000;Rausch et al., 1998;Servos et al., 1998), scratching of the hand palm (Hoeller et al., 2002), vibration (Gelnar et al., 1998b;Golaszewski et al., 2002;Golaszewski et al., 2006;Golaszewski et al., 2002;Hodge et al., 1998), electrical stimulation (Arthurs et al., 2000;Backes et al., 2000;Korvenoja et al., 1999;Krause et al., 2001;Kurth et al., 1998;Takanashi et al., 2001), noxious stimuli (Apkarian et al., 2000;Peyron et al., 2000), and proprioception induced by passive joint movement (Rausch et al., 1998) were used. Usually, the primary somatosensory cortex in the postcentral gyrus and the secondary somatosensory cortex in the parietal operculum, insula, and more posterior ventral parietal areas are activated. A clear somatotopic organization in the primary somatosensory cortex could be demonstrated, whereas this somatotopic organization could not be clearly shown in the secondary somatosensory area (Disbrow et al., 2000;Gelnar et al., 1998b;Hodge et al., 1998;Krause et al., 2001;Kurth et al., 1998;Servos et al., 1998). An evident somatotopy also in the secondary somatosensory area was demonstrated in a study by Gelnar et al. (Gelnar et al., 1998c). A vibratory stimulus was applied to an individual digit tip (digit 1, 2, or 5) on the right hand of healthy adults which led to a BOLD response in cortical regions located on the upper bank of the Sylvian fissure, the insula, and the posterior parietal cortices. Multiple digit representations were observed in the primary somatosensory cortex, corresponding to the four anatomic subdivisions areas 3a, 3b, 1, and 2. There was no simple medial to lateral somatotopic representation in individual fMRI maps but a clear spatial distance between digit 1 and digit 5 was seen on the cortex in both the primary and secondary somatosensory regions. Ruben et al. was able to demonstrate a somatotopic organization of the secondary somatosensory area with electrical stimulation of the right hallux, the index and the fifth finger (Ruben et al., 2001). They were not able to observe separate representations of digit 2 and 5 in the secondary somatosensory area, but a somatotopic representation between the fingers and the hallux could be detected bilaterally within the secondary somatosensory region. Kurth et al. demonstrated a somatotopy in the primary somatosensory cortex by using electrical finger stimulation (Kurth et al., 2000). Functional MRI detected separate representations for all five fingers in the primary somatosensory cortex. Responses were located in the posterior wall of the deep central sulcus (corresponding to Brodmann area 3b), and the anterior (Brodmann area 1) or the posterior crown of the postcentral gyrus (Brodmann area 2) with rare activations in Brodmann area 3a and 4. In Brodmann area 3b, a regular somatotopic mediolateral digit arrangement for fingers 5 to 1 with a mean Euclidean distance of 16 mm between fingers 1 and 5 was found. In contrast, Brodmann area 1 and 2 showed a greater number of adjacent activation foci with a significantly greater overlap and partly even reversed ordering of the neighboring fingers. This paradigm can be used to localize the central sulcus preoperatively (Kurth et al., 1998) and it is applicable even in patients with severe hemiparesis without severe hemianesthesia.

In many studies investigating the primary somatosensory cortex, only a contralateral BOLD response could be elicited, whereas the secondary somatosensory areas were activated bilaterally (Backes et al., 2000;Disbrow et al., 2001;Korvenoja et al., 1999). It is still uncertain, what stimulus leads to the most robust BOLD response within the somatosensory cortex. There is evidence that pain stimuli are less reliable than vibrotactile or electrical stimuli for evoking primary somatosensory activation (Backes et al., 2000;Disbrow et al., 2001;Korvenoja et al., 1999;Peyron et al., 2000). Activation magnitude in the primary somatosensory cortex depends on the intensity of stimulation (Arthurs et al., 2000;Krause et al., 2001), the size of the stimulated body surface (Apkarian et al., 2000;Peyron et al., 2000), and the rate of stimulation (Apkarian et al., 2000;Peyron et al., 2000;Takanashi et al., 2001). Nelson et al. demonstrated an increasing stimulus-response relationship between the amplitude of vibrotactile stimuli delivered to the volar surface of the right index finger and BOLD activity in the primary somatosensory area that persisted during an attention-demanding tactile tracking task (Nelson et al., 2004). The secondary somatosensory cortex did not show any clear relationship with the vibration amplitude, but was more often activated during the attention demanding tracking task compared with passive vibration. Responses in secondary areas seem to be less influenced by these variables, but are probably more dependant of the level of attention directed to the stimulus (Apkarian et al., 2000;Backes et al., 2000;Peyron et al., 2000;Takanashi et al., 2001) and on whether stimulation is delivered uni- or bilaterally (Apkarian et al., 2000;Backes et al., 2000;Disbrow et al., 2001;Peyron et al., 2000;Takanashi et al., 2001). Regarding attentional phenomena interfering with somatosensory processing, tactile processing while varying the focus of attention was studied. Activations were contrasted between attend and ignore conditions, both of which employed identical stimulation characteristics and an active task. Random effects analysis revealed significant attention effects in the primary somatosensory area. The blood oxygenation level-dependent response was greater for attended than for ignored stimuli. Modulations were also found in the secondary somatosensory cortex and the middle temporal gyrus. These findings suggest that the stimulus processing at the level of the primary representations in the primary somatosensory area is modulated by attention (Sterr et al., 2007).

Somatosensory stimulation has the advantage of not requiring movement which may cause artifacts. With somatosensory stimulation (repetitive brushing of the hand palm) in brain tumor patients, a lower incidence of severe movement artifacts was found compared to an active motor paradigm (finger-to-thumb-tapping), however, the motor paradigm elicited a significantly higher percentage of signal increases. (Apkarian et al., 2000;Backes et al., 2000;Disbrow et al., 2001;Hoeller et al., 2002;Peyron et al., 2000;Takanashi et al., 2001). Several fMRI studies discovered a similar functional localisation comparing somatosensory stimulation and active motor paradigms (Golaszewski et al., 2002;Golaszewski et al., 2006;Golaszewski et al., 2002;Lee et al., 1998). Lee et al. (1998) demonstrated in an fMRI study similar results with active and passive activation tasks by comparing palm-finger brushing with sponge-squeezing and active finger movements according to their functional localisation. The sensorimotor and somatosensory BOLD responses were located to a large extent in the postcentral gyrus, and their spatial locations were not significantly different. Golaszewski et al. showed largely similar functional maps by active finger-to-thumb tapping and vibration of the hand palm (Golaszewski et al., 2002a;Golaszewski et al., 2002b). In patients who are physically unable to perform active finger-to-thumb-tapping, hand-squeezing or fist clenching as sensorimotor activation tasks the vibration of the hand palm can be regarded as a proper paradigm in presurgical fMRI mapping of the sensorimotor hand area.

In an fMRI study with a piezoelectric vibration device Francis et al. found a frequency dependence of the primary and secondary somatosensory area (Francis et al., 2000). With both frequencies applied to the index finger during the same scanning session, an increase in the vibration frequency from 30 to 80 Hz showed a significant increase of the BOLD response within the secondary somatosensory area and the posterior insula, while the number of pixels activated in the primary somatosensory area declined.

Moreover, functional imaging studies are important for the monitoring of rehabilitation and the understanding of motor recovery after cortical strokes (Cramer et al., 2000). Functional MRI was used to compare sensory and motor maps obtained in normal controls with functional maps from two patients with good recovery six months after a cortical stroke. Cortical map reorganization along the detected infarct rim might be an important contributor to recovery of motor and sensory function after stroke. Moreover, functional imaging studies with somatosensory stimulation are also important for the monitoring of the rehabilitation after extremity transplantations (Piza, 2000). A close relationship between the intensity of phantom limb pain in amputees and the amount of reorganization of the somatosensory cortex was reported in fMRI studies (Flor et al., 2001;Hamzei et al., 2001;Koppelstaetter et al., 2007).

Functional MRI was also used to investigate brain activations underlying menthol-induced cold allodynia (Seifert and Maihöfner, 2007). Healthy volunteers were investigated using a block-design fMRI approach. Brain activity was measured during application of innocuous cold stimuli (5°C above cold pain threshold) and noxious cold stimuli (5°C below cold pain threshold) to the skin of the forearm using a peltier-driven thermostimulator. The stimuli were adjusted to the individual cold pain threshold. Cold allodynia was induced by topical menthol and cortical activations were measured during previously innocuous cold stimulation (5°C) that was at this situation perceived as painful. On a numeric rating scale for pain (0-10) innocuous cold, cold pain and cold allodynia were rated. Sensory and affective components of allodynia and cold pain were equal in the McGill pain questionnaire (Roelcke et al., 1997b). All tested conditions (innocuous cold, noxious cold and cold allodynia) led to significant activations of the bilateral insular cortices, the bilateral frontal cortices and the anterior cingulate cortex. When compared with innocuous cold, noxious cold led to significantly more activations of the posterior insula and to less activations of the ipsilateral insular cortex.

Significantly increased activations in bilateral dorsolateral prefrontal cortices and brainstem (ipsilateral parabrachial nucleus) were found during cold allodynia when compared with equally intense cold pain conditions. Cold allodynia led to significantly more activations of the bilateral anterior insula, whereas the activation of the contralateral posterior insula was equal. It was concluded that cold allodynia activates a network similar to that of normal cold pain, but additionally recruits bilateral dorsolateral prefrontal cortex and the midbrain, suggesting that these brain areas are involved in central nociceptive sensitization processes.

In the authors' facility, somatosensory stimulation is also used in the clinical routine to assess patients with chronic disorders of consciousness (unresponsive wakefulness syndrome, minimally conscious state) in fMRI (unpublished data). In a series of 22 consecutive patients with chronic disorders of consciousness, seven patients showed reliable response in typical brain areas using a pneumatic activation device (Figure 3, 4, 6). The above-mentioned somatosensory assessment combined with cognitive testing in functional neuroimaging is routinely acquired in patients with chronic disorders of consciousness for the planning of neurorehabilitation and estimation of prognosis.

4. Current devices for somatosensory stimulation

Next to the classical electrical nerve stimulation, vibrotactile stimulation has become very common in functional brain imaging. Vibrotactile stimulation has several advantages over electrical stimulation. First, the stimuli are not painful and therefore a certain stimulus can be presented over a long time period. This is often necessary to obtain a stable cortical response. Second, by selecting the site and frequency of the stimulus, the different receptor types (cutaneous mechanoreceptors, proprioceptors, thermo receptors) can be specifically excited and their functional integration at the cortical level can be studied. Third, the stimulus response underlies adaptation which can be used to analyze the somatosensory information processing, its influence to cortical structures, and the modulation by other brain regions (Giabbiconi et al., 2007). On the other hand, a cortical response may be affected adversely by somatosensory adaptation phenomena. This has to be considered when designing a specific stimulation protocol.

In clinical routine, the vibrotactile sense is assessed by brushing on a certain body region (Frey hair) or by using a tuning fork. These manual stimulations were used in the earlier studies of somatotopic mapping (Polonara et al., 1999). However, for more complex stimulation designs, it is more convenient to use quantitative testing equipment. Within the past ten years, various prototypes of stimulation devices have been tested for somatotopic mapping. Among these devices, pneumatically driven air bags were introduced (Gelnar et al., 1998b;Golaszewski et al., 2002a;Stippich et al., 1999b), as well as piezodisks (Harrington et al., 2000b;Maldjian et al., 1999b), cable driven rotating masses (Golaszewski et al., 2002b) and even coil designs using the static magnetic field of an MR scanner (Graham et al., 2001). As most of these devices were used in fMRI-paradigms, the interactions between MRI and the certain stimulation device must be considered. In this chapter, we first focus on the MR compatibility and the MR safety and subsequently give an overview on the different types of devices.

4.1 MR compatibility and MR safety

According to the safety guidelines by General Electric (GE) Medical Systems (GE-Medical Systems, 1997), a device is considered to be MR save, if it can be demonstrated that it does not lead to an increased safety risk towards the patient and the staff, when the device is introduced or used in the MR scanner room. For a certain device to be labeled MR compatible, it has to be demonstrated that it performs in its intended function without performance degradation. For the MR compatibility, effects on the devices and effects on the imaging have to be differentiated (Chinzei et al., 1999). These devices are influenced by induced static magnetization as well as torque and translational forces (see Figure 1). Both effects influence the performance of devices containing ferromagnetic materials. Standard springs made of metal do not function as expected. According to the guidelines mentioned above, devices containing ferromagnetic materials should be operated behind the 20-mT line. In this zone, the effects on the devices are irrelevant. However, the risk that such a device is pulled towards the scanner bore (projectile effect) still is high. For safety reasons, not permanently fixed electromagnetic devices should be operated only behind the 5-mT line. The imaging quality is degraded by field inhomogenities and RF (radio frequency) emission (see Figure 1). Static field inhomogenities come from the ferromagnetic materials contained in the devices, but in most cases the image quality can be restored after shimming the magnet. RF is typically produced by pulsed electronics and the digital hardware emitted by the cables of the device. As MRI is highly sensitive to RF noise, such devices have to be operated outside the MR scanner room. On the other hand, small amplitude electromagnetic fields up to some hundred Hz, as produced by some vibrotactile stimulation devices, only showed minor effects on imaging.

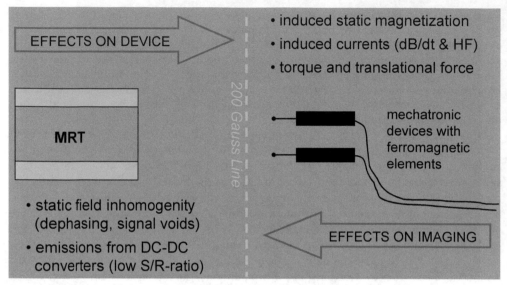

Fig. 1. Overview on MR-compatibility (GE Medical Systems. MR safety and MR compatibility. http://www.ge.com/medical/mr/iomri/safety.htm; 1997).

4.2 Principles and technical designs

For somatosensory mapping, well-controlled and reproducible stimuli are required. Principally, this can be achieved by using pneumatic, piezoceramic and electromechanical devices. Concerning MR compatibility and safety, pneumatic devices are the best choice. The hardware of a pneumatic stimulation device typically consists of a pressure source, a valve for converting the air stream into the desired pressure oscillations and a vibrotactile display to deliver the stimuli to the skin surface. As vibrotactile probe, a latex balloon, a pickup with an integrated rubber membrane (Briggs et al., 2004), or an injector element to produce air puffs was described (Huang and Sereno, 2007). The pressure oscillations are transmitted to the vibrotactile display via long plastic tubes so that all other components of the device can be operated outside of the MR scanner room. However, pneumatic systems have the disadvantage of limited vibration frequencies. Due to the mechanical damping of the pressure oscillations in the plastic tubes the stimulus frequency is limited to about 30 Hz. Higher stimulation frequencies can be achieved by using nonmagnetic valves, suited for operation inside the MR scanner room. Multi-channel stimulation designs are feasible with multiple valves and pickups (Wienbruch et al., 2006). Pneumatic devices have shown to cause somatosensory brain activation, but failed to additionally activate motor cortical areas in somatosensory paradigms.

Piezoceramic devices provide a wide range of frequencies, but only have small displacement amplitudes, which limits their application to the skin receptors. Stimulation frequencies up to 1000 Hz can be obtained. The vibration amplitude achieved by these devices is limited to some hundred μm and even for this relative high operation voltages (up to 200 Volts) are necessary. Because these devices are nonmagnetic, they can be operated inside the MR scanner room. Basically, bar- and disk-like actuators as well as piezomotors are available. The bar- and the disk-like actuators directly convert the electrical signal into bending motions (Piezomechanik Gmbh, 2002). For stimulation applications, these devices can either be held between the fingertips (Harrington et al., 2000b) or touched by the fingertips (Maldjian et al., 1999b). Functional MRI with piezoceramic vibrators showed brain activation within the somatosensory cortex but not within motor cortical areas (Harrington et al., 2000a). It is important to avoid loops in the cables, because this may lead to currents from the RF- and gradient coils. These may cause heat and even fire hazard. There is less data with piezomotors. Basically, piezomotors are well suited for construction of MR compatible robotic stimulation devices, for example to induce passive limb motions. For their operation, high driving frequencies (> 40 kHz) are necessary, therefore effects on the MR imaging have to be considered, when using such devices (Chinzei et al., 1999).

Electromagnetic stimulation devices may be classified into three groups depending on the vicinity to the MR scanner at their operation. In the first group, there is common standard equipment containing motors or actuators with pulsed electronics. Such equipment causes RF-emission and therefore has to be operated outside the shielded area of the MR scanner room. For vibrotactile stimulation long cables are needed to transmit the stimulus from the outside to the subject. Cable driven rotating eccentric masses are an example for such type of stimulation device. A frequency range between 1–130 Hz and displacement amplitudes up to 4 mm can be reached. In an fMRI study implementing this technique, BOLD responses within the somatosensory as well as the motor cortical areas could be demonstrated (Golaszewski et al., 2002b). The second group consists of non-switched moving magnet, and moving coil devices, which can be operated inside the scanner behind the 20-mT line (Golaszewski et al., 2006;Gallasch et al., 2006). With this technique, the parameters of a stimulus (amplitude, frequency, waveform) can be selected within a wide range, which is advantageous for basic investigations. On the other hand, these devices also need some mechanics for translating the stimulus to the subject under investigation. When these mechanic parts are made of metallic materials, the device will also influence the imaging and itself be influenced by the magnetic field. In the third group of somatosensory stimulation, the devices comprise coil actuators utilizing the static magnetic field of the MR scanner. By applying currents to a coil, Lorenz forces generate vibration (Graham et al., 2001), as well as load and movement (Riener et al., 2005). This type of actuator-stimulator is suited for the operation inside the MR scanner, but it is important to be careful in order to prevent heating of the coils due to induced currents.

4.3 Device for stimulation of the foot sole

A recently developed stimulator for the foot sole is described here as an example for an electromechanical device to be operated inside the scanner room (Gallasch et al., 2006). It consists of two moving magnet actuators rigidly connected on a platform by two non-magnetic adjustable stands (see Figure 2). To preserve MR compatibility (operation behind the 20-mT line) the foot sole is contacted via long indentors (30 cm). Further, to avoid effects on imaging, the actuators are powered by non-pulsed servo amplifiers. All other components containing pulsed electronics (digital controller and PC) are operated outside the MR scanner room. For stimulation of slowly and rapid adapting mechanoreceptors a mixed open and closed loop control scheme was implemented. Slowly adapting receptors respond to nearly static loading (0 - 1 Hz). This is achieved by an open loop programming of the contact force (0- 20 N). Rapid adapting receptors respond to vibration, which is achieved by the closed loop control scheme. With the implemented controller arbitrary vibration waveforms within the frequency band of 20 to 100 Hz can be generated. A computer is used for stimulus synthesis, sequencing of the stimuli and synchronization with the MR scans. The first MRI studies with this device show that specially designed electromagnetic devices are well suited for somatotopic mapping.

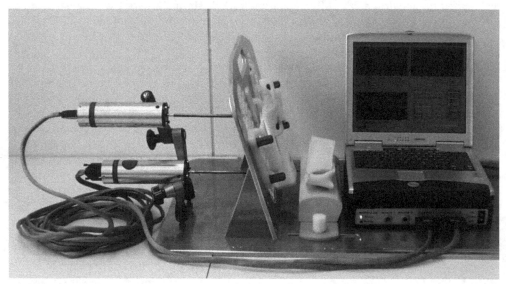

Fig. 2. Example of an electromagnetic vibrotactile stimulation system (Gallasch et al., 2006).

4.4 Perspectives

Recently, various types of stimulation devices were evaluated for somatotopic mapping. Although substantial physiological results have been obtained with some of these devices, this technology still needs to be improved. Clinicians expect equipment for quantitative sensory testing, which is safe and simple to use. Other systems will be needed for stimulation of the entire spectrum of somatosensory fibers. These are the large diameter A-beta fibers mediating touch and vibration, the smaller A-delta fibers mediating cool sensation and the first signs of pain, and the small diameter C-fibers mediating sensation of heat and pain. We therefore suggest a bimodal stimulation system to deliver with both vibrotactile and temperature stimuli. For the sole of the foot, such a system may have an arrangement as shown in Figure 2 with additional Peltier elements on the tip of the indentors, however with pneumatic actuators instead of the electromagnetic ones. For hand and fingers wearable stimulation devices are prospective, e.g. pneumatic finger or toe cuffs (Gallasch et al., 2010;Figure 3, 4, 5) or some kind of stimulation glove with pressurized sections at the fingertips including flat shaped heat pipes for quick cooling and warming. For the usage as a clinical tool, further multicenter studies with standardized stimulation protocols have to be carried out. Such studies are necessary to establish stable stimulus-response relationships independent of a certain scanner type.

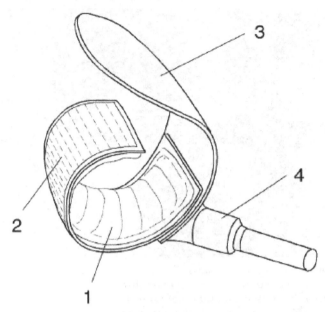

Fig. 3. Drawing of finger cuff with inflatable air bladder (1), flexible Welco strips (2, 3) and air connector (4)

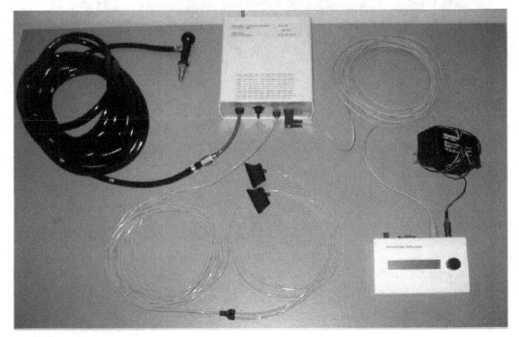

Fig. 4. Stimulator system consisting of twin finger cuff, valve box and microprocessor unit.

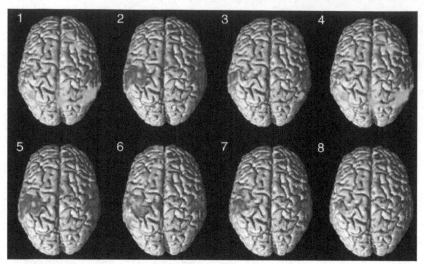

Fig. 5. Single subject analysis: fMRI maps of eight single subjects (1-8) applying pneumatic cuff somatosensory finger stimulation with fixed (fixed simulation FS, green) and random (random stimulation RS, red) presentation of vibrotactile stimuli with a mean frequency of 4 Hz over all blocks. Yellow spots represent activation overlap between FS and RS maps

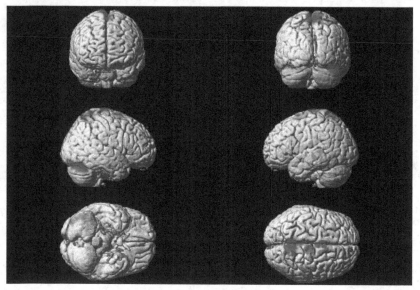

Fig. 6. Patient in vegetative state 14 days post hypoxia. Vibration stimulation with a moving magnet actuator system delivered to the sole of the left foot (Gallasch et al., 2006;Golaszewski et al., 2006) elicits brain activation contra- and ipsilaterally within the primary and secondary sensorimotor cortex and especially within the premotor cortex, the center for predefined movement loops, and the supplementary motor area that represents the superior center for motor planning. Functional brain mapping in this patient proved an intact somatosensory channel to the sensorimotor system for a targeted therapeutic approach in neurorehabilitation.

5. Perspective of the application of somatosensory stimulation within the clinical environment

In the studies of Gelnar, Harrington, and Stippich et al., brain activation within the postcentral gyrus and superior and inferior parietal lobule have been found (Gelnar et al., 1998a;Harrington et al., 2000a;Stippich et al., 1999a). Furthermore, brain activation within Brodmann area 3a was detected due to somatosensory stimulation (Geyer et al., 1999;Geyer et al., 2000;Kurth et al., 2000), which can be explained by the fact that Brodmann area 3a receives input from the deep and from the proprioceptive receptors (Ibanez et al., 1989;Iwamura et al., 1993;Kaas et al., 1979;Maldjian et al., 1999a;Recanzone et al., 1992;Tharin and Golby, 2007). BOLD response in the primary motor cortex due to vibrotactile stimulation is an important finding, because the stimulation does not require the collaboration of the subject under examination. In an fMRI study with mechanical vibration, BOLD response in primary sensorimotor cortex was found in all of the investigations (Golaszewski et al., 2002a,b). Motor cortical activation caused by vibration, is presumably based on the co-stimulation of cutaneous mechanoreceptors and muscle spindles that requires sufficient displacement amplitudes and vibration frequencies. Similar to the finger-to-thumb-tapping paradigm, vibration led to contralateral brain activity in postcentral gyrus in ten out of ten subjects. Vibration stimulation failed to consistently activate supplementary motor area and anterior cingular cortex since it represents a passive paradigm that does not involve motor cortical areas for planning of volitional movements. Vibratory stimuli are transmitted via the large afferents of the dorsal column to the thalamus and are relayed there to the brain cortex. This "information" originates from the extra personnel space that might be an explanation, why Brodmann area 9 in superior frontal gyrus responds with activation in some cases.

In functional brain imaging with certain somatosensory stimulation protocols the whole sensorimotor cortex can be addressed for functional brain mapping that offers the possibility of several clinical applications for somatosensory paradigms in Neuroradiology. Somatosensory paradigms can be used for preoperative functional brain mapping of the sensorimotor cortex in patients with perirolandic lesions. Further applications include the investigation of brain plasticity and reorganization (Pons et al., 1992) and investigation of patients in comatose and vegetative state (Kampfl et al., 1998).

6. References

Apkarian, A.V., Gelnar, P.A., Krauss, B.R., and Szeverenyi, N.M. (2000). Cortical responses to thermal pain depend on stimulus size: a functional MRI study. J Neurophysiol 83, 3113-22.

Arthurs, O.J., Williams, E.J., Carpenter, T.A., Pickard, J.D., and Boniface, S.J. (2000). Linear coupling between functional magnetic resonance imaging and evoked potential amplitude in human somatosensory cortex. Neuroscience 101, 803-6.

Backes, W.H., Mess, W.H., van Kranen-Mastenbroek, V., and Reulen, J.P. (2000). Somatosensory cortex responses to median nerve stimulation: fMRI effects of current amplitude and selective attention. Clin Neurophysiol 111, 1738-44.

Bittar, R.G., Olivier, A., Sadikot, A.F., Andermann, F., Comeau, R.M., Cyr, M., Peters, T.M., and Reutens, D.C. (1999a). Localization of somatosensory function by using positron emission tomography scanning: a comparison with intraoperative cortical stimulation. J Neurosurg *90*, 478-83.

Bittar, R.G., Olivier, A., Sadikot, A.F., Andermann, F., Pike, G.B., and Reutens, D.C. (1999b). Presurgical motor and somatosensory cortex mapping with functional magnetic resonance imaging and positron emission tomography. J Neurosurg *91*, 915-21.

Boecker, H., Ceballos-Baumann, A., Bartenstein, P., Weindl, A., Siebner, H.R., Fassbender, T., Munz, F., Schwaiger, M., and Conrad, B. (1999). Sensory processing in Parkinson's and Huntington's disease: investigations with 3D H(2)(15)O-PET. Brain *122 (Pt 9)*, 1651-65.

Briggs, R.W., Dy-Liacco, I., Malcolm, M.P., Lee, H., Peck, K.K., Gopinath, K.S., Himes, N.C., Soltysik, D.A., Browne, P., and Tran-Son-Tay, R. (2004). A pneumatic vibrotactile stimulation device for fMRI. Magn Reson Med *51*, 640-3.

Burton, H., MacLeod, A.M., Videen, T.O., and Raichle, M.E. (1997). Multiple foci in parietal and frontal cortex activated by rubbing embossed grating patterns across fingerpads: a positron emission tomography study in humans. Cereb Cortex *7*, 3-17.

Casey, K.L., Minoshima, S., Berger, K.L., Koeppe, R.A., Morrow, T.J., and Frey, K.A. (1994). Positron emission tomographic analysis of cerebral structures activated specifically by repetitive noxious heat stimuli. J Neurophysiol *71*, 802-7.

Casey, K.L., Minoshima, S., Morrow, T.J., and Koeppe, R.A. (1996). Comparison of human cerebral activation pattern during cutaneous warmth, heat pain, and deep cold pain. J Neurophysiol *76*, 571-81.

Chinzei, K., Kikinis, R., and Jolesz, F. (1999). MR compatibility of mechanotronic devices, design criteria. In Proc MICCA 99, Lecture Notes in Computer Science *1679*, 1020-1031.

Cramer, S.C., Moore, C.I., Finklestein, S.P., and Rosen, B.R. (2000). A pilot study of somatotopic mapping after cortical infarct. Stroke *31*, 668-71.

Derbyshire, S.W., Jones, A.K., Gyulai, F., Clark, S., Townsend, D., and Firestone, L.L. (1997). Pain processing during three levels of noxious stimulation produces differential patterns of central activity. Pain *73*, 431-45.

Disbrow, E., Roberts, T., and Krubitzer, L. (2000). Somatotopic organization of cortical fields in the lateral sulcus of Homo sapiens: evidence for SII and PV. J Comp Neurol *418*, 1-21.

Disbrow, E., Roberts, T., Poeppel, D., and Krubitzer, L. (2001). Evidence for interhemispheric processing of inputs from the hands in human S2 and PV. J Neurophysiol *85*, 2236-44.

Drevets, W.C., Burton, H., Videen, T.O., Snyder, A.Z., Simpson, J.R. Jr, and Raichle, M.E. (1995). Blood flow changes in human somatosensory cortex during anticipated stimulation. Nature *373*, 249-52.

Flor, H., Denke, C., Schaefer, M., and Grusser, S. (2001). Effect of sensory discrimination training on cortical reorganisation and phantom limb pain. Lancet *357*, 1763-4.

Fox, P.T., Burton, H., and Raichle, M.E. (1987). Mapping human somatosensory cortex with positron emission tomography. J Neurosurg *67*, 34-43.

Francis, S.T., Kelly, E.F., Bowtell, R., Dunseath, W.J., Folger, S.E., and McGlone, F. (2000). fMRI of the responses to vibratory stimulation of digit tips. Neuroimage *11*, 188-202.

Gallasch, E., Fend, M., Rafolt, D., Nardone, R., Kunz, A., Kronbichler, M., Beisteiner, R., and Golaszewski, S. (2010). Cuff-type pneumatic stimulator for studying somatosensory evoked responses with fMRI. Neuroimage *50*, 1067-73.

Gallasch, E., Golaszewski, S.M., Fend, M., Siedentopf, C.M., Koppelstaetter, F., Eisner, W., Gerstenbrand, F., and Felber, S.R. (2006). Contact force- and amplitude-controllable vibrating probe for somatosensory mapping of plantar afferences with fMRI. J Magn Reson Imaging 24, 1177-82.

GE Medical Systems. MR safety and MR compatibility. http://www.ge.com/medical/mr/iomri/safety.htm; 1997.

Gelnar, P.A., Krauss, B.R., Szeverenyi, N.M., and Apkarian, A.V. (1998a). Fingertip representation in the human somatosensory cortex: an fMRI study. Neuroimage 7, 261-83.

Gelnar, P.A., Krauss, B.R., Szeverenyi, N.M., and Apkarian, A.V. (1998b). Fingertip representation in the human somatosensory cortex: an fMRI study. Neuroimage 7, 261-83.

Gelnar, P.A., Krauss, B.R., Szeverenyi, N.M., and Apkarian, A.V. (1998c). Fingertip representation in the human somatosensory cortex: an fMRI study. Neuroimage 7, 261-83.

Geyer, S., Schleicher, A., and Zilles, K. (1999). Areas 3a, 3b, and 1 of human primary somatosensory cortex. Neuroimage 10, 63-83.

Geyer, S., Schormann, T., Mohlberg, H., and Zilles, K. (2000). Areas 3a, 3b, and 1 of human primary somatosensory cortex. Part 2. Spatial normalization to standard anatomical space. Neuroimage 11, 684-96.

Giabbiconi, C.M., Trujillo-Barreto, N.J., Gruber, T., and Muller, M.M. (2007). Sustained spatial attention to vibration is mediated in primary somatosensory cortex. Neuroimage 35, 255-62.

Golaszewski, S.M., Siedentopf, C.M., Baldauf, E., Koppelstaetter, F., Eisner, W., Unterrainer, J., Guendisch, G.M., Mottaghy, F.M., and Felber, S.R. (2002b). Functional magnetic resonance imaging of the human sensorimotor cortex using a novel vibrotactile stimulator. Neuroimage 17, 421-30.

Golaszewski, S.M., Siedentopf, C.M., Baldauf, E., Koppelstaetter, F., Eisner, W., Unterrainer, J., Guendisch, G.M., Mottaghy, F.M., and Felber, S.R. (2002). Functional magnetic resonance imaging of the human sensorimotor cortex using a novel vibrotactile stimulator. Neuroimage 17, 421-30.

Golaszewski, S.M., Siedentopf, C.M., Koppelstaetter, F., Fend, M., Ischebeck, A., Gonzalez-Felipe, V., Haala, I., Struhal, W., Mottaghy, F.M., Gallasch, E., Felber, S.R., and Gerstenbrand, F. (2006). Human brain structures related to plantar vibrotactile stimulation: a functional magnetic resonance imaging study. Neuroimage 29, 923-9.

Golaszewski, S.M., Zschiegner, F., Siedentopf, C.M., Unterrainer, J., Sweeney, R.A., Eisner, W., Lechner-Steinleitner, S., Mottaghy, F.M., and Felber, S. (2002a). A new pneumatic vibrator for functional magnetic resonance imaging of the human sensorimotor cortex. Neurosci Lett 324, 125-8.

Golaszewski, S.M., Zschiegner, F., Siedentopf, C.M., Unterrainer, J., Sweeney, R.A., Eisner, W., Lechner-Steinleitner, S., Mottaghy, F.M., and Felber, S. (2002). A new pneumatic vibrator for functional magnetic resonance imaging of the human sensorimotor cortex. Neurosci Lett 324, 125-8.

Graham, S.J., Staines, W.R., Nelson, A., Plewes, D.B., and McIlroy, W.E. (2001). New devices to deliver somatosensory stimuli during functional MRI. Magn Reson Med 46, 436-42.

Hamzei, F., Liepert, J., Dettmers, C., Adler, T., Kiebel, S., Rijntjes, M., and Weiller, C. (2001). Structural and functional cortical abnormalities after upper limb amputation during childhood. Neuroreport 12, 957-62.

Harrington, G.S., Wright, C.T., and Downs, J.H. 3rd (2000a). A new vibrotactile stimulator for functional MRI. Hum Brain Mapp 10, 140-5.

Harrington, G.S., Wright, C.T., and Downs, J.H. 3rd (2000b). A new vibrotactile stimulator for functional MRI. Hum Brain Mapp 10, 140-5.

Hodge, C.J. Jr, Huckins, S.C., Szeverenyi, N.M., Fonte, M.M., Dubroff, J.G., and Davuluri, K. (1998). Patterns of lateral sensory cortical activation determined using functional magnetic resonance imaging. J Neurosurg 89, 769-79.

Hoeller, M., Krings, T., Reinges, M.H., Hans, F.J., Gilsbach, J.M., and Thron, A. (2002). Movement artefacts and MR BOLD signal increase during different paradigms for mapping the sensorimotor cortex. Acta Neurochir (Wien) 144, 279-84; discussion 284.

Huang, R.S. and Sereno, M.I. (2007). Dodecapus: An MR-compatible system for somatosensory stimulation. Neuroimage 34, 1060-73.

Ibanez, V., Deiber, M.P., and Mauguiere, F. (1989). Interference of vibrations with input transmission in dorsal horn and cuneate nucleus in man: a study of somatosensory evoked potentials (SEPs) to electrical stimulation of median nerve and fingers. Exp Brain Res 75, 599-610.

Ibanez, V., Deiber, M.P., Sadato, N., Toro, C., Grissom, J., Woods, R.P., Mazziotta, J.C., and Hallett, M. (1995). Effects of stimulus rate on regional cerebral blood flow after median nerve stimulation. Brain 118 (Pt 5), 1339-51.

Iwamura, Y., Tanaka, M., Sakamoto, M., and Hikosaka, O. (1993). Rostrocaudal gradients in the neuronal receptive field complexity in the finger region of the alert monkey's postcentral gyrus. Exp Brain Res 92, 360-8.

Kaas, J.H., Nelson, R.J., Sur, M., Lin, C.S., and Merzenich, M.M. (1979). Multiple representations of the body within the primary somatosensory cortex of primates. Science 204, 521-3.

Kampfl, A., Schmutzhard, E., Franz, G., Pfausler, B., Haring, H.P., Ulmer, H., Felber, S., Golaszewski, S., and Aichner, F. (1998). Prediction of recovery from post-traumatic vegetative state with cerebral magnetic-resonance imaging. Lancet 351, 1763-7.

Kassubek, J., Juengling, F.D., Els, T., Spreer, J., Herpers, M., Krause, T., Moser, E., and Lucking, C.H. (2003). Activation of a residual cortical network during painful stimulation in long-term postanoxic vegetative state: a 15O-H2O PET study. J Neurol Sci 212, 85-91.

Koppelstaetter, F., Siedentopf, C.M., Rhomberg, P., Lechner-Steinleitner, S., Eisner, W., and Golaszewski, S.M. (2007). FMRT vor Motorkortexstimulation bei Phantomschmerz: Ein Fallbericht. Nervenarzt.

Korvenoja, A., Huttunen, J., Salli, E., Pohjonen, H., Martinkauppi, S., Palva, J.M., Lauronen, L., Virtanen, J., Ilmoniemi, R.J., and Aronen, H.J. (1999). Activation of multiple cortical areas in response to somatosensory stimulation: combined magnetoencephalographic and functional magnetic resonance imaging. Hum Brain Mapp 8, 13-27.

Krause, T., Kurth, R., Ruben, J., Schwiemann, J., Villringer, K., Deuchert, M., Moosmann, M., Brandt, S., Wolf, K., Curio, G., and Villringer, A. (2001). Representational overlap of adjacent fingers in multiple areas of human primary somatosensory cortex depends on electrical stimulus intensity: an fMRI study. Brain Res 899, 36-46.

Kurth, R., Villringer, K., Curio, G., Wolf, K.J., Krause, T., Repenthin, J., Schwiemann, J., Deuchert, M., and Villringer, A. (2000). fMRI shows multiple somatotopic digit representations in human primary somatosensory cortex. Neuroreport 11, 1487-91.

Kurth, R., Villringer, K., Mackert, B.M., Schwiemann, J., Braun, J., Curio, G., Villringer, A., and Wolf, K.J. (1998). fMRI assessment of somatotopy in human Brodmann area 3b by electrical finger stimulation. Neuroreport 9, 207-12.

Laureys, S., Faymonville, M.E., Peigneux, P., Damas, P., Lambermont, B., Del Fiore, G., Degueldre, C., Aerts, J., Luxen, A., Franck, G., Lamy, M., Moonen, G., and Maquet, P. (2002). Cortical processing of noxious somatosensory stimuli in the persistent vegetative state. Neuroimage *17*, 732-41.

Lee, C.C., Jack, C.R. Jr, and Riederer, S.J. (1998). Mapping of the central sulcus with functional MR: active versus passive activation tasks. AJNR Am J Neuroradiol *19*, 847-52.

Maldjian, J.A., Gottschalk, A., Patel, R.S., Detre, J.A., and Alsop, D.C. (1999a). The sensory somatotopic map of the human hand demonstrated at 4 Tesla. Neuroimage *10*, 55-62.

Maldjian, J.A., Gottschalk, A., Patel, R.S., Pincus, D., Detre, J.A., and Alsop, D.C. (1999b). Mapping of secondary somatosensory cortex activation induced by vibrational stimulation: an fMRI study. Brain Res *824*, 291-5.

Mazziotta, J.C.a.T.A.W. (2000). Brain Mapping: The methods. Academic Press).

Mima, T., Sadato, N., Yazawa, S., Hanakawa, T., Fukuyama, H., Yonekura, Y., and Shibasaki, H. (1999). Brain structures related to active and passive finger movements in man. Brain *122 (Pt 10)*, 1989-97.

Moore, C.I., Stern, C.E., Corkin, S., Fischl, B., Gray, A.C., Rosen, B.R., and Dale, A.M. (2000). Segregation of somatosensory activation in the human rolandic cortex using fMRI. J Neurophysiol *84*, 558-69.

Nelson, A.J., Staines, W.R., Graham, S.J., and McIlroy, W.E. (2004). Activation in SI and SII: the influence of vibrotactile amplitude during passive and task-relevant stimulation. Brain Res Cogn Brain Res *19*, 174-84.

Ogawa, S., Lee, T.M., Kay, A.R., and Tank, D.W. (1990). Brain magnetic resonance imaging with contrast dependent on blood oxygenation. Proc Natl Acad Sci U S A *87*, 9868-72.

Ogawa, S., Tank, D.W., Menon, R., Ellermann, J.M., Kim, S.G., Merkle, H., and Ugurbil, K. (1992). Intrinsic signal changes accompanying sensory stimulation: functional brain mapping with magnetic resonance imaging. Proc Natl Acad Sci U S A *89*, 5951-5.

Penfield, W.a.B.E. (1937). Somatic motor and sensory representation in the cerebral cortex of man as studied by electrical stimulation. Brain *60*, 389-443.

Peyron, R., Laurent, B., and Garcia-Larrea, L. (2000). Functional imaging of brain responses to pain. A review and meta-analysis (2000). Neurophysiol Clin *30*, 263-88.

Piezomechanik Gmbh (ed). (2002). Piezoelectric bending actuators. http://www.piezomechanik.com.

Piza, H. (2000). [Transplantation of hands in Innsbruck]. Wien Klin Wochenschr *112*, 563-5.

Polonara, G., Fabri, M., Manzoni, T., and Salvolini, U. (1999). Localization of the first and second somatosensory areas in the human cerebral cortex with functional MR imaging. AJNR Am J Neuroradiol *20*, 199-205.

Pons, T.P., Garraghty, P.E., and Mishkin, M. (1992). Serial and parallel processing of tactual information in somatosensory cortex of rhesus monkeys. J Neurophysiol *68*, 518-27.

Rausch, M., Spengler, F., and Eysel, U.T. (1998). Proprioception acts as the main source of input in human S-I activation experiments: a functional MRI study. Neuroreport *9*, 2865-8.

Recanzone, G.H., Merzenich, M.M., and Jenkins, W.M. (1992). Frequency discrimination training engaging a restricted skin surface results in an emergence of a cutaneous response zone in cortical area 3a. J Neurophysiol *67*, 1057-70.

Riener, R., Villgrattner, T., Kleiser, R., Nef, T., and Kollias, S. (2005). fMRI compatible electromagnetic haptic device. Conf Proc IEEE Eng Med Soc 2005. Conf Proceedings 7024-7027.

Roelcke, U., Curt, A., Otte, A., Missimer, J., Maguire, R.P., Dietz, V., and Leenders, K.L. (1997a). Influence of spinal cord injury on cerebral sensorimotor systems: a PET study. J Neurol Neurosurg Psychiatry 62, 61-5.

Roelcke, U., Curt, A., Otte, A., Missimer, J., Maguire, R.P., Dietz, V., and Leenders, K.L. (1997b). Influence of spinal cord injury on cerebral sensorimotor systems: a PET study. J Neurol Neurosurg Psychiatry 62, 61-5.

Ruben, J., Schwiemann, J., Deuchert, M., Meyer, R., Krause, T., Curio, G., Villringer, K., Kurth, R., and Villringer, A. (2001). Somatotopic organization of human secondary somatosensory cortex. Cereb Cortex 11, 463-73.

Seifert, F. and Maihofner, C. (2007). Representation of cold allodynia in the human brain--a functional MRI study. Neuroimage 35, 1168-80.

Seitz, R.J. and Roland, P.E. (1992). Vibratory stimulation increases and decreases the regional cerebral blood flow and oxidative metabolism: a positron emission tomography (PET) study. Acta Neurol Scand 86, 60-7.

Servos, P., Zacks, J., Rumelhart, D.E., and Glover, G.H. (1998). Somatotopy of the human arm using fMRI. Neuroreport 9, 605-9.

Sterr, A., Shen, S., Zaman, A., Roberts, N., and Szameitat, A. (2007). Activation of SI is modulated by attention: a random effects fMRI study using mechanical stimuli. Neuroreport 18, 607-11.

Stippich, C., Hofmann, R., Kapfer, D., Hempel, E., Heiland, S., Jansen, O., and Sartor, K. (1999a). Somatotopic mapping of the human primary somatosensory cortex by fully automated tactile stimulation using functional magnetic resonance imaging. Neurosci Lett 277, 25-8.

Stippich, C., Hofmann, R., Kapfer, D., Hempel, E., Heiland, S., Jansen, O., and Sartor, K. (1999b). Somatotopic mapping of the human primary somatosensory cortex by fully automated tactile stimulation using functional magnetic resonance imaging. Neurosci Lett 277, 25-8.

Takanashi, M., Abe, K., Yanagihara, T., Oshiro, Y., Watanabe, Y., Tanaka, H., Hirabuki, N., Nakamura, H., and Fujita, N. (2001). Effects of stimulus presentation rate on the activity of primary somatosensory cortex: a functional magnetic resonance imaging study in humans. Brain Res Bull 54, 125-9.

Tempel, L.W. and Perlmutter, J.S. (1990). Abnormal vibration-induced cerebral blood flow responses in idiopathic dystonia. Brain 113 (Pt 3), 691-707.

Tempel, L.W. and Perlmutter, J.S. (1992). Vibration-induced regional cerebral blood flow responses in normal aging. J Cereb Blood Flow Metab 12, 554-61.

Tharin, S. and Golby, A. (2007). Functional brain mapping and its applications to neurosurgery. Neurosurgery 60, 185-201; discussion 201-2.

Toga, A. W. and Mazziotta, J. C. Brain Mapping. The Methods. Second Edition. Academic Press, San Diego, CA, 2002.

Wienbruch, C., Candia, V., Svensson, J., Kleiser, R., and Kollias, S.S. (2006). A portable and low-cost fMRI compatible pneumatic system for the investigation of the somatosensory system in clinical and research environments. Neurosci Lett 398, 183-8.

Xu, X., Fukuyama, H., Yazawa, S., Mima, T., Hanakawa, T., Magata, Y., Kanda, M., Fujiwara, N., Shindo, K., Nagamine, T., and Shibasaki, H. (1997). Functional localization of pain perception in the human brain studied by PET. Neuroreport 8, 555-9.

7

Graphical Models of Functional MRI Data for Assessing Brain Connectivity

Junning Li[1], Z. Jane Wang[1] and Martin J. McKeown[2]
[1]Department of Electrical and Computer Engineering
[2]Department of Medicine (Neurology), Pacific Parkinson's Research Centre
University of British Columbia
Canada

1. Introduction

1.1 Brain connectivity and fMRI

Modern neuroimaging technologies have allowed researchers to non-invasively observe indirect markers of brain activity *in vivo* (Fig. 1). This has resulted in a rapid growth of studies trying to ascertain what brain loci are associated with certain cognitive, sensory and motor tasks. In particular, the recent development of functional magnetic resonance imaging (fMRI) has allowed researchers to non-invasively investigate brain activity at excellent spatial resolution and relatively good temporal resolution. While probing aspects of brain function is typically under the domain of neuroscientists, fMRI work is inherently interdisciplinary: it involves MR physicists who determine MRI sequences sensitive to small changes in the brain, neuroscientists who design the behavioural experiments and interpret the observations, statisticians to assess significance of changes, and increasingly, people with signal processing expertise to derive more and more information from the time series extracted.

Analysis of fMRI data sets represents a special challenge for traditional statistical methods that were originally designed for a large number of samples of low-dimensional data points. The number of "voxels" (ie. representing a specific locus in the brain) to be analyzed are large ($\approx 10^5$), yet the number of time points ($\approx 10^2$) is relatively small. Most early fMRI analysis methods were designed to ascertain the regions where brain functions are localized by performing voxel-wise analysis.

Even when simple tasks are performed in the MRI scanner, widespread activation can be observed in the brain with fMRI. These and other studies suggest that the brain is active at multiple spatial and time scales supporting both segregated and distributed information processing (Bassett & Bullmore, 2006). In fact, the advent of non-invasive functional neuroimaging has re-ignited a centuries-old debate about whether or not cognitive and motor tasks are encoded in discrete loci or are more diffusely and fluidly represented, the latter emphasizing the importance of assessing brain connectivity (Catani & ffytche, 2005).

While connectivity appears to be of critical importance for understanding and assessment of brain function, it can be difficult to define in a rigorous sense with current technologies that can only probe brain activity at certain spatial and temporal scales (see Fig. 1). Conventionally, brain connectivity can be studied at three levels: anatomical, functional, and effective connectivity (see Fig. 2). Anatomical connectivity refers to actual physical connections

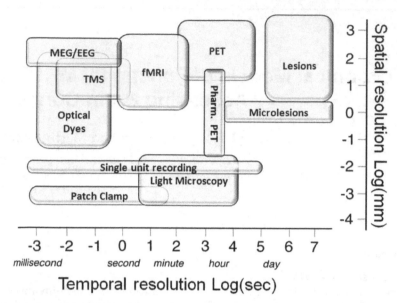

Fig. 1. Temporal and spatial resolution of current neuro-imaging technology. TMS: transcranial magnetic stimulation, MEG: magnetoencephalography, EEG: electroencephalography, PET: positron emission tomography, and Pharm.: pharmacological. (Adapted from: Churchland, Patricia, and Terrence Sejnowski (1992) The Computational Brain. Cambridge, MA: MIT Press.)

between brain structures. It can be determined with the help of rich anatomical studies that have been developed over decades, or more recently, using MR techniques such as Diffusion Tensor Imaging (DTI). Functional connectivity is defined as the significant mutual information between the time series found at distinct loci in the brain. However this raises several problems. If two regions have similarities between their respective time series, is this because one region influences the other, or there is a third region affecting both (Figs. 4 and 5)? Thus the term effective connectivity has been used to imply the causal influence that activity in one brain region exerts over the activity of another. The importance of assessing brain effective connectivity is also related to the fact that brain connectivity impairments are associated with many neuropsychiatric diseases such as depression (Schlösser et al., 2008), schizophrenia (Schlösser et al., 2008), Alzheimer's (Supekar et al., 2008) and Parkinson's disease (Palmer et al., 2009).

1.2 Graphical models for brain effective connectivity
Many methods for inferring connectivity from the four-dimensional fMRI data (three spatial dimensions and one temporal dimension) have been suggested. Proposed methods include correlation thresholding (Cao & Worsley, 1999), linear decomposition (Calhoun et al., 2001; McKeown, 2000), structural equation models (SEM) (Bollen, 1989), multi-variate auto-regression (Valdes-Sosa et al., 2005), dynamic causal models (Friston et al., 2003), Bayesian networks (Li et al., 2008; Zheng & Rajapakse, 2006), wavelet analysis (Bullmore et al., 2004), and clustering (Heller et al., 2006).

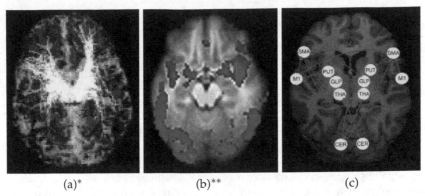

(a)*   (b)**   (c)

Fig. 2. Conventionally, brain connectivity is studied at three levels: (a) anatomical, (b) functional, and (c) effective connectivity. Anatomical connectivity is actual physical connections between brain structures. Functional connectivity is defined as the significant mutual information between the time series found at distinct loci in the brain. Effective connectivity has been used to imply the causal influence that activity in one brain region exerts over the activity of another. * Sub-figure (a) is from P. Hagmann, J.-P. Thiran, L. Jonasson, P. Vandergheynst, S. Clarke, P. Maeder and R. Meuli (2003) DTI mapping of human brain connectivity: statistical fibre tracking and virtual dissection, NeuroImage 19(3): 545–554. ** Sub-figure (b) is from Daniel S. Margulies, A.M. Clare Kelly, Lucina Q. Uddin, Bharat B. Biswal, F. Xavier Castellanos and Michael P. Milham (2007) NeuroImage 37(2): 579–588.

Correlation thresholding (Cao & Worsley, 1999) directly examines the correlation between the activities of brain regions. If the correlation is so strong that it is extremely unlikely based on chance, then the two regions are considered connected, though not necessarily directly. Linear decomposition approaches, e.g. principal component analysis and independent component analysis (ICA) (Calhoun et al., 2001; McKeown, 2000), assume that observed brain activities are a combination of underlying psychological processes that spatially recruit different brain regions or temporally have unrelated behaviours. Regions involved in the same psychological process as revealed by the decomposition is considered as connected, though not necessarily directly. Both correlation thresholding and linear decomposition are designed for discovering functional connectivity, and neither can distinguish whether two regions interact directly or indirectly through a third region (Kaminski, 2005). Though correlation thresholding and linear decomposition are generally not considered as graphical model, actually both can be related to graphical models (Roweis & Ghahramani, 1999).

Unlike correlation thresholding and linear decomposition whose results can be visualized as brain images at the voxel level, structure equation models[1](Bollen, 1989), dynamic causal models (Friston et al., 2003), multivariate auto-regression (Valdes-Sosa et al., 2005), and Bayesian networks (Zheng & Rajapakse, 2006), are another category of methods that normally work at the level of regions, and whose results can be visualized as graphs where nodes usually represent brain regions and edges represent connections. The brain regions are typically defined anatomically, and some automatic or manual segmentation of brain

---

[1] Structure equation models allow reciprocal connections, and normally are not considered as classical graphical models. As advanced graphical models, their Markov property and equivalence classes have been explored in (Ali et al., 2009; Richardson, 2003; Spirtes et al., 1998).

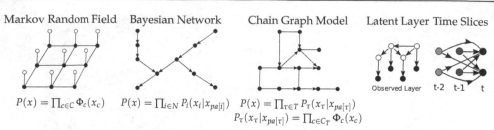

Markov Random Field   Bayesian Network   Chain Graph Model   Latent Layer Time Slices

$$P(x) = \prod_{c \in C} \Phi_c(x_c) \qquad P(x) = \prod_{i \in N} P_i(x_i | x_{pa[i]}) \qquad \begin{aligned} P(x) &= \prod_{\tau \in T} P_\tau(x_\tau | x_{pa[\tau]}) \\ P_\tau(x_\tau | x_{pa[\tau]}) &= \prod_{c \in C_T} \Phi_c(x_c) \end{aligned}$$

Fig. 3. Examples of the structures of classical graphical models. The structure of a Markov random field is an undirected graph. The joint probability is decomposed as the product of clique potential functions $\Phi_c(x_c)$ where c is a clique in the graph and x_c is the variables associated with the nodes in c. The structure of a Bayesian network is a directed acyclic graph. The joint probability is decomposed as the product of node conditional probabilities $P_i(x_i | x_{pa[i]})$ where i is a node in the graph and $pa[i]$ is the parent nodes of node i. Chain graph models unify Markov random fields and Bayesian networks. They allow both directed and undirected edges, but forbid directed cycles. The joint probability is decomposed as the product of chain-component conditional probabilities $P_\tau(x_\tau | x_{pa[\tau]})$ where τ is a chain component and $pa[\tau]$ is the parent nodes of the component. The chain-component conditional probability $P_\tau(x_\tau | x_{pa[\tau]})$ can be further decomposed as clique potential functions $\Phi_c(x_c)$ where c is a clique in the moral graph derived from the chain component τ. Dynamic causal models (Friston et al., 2003) can be regarded as non-linear Bayesian networks with an observed layer and a latent layer. Multi-variate auto-regression (Valdes-Sosa et al., 2005) can be regarded as linear Bayesian networks with many time slices and directed edges from slices at time $t - 1, t - 2, \cdots$ pointing to the slice at time t.

structures is required to act as nodes in the model. According to the interaction relationships specified by the graph, the joint probability of node random variables can be decomposed as the product of many local potential functions or local conditional probabilities, as shown in Fig. 3. A node variable usually depends on its neighbor variables and/or parent variables. For example, in Bayesian networks, the activity of a region A is usually modeled as a stochastic function of the activities of its "parent" regions, as in Eq. (1)

$$X_A = f(X_{pa_1[A]}, X_{pa_2[A]}, \ldots, X_{pa_n[A]}) \qquad (1)$$

where X_A is the activity of region A and $pa_i[A]$s are the parent nodes of A in the graph. The graph structure of the model is not just for visualization, but encodes conditional-independence relationships among the activities of brain regions. A network structure can be translated to a set of conditional-independence relationships according to the Markov properties and vice versa, with certain assumptions, a set of conditional-independence relationships can also be encoded by a network structure (Lauritzen, 1996).

1.3 Pair-wise and conditional correlation

Graphical models are suitable for modelling brain connectivity, not only because their structures can be easily visualized as a network, but more importantly, their fundamental feature, namely conditional independence, is a key concept for differentiating effective connectivity from functional connectivity. When two brain regions show similar activation patterns, they can be somehow connected with several underlying possibilities, as illustrated in Fig. 4:

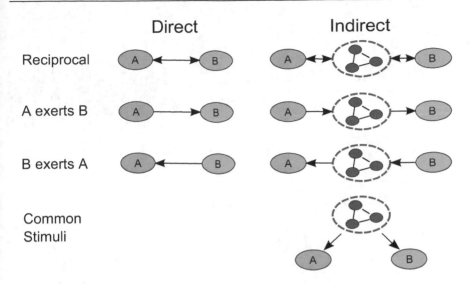

Fig. 4. When two brain regions show similar activation patterns, they can be connected with different underlying possibilities: (1) they directly reciprocally communicate with each other; (2) one region directly exerts the other; (3) they indirectly reciprocally communicate with each other via other brain regions; (4) one indirectly exerts the other via other regions; (5) they both are driven other regions; (6) they communicate with a combination of (1)–(5).

1. they directly reciprocally communicate with each other;

2. one region directly exerts the other;

3. they indirectly reciprocally communicate with each other via other brain regions;

4. one indirectly exerts the other via other regions;

5. they both are driven other regions;

6. they communicate by a combination of the above possibilities.

Pair-wise correlation can only tell that two regions is probably connected, but cannot distinguish among the above possibilities. To distinguish between direct and indirect connections, conditional independence must be considered. The example in Fig. 5 clearly explains this motivation. The two signals A and B show strong pair-wise correlation, but if we consider a third signal C, then the residuals of A and B after C is extracted from them hardly show any correlation. In this example, A and B are conditionally independent if given C, and maybe both are driven by C, as illustrated in the indirect common-stimuli case in Fig. 4. It must be noted that conditional independence alone without temporal information is not enough to determine causal relationships, ie. the direction of connections. To infer the direction, criteria considering temporal information, such as Granger causality (Granger, Aug., 1969), can be employed.

1.4 Challenges in modeling brain connectivity

Biomedical research explores the highly complex and diverse realm of living organisms and often incorporates clinical needs such as diagnosis and treatment design. Analysis

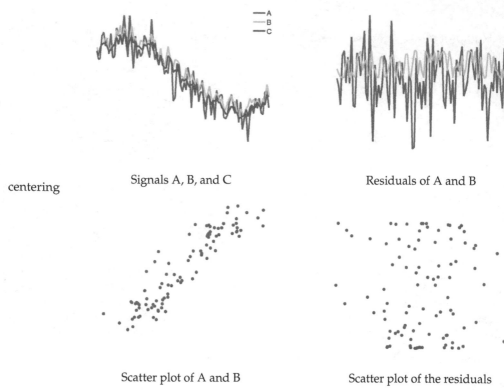

centering

Signals A, B, and C   Residuals of A and B

Scatter plot of A and B   Scatter plot of the residuals

Fig. 5. Two signals A (blue) and B (green) show strong pair-wise correlation, but with a third signal C (red) being considered, the residuals of A and B after removing the projection onto C hardly show any correlation.

of biomedical data typically emphasizes such features of reliability, interpretability and generality of reported results.

For example, when brain connections are reported, it is important to control or assess error rates in the claimed discoveries, addressing questions such as "how many among the reported connections are actually true connections?" and "how many true connections can be detected?"

Additionally, the ultimate goal of a biomedical experiment is usually a population inference applicable to a group of people, such as patients with a particular disease. However, subjects classified to the same experimental group according to the factor of interest can still be highly diverse with respect to other factors, such as gender, age, or race. Even repetitive experiments with the same subject can still be affected by various physical or psychological factors, such as drowsiness or stress. It is therefore important to integrate the information from separate experiments to make inference on the target topic, and to keep a balance between commonality and diversity.

Finally, as a multidisciplinary field, end users of connectivity analysis reports are often biomedical researchers or clinicians who focus on the biological implication of the results and the effects of medication. Therefore, it is undesirable to simply generate a vast network of potential connections or just report abstract statistical scores, without providing an intuitive interpretation. Rather, clinicians prefer interpretable, informative and human-understandable results, for example, which brain regions play the central role in conducting a functional task, or which connections are normalized by a pharmacological manipulation. These considerations have implications for interpretation and feature extraction from graphical models.

As a response to the above common challenges in biomedical research (ie. reliability, generality and interpretability), in the following sections, we will focus on three topics: error control in learning brain connectivity, group analysis taking into account the enhanced inter-subject variability typically seen in patient populations, and brain network analysis. Finally, for completeness, we also briefly overview several popular software packages suitable for assessing fMRI brain connectivity in the Appendix.

2. Error control in structure learning

In real world applications, especially in modelling brain connectivity, graphical models are not only a tool for operations such as classification or prediction, but more often than not, it is the network structure of the model itself which is of particular interest. Thus a desirable graphical model of fMRI data should not only statistically fit the overall data well, but also accurately reflect the internal brain connectivity structure. Structure-learning algorithms must therefore control or assess the error rate of the connections/edges detected by them.

2.1 Criteria for error control

There are two basic types of statistical errors: type I errors, ie. falsely claiming connections when they actually do not exist; and type II errors, ie. failure in detecting connections that truly exist. Since real data are not free from noise, limited samples may appear to support the existence of a connection when it does not exist, or vice versa. It is therefore impossible to absolutely prevent the two types of errors simultaneously, but rather keep a balance between them. This can be done by, for example, minimizing a loss function associated with the two types of errors according to Bayesian decision theory.

There are several criteria available for error-rate control (see Table 2). Generally there is no single criteria that is universally superior if the research scenario is not specified. Selecting the error rate is largely not an abstract question "which error rate is superior over others?", but a practical question "which error rate is the researchers' concern?". One error-rate criterion may be favored in one scenario while another may be right in a different scenario, for example:

- We are diagnosing a serious disease whose treatment has serious potential side effects. Due to the risk of the treatment, we hope that less than 0.01% of healthy people will be falsely diagnosed as affected by the disease. In this case, the type I error rate should be controlled under 0.01%.

- We are diagnosing a disease with high mortality, e.g. a type of cancer. Because failure in detecting the disease will have catastrophic consequences, we hope that 95% of subjects with the disease will be correctly detected. In this case, the type II error rate should be controlled under 5%.

- In a pilot study, we are selecting candidate genes for a genetic research on Parkinson's disease. Because of limited funding, we can only study a limited number of genes, so when selecting candidate genes in the pilot study, we hope that 95% of the selections are

Test Results	Truth		
	Negative	Positive	Total
Negative	TN (true negative)	FN (false negative)	R_1
Positive	FP (false positive)	TP (true positive)	R_2
Total	T_1	T_2	

Table 1. Results of multiple hypothesis testing, categorized according to the claimed results and the truth.

Full Name	Abbrev.	Definition
False Discovery Rate (Benjamini & Yekutieli, 2001)	FDR	$E(FP/R_2)$*
Positive False Discovery Rate (Storey, 2002)	pFDR	$E(FP/R_2 \mid R_2 > 0)$
Family-Wise Error Rate	FWER	$P(FP \geq 1)$
Type I Error Rate (False Positive Rate)	α	$E(FP/T_1)$
Specificity (True Negative Rate)	$1 - \alpha$	$E(TN/T_1)$
Type II Error Rate (False Negative Rate)	β	$E(FN/T_2)$
Power (Sensitivity, True Positive Rate)	$1 - \beta$	$E(TP/T_2)$
Positive Predictive Value	PPV	$E(TP/R_2)$

Table 2. Criteria for multiple hypothesis testing. Here $E(x)$ means the expected value of x, and $P(\mathcal{A})$ means the probability of event $\mathcal{A}$. Please refer to Table 1 for related notations. * If $R_2 = 0$, FP/R_2 is defined to be 0.

truly associated with the disease. In this case, the FDR will be chosen as the error rate of interest and should be controlled under 5%.

- We are selecting electronic components to make a device. Any error in any component will cause the device to run out of order. To guarantee the device functions well with a probability higher than 99%, the family-wise error rate should be controlled under 1%.

Since the scenario favoring the false discovery rate (FDR) (Benjamini & Yekutieli, 2001; Storey, 2002) is common in exploratory research, the FDR has become an important and widely used criterion in many fields, such as in inferring brain connectivity. Simply controlling the type I and type II error rates at specified levels does not necessarily keep the FDR sufficiently low, especially in the case of large and sparse networks. For example, suppose a network includes 40 nodes where each interact in average with 3 other nodes, i.e. there are 60 edges in the network. Then an algorithm with the *realized* type I error rate = 5% and the *realized* power = 90% (i.e. the *realized* type II error rate = 10%) will recover a network with 60×90% = 54 correct connections and $[40 \times (40 - 1)/2 - 60] \times 5\% = 36$ false connections, which means that $36/(36 + 54) = 40\%$ of the claimed connections do not exist in the true network.

2.2 Structure-learning methods with error controlled

Score-based search methods (Heckerman et al., 1995) look for a suitable network structure by optimizing a certain criterion of goodness-of-fit, such as the Akaike information criterion (AIC) (Akaike, 1974), the Bayesian information criterion (BIC) (Schwarz, 1978), or the Bayesian Dirichlet likelihood equivalent metric (BDE) (Heckerman et al., 1995)), with a random walk (*e.g.* simulated annealing) or a greedy walk (*e.g.* hill-climbing). However, scores do not explicitly reflect the error rate of edges, and the sample sizes in real world applications are usually not enough to guarantee asymptotic performance.

Both classical and Bayesian approaches are available for controlling errors during network learning (Listgarten & Heckerman, 2007). Classical approaches are based on the Markov property of graphical models, and treat error control as a problem of multiple testing. Since a graphical model is a graphical encoding of conditional-independence relationships, the non-adjacency between two nodes is tested by inspecting their conditional independence given other nodes. Conditional-independence relationships among node variables are tested one by one in a certain order, and p-values about the existence of each edge are estimated. Error control procedures, such as Bonferroni correction for the family-wise error rate, or the Benjamini-Hochberg procedure for the FDR, or without-correction for the type-I error rate, are applied to the p-values to set the cut-off threshold of accepting or rejecting the existence of edges.

Recently, a series of papers have addressed the problem using the classical approach. Listgarten and Heckman (Listgarten & Heckerman, 2007) proposed a permutation method to estimate the number of spurious connections in a graph learned from data. The basic idea is to repetitively apply a structure learning algorithm to data simulated from the null hypotheses with permutation. In general, this method will work with any structure learning method, but permutation may make the already time-consuming structure learning problem even more computationally expensive, limiting its practical usage. Kalisch and Bühlmann (Kalisch & Bühlmann, 2007) in 2007 proved that for Gaussian Bayesian networks, by adaptively decreasing the type I error rate, as the sample size approaches infinity, the PC algorithm (Spirtes et al., 2001) can, without errors, recover the equivalence class of the underlying sparse directed acyclic graphs, even if the number of nodes grows exponentially as the sample size does. Tsamardinos and Brown (Tsamardinos & Brown, July, 2008) in 2008 applied the FDR-procedure separately to edges related to each node. Li and Wang (Li & Wang, 2009) in 2009 applied FDR-control procedures globally to all connections of interest, and proved that with mild conditions, their method is able to asymptotically control the FDR of the "claimed" edges. They showed by empirical experiments that in the cases of moderate sample size (about several hundred), the method is still able to control the FDR under the user-specified level.

Bayesian approaches control errors by inferring the posterior probability of edges given the data. If G is the learned graph and G_i is the true graph, then the spurious edges in G are those of $G \setminus G_i$, ie. the sub-graph of G after edges in G_i are removed. In this case, the *realized* FDR is $|G \setminus G_i| / |G|$ where $|\bullet|$ denotes the number of edges in a graph, and the *realized* type-I error rate in this case is $|G \setminus G_i| / |G_{full} \setminus G_i|$ where G_{full} is the fully connected graph. Since Bayesian inference assigns a probability to each possible model, the error rate of G given data D should be integrated over all possible G_i according to their posterior possibilities (Listgarten & Heckerman, 2007). Therefore we have:

$$FDR(G|D) = \sum_{G_i} \frac{|G \setminus G_i|}{|G|} P(G_i|D), \tag{2}$$

where $P(G_i|D)$ is the probability of a model structure G_i given data D. Similarly the posterior type-I error rate is:

$$\alpha(G|D) = \sum_{G_i} \frac{|G \setminus G_i|}{|G_{full} \setminus G_i|} P(G_i|D). \tag{3}$$

As in many other Bayesian procedures, the most difficult part of the inference is not the formulation, but rather the calculation, and especially the integration. Because the number of possible graphs increases super-exponentially as the number of nodes increases (Steinsky, 2003), it is impractical to enumerate all the possibilities and sum them up. For certain prior distributions, given the order of nodes, Friedman and Koller (Friedman & Koller, 2003) in

2003 derived a formula that can calculate the exact posterior probability of a structure feature with the computational complexity bounded by $O(N^{D_{in}+1})$, where N is the number of nodes and D_{in} is the upper bound of node in-degrees. Considering similar prior distributions, but without the restriction on the order of nodes, Koivisto and Sood (Koivisto & Sood, 2004) in 2004 developed a fast exact Bayesian inference algorithm based on dynamic programming that is able to compute the exact posterior probability of a sub-network with the computational complexity bounded by approximately $O(N2^N)$. In practice, this algorithm runs fairly fast when the number of nodes is less than 25. For networks with more than about 30 vertices, the authors suggested setting more restrictions or combining with inexact techniques. For general situations, the posterior probability of a structure feature can be estimated with Markov chain Monte Carlo (MCMC) methods (Madigan et al., 1995). As a versatile implementation of Bayesian inference, the MCMC method can estimate the posterior probability given any prior probability distribution. However, MCMC usually requires intensive computation and the results may depend on the initial state.

In Listgarten and Heckman's simulation (2007) (Listgarten & Heckerman, 2007), the error-control curves of the Bayesian approach was smoother and more favorable than those of the classical approach, as show in Fig. 6-A and Fig. 6-B. However, it was also pointed out that in practice the expected FDR of interest usually is very small, within a narrow range near 0, and that the classical approach showed reasonable performance in this range. (The axes of Fig. 6-A and Fig. 6-B are marked with the positive predictive value (PPV) instead of the FDR. The relationship between PPV and FDR is $PPV = 1 - FDR$, as in Table 2.) In Li and Wang's simulation (2009) (Li & Wang, 2009), to control the FDR at the conventional level of 5%, their classical approaches, the PC_{fdr} algorithm and its heuristic modification, the PC_{fdr*} algorithm, controlled the FDR satisfactorily around the expected level 5%, as shown in Fig. 6-C. For inferring brain connectivity, since brain regions are not just algebraically isolated variables, but rather located in a three-dimension space with complex geometric structure, it may be important in the future to exploit such geometric information for improving error control.

3. Group analysis

Biomedical experiments are usually conducted to verify or discover knowledge about a population characterized by health or certain disease state. However, subjects classified to the same group can still be highly diverse with respect to factors such as gender, age, or race. With careful experiment design, the effect of these confounding factors can be reduced, but inter-subject variability still plays an important role and remains a challenge. Even studies on a single subject may still face challenges related to variability. For example, EEG recordings conducted at different times from the same subject can be affected by the subject's physical or psychological state, such as drowsiness or stress. Thus in this paper, the term "group analysis" is not restricted to the analysis of a group of people, but generalized to the inference by integrating the information distributed in separate experiments and affected by cross-experiment variability.

3.1 Commonality and diversity at different levels

Two basic concepts in group analysis are *commonality and* diversity. For example, all doctors learn professional knowledge related to medicine, but a doctor could be a pediatrician, a surgeon or a physician. Each one has their own speciality and this is the diversity among them. Commonality and diversity usually co-exist, and are revealed at different levels, depending on the perspective and scale we study the problem.

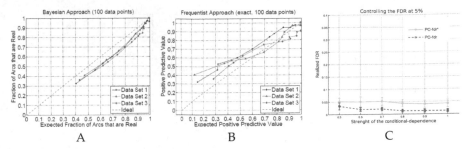

A   B   C

Fig. 6. Simulation results of the FDR control with the Bayesian and classical approaches. Sub-figure A and B are results in (Listgarten & Heckerman, 2007). Their x-axes and y-axes are the expected and realized positive predictive values (PPV) respectively. (The relationship between PPV and FDR is PPV = 1 - FDR.) The curves of the Bayesian approach was smoother and more favorable than those of the classical approach. When the expected PPV is high, or equivalently the expected FDR is low, the classical approach performed reasonably well. Sub-figure C is the result in (Li & Wang, 2009) to control the FDR at the conventional level of 5% with the classical approach. The x-axis is the strength of the conditional-dependence relationships among node variables, and the y-axis is the realized FDR. The PC_{fdr} algorithm controlled the FDR under 5%, and its heuristic modification, the PC_{fdr*} algorithm, controlled the FDR satisfactorily around 5%. For details of the two simulation studies, please refer to (Listgarten & Heckerman, 2007) and (Li & Wang, 2009).

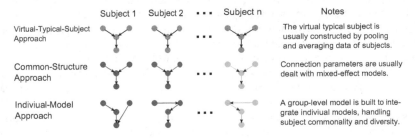

Fig. 7. Three broad categories of group-analysis methods. The "virtual typical" approach constructs a typical subject to represent the whole group, usually by pooling or averaging data of subjects. The "common-structure" approach imposes the same network structure to the model of every subject, and usually uses mixed-effect models to handle the parameter variability among subjects. The "individual-model" approach allows each individual subject to have its own model, and integrates the individual models with a group-level model.

Since graphical models combine network structures and probability descriptions, the group analysis needs also accommodate commonality and diversity with both model structures and probability parameters. A review of the literature shows that current group-analysis methods based on graphical models can be classified into three broad categories (see Fig. 7), as discussed as follows (Li et al., 2008).

First, we could ignore subject diversity, and assume that the brains of all the subjects are structured and function in a similar way, as if there is a virtual typical subject able to satisfactorily represent the whole group. This can be called the "virtual typical subject" approach. In this approach, the model for every subject has the same structure, and the

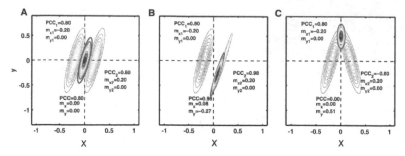

Fig. 8. Product of two Gaussian distributions. Thin lines are the contour of two bivariate Gaussian distributions, and the bold lines are the contour of their product. If the parameter likelihood for the data of two subjects is the two bivariate Gaussian distributions, then the parameter likelihood for the pooled data is the product distribution. In sub-figures B and C, the center of the product distribution is located off the x-axis, while neither of the two bivariate Gaussian distributions is centred off the x-axis. This is an undesirable and misleading phenomenon for data pooling. PPC is the abbreviation for partial correlation coefficient; m_x is the mean of x, and m_y is that of y. This figure is from (Kasess et al., 2010).

same parameters as well. The "virtual-typical" subject is usually constructed by pooling or averaging the group data, and then one model is learned from the data. Technically this degrades group analysis to learning a model for a single subject, for which both classical (Heckerman et al., 1995) and Bayesian (Neumann & Lohmann, 2003) approaches have been developed. When the group is homogeneous or inter-subject variability follows certain regular distributions, this approach could increase detection sensitivity, because pooling can build a relatively large data set, and averaging can enhance the signal-to-noise ratio (Kasess et al., 2010). However, when the group becomes more heterogeneous, this approach could lead to undesirable and misleading results (Kasess et al., 2010). Fig. 8 shows that by pooling data together, the group estimation of connection parameters could be located far way from the center of individual estimations.

The other extreme is that we assume subjects can be completely different from each other – the "individual-model approach". In this approach, the model of each subject can be completely different. This approach is related to the concept of functional degeneracy, ie. "the ability of elements that are structurally different to perform the same function or yield the same output" (Edelman & Gally, 2001), or more plainly "there are multiple ways of completing the same task" (Price & Friston, 2002). Because subjects in the same group are considered to share similarity, their individual models must be linked together in a certain way, usually by a second-level group model built over the individual models.

The most straight-forward implementation of the "individual-model approach" is to directly input separately learned individual models as subject features into a second-level analysis. For example, structural features of the network of individual models can be selected with classification and cross-validation procedures at the group level, as applied in (Li et al., 2008). A theoretically elegant approach is to build a group-level model to describe the diversity distribution in a group, and the group-level and the individual-level models form a big model over the group data. Usually this big integrated model should be learned from the batch of group data, which would require an intensive computation. The Bayesian group model proposed by Stefan, etc. (Stephan et al., 2009) provides a rigorous theoretical background and is able to break the model learning into two separate stages, the individual and group stages.

This property allow the group to be updated incrementally without re-learning individual models when new data are added. Niculescu-Mizil and Caruana proposed a heuristic method to link individual models (Niculescu-Mizil & Caruana, 2007). They allow network structures to be different across subjects, and punish excessive diversity among the structures with a tunable parameter.

A trade-off between the two extremes is assuming that subjects' brains are structured similarly, but function with considerable difference. This can be referred as the "common-structure" approach (Mechelli et al., 2002). In this approach, the model of every subject share the same network structure, but the parameters can be different from subject to subject. When the common model structure is specified, this approach focuses on dealing with the model parameters across subjects. The standard method is the mixed-effect model (Mumford & Nichols, 2006) as follows. Consider an experiment where there are n subjects and for each subject, indexed by k, a regression parameter β_k modeling the relationship between a response variable Y_k and an explanatory variables X_k. The first-level model for each individual subject is

$$Y_k = X_k \beta_k + \epsilon_k, \text{ for } k = 1, 2, \cdots, n, \tag{4}$$

where ϵ_k is the within-subject randomness following Gaussian distribution $N(0, V_k)$. The second-level model for group parameters is

$$\beta = \begin{bmatrix} \beta_1 \\ \vdots \\ \beta_n \end{bmatrix} = X_g \beta_g + \epsilon_g, \tag{5}$$

where β_g is the group-level parameter, X_g is the group design matrix and ϵ_g is the cross-subject randomness following Gaussian distribution $N(0, V_g)$. The combination of Eqs. (4) and (5) is called a mixed model, because both the within-subject and the cross-subject randomness are considered in the model. A notable issue in mixed-effect models is that the cross-subject variance V_g could be negative in maximum likelihood estimation. To avoid this undesirable and counter-intuition phenomenon, the random-effect variance is usually enforced to be positive. The mixed-effect model in practice usually is solved with the summary-statistics approach that reformulates the model as Eqs. (6) and (7):

$$\hat{\beta}_k = (X_k^T V_k^{-1} X_k)^{-1} X_k^T V_k^{-1} Y_k, \tag{6}$$

$$\hat{\beta} = \begin{bmatrix} \hat{\beta}_1 \\ \vdots \\ \hat{\beta}_n \end{bmatrix} = X_g \beta_g + \epsilon_g + \hat{\beta} - \beta \tag{7}$$

$$= X_g \beta_g + \epsilon_g^*,$$

where $\hat{\beta}_k$ is the least-square-estimation of the parameter for each subject, and $\epsilon_g^* = \epsilon_g + \hat{\beta} - \beta$ following $N(0, V_g^*)$. Given V_g^* (the variance of ϵ_g^*), β_g can be solved from the estimation of β_ks, unnecessarily from β_ks. The summary-statistics approach decomposes a complicated model into two relatively easy stages, and retains the estimation for each single subject even when new subjects are added into the analysis. The summary-statistics approach assumes that V_g^* is known, but in practice it should be estimated from the data. The estimation, including both its value and its degree of freedom, is challenging and has attracted much research attention. Methods such as Restricted Maximum Likelihood (Harville, 1977), Smoothing with fixed-effect model (Worsley et al., 2002) , and Markov Chain Monte Carlo (Woolrich et al., 2004) have been developed.

Though the aforementioned methods deal with group commonality and diversity with various techniques, most take or can be considered to be in a two-level framework: a lower level of models for each individual subject, and a group level integrating individual models and describing inter inter-subject commonality and diversity. The group level could enforce strong commonality, like the "virtual-typical" approach, or model group diversity probabilistically, like the "individual-model" approach in (Stephan et al., 2009). Models able to technically decouple the computation of the individual and the group levels are favoured.

3.2 Desirable features of graph analysis methods

To set clear goals for the future development of more advanced group-analysis methods, we suggest three highly desirable features: being modular, being incrementally updatable, and being scalable. Being modular means that a group-analysis method is not only designed for a particular type of single-subject model, but versatile and applicable to different types of single-subject models. For example, both Bayesian networks and structural equation models are applicable at the subject level, so the group-analysis method should not be restricted to only one of them, but should be able to work with both of them, though not necessarily with a mixture of them. If the group-level model just needs inputs such as the likelihood of individual models, then it is free from the specific format of the individual models. If a group-analysis model can be a module of itself, then it will be able to handle multi-level hierarchical group structures.

Being incrementally updatable means that group-inference results can be summarized as summary statistics and used for further analysis involving newly collected data. This feature is very useful in research practice because experimental data are usually collected incrementally. For example, after a study on eighty subjects half a year ago, twenty more subjects might be recruited. In this case, it may require cumbersome computation to analyze the entire data of one hundred subjects. However, if the group inference is incrementally updatable, it may need much less computation to include the additional twenty subjects.

Being scalable means that a group-analysis method can handle fast growing diversity among subjects. Because modern exploratory research usually involves investigation of a large number of candidate models, scalability has become a highly desirable feature for group analysis. For example, if the connectivity between ten brain regions is studied with Bayesian networks, then a group-analysis method should be able to handle the diversity of about 3.1×10^{17} (Steinsky, 2003) possible network structures.

4. Network analysis

Modelling is only the first step to investigate a system, following which human-understandable information should be further extracted from models to provide insightful understanding. For example, as final readers of a report on brain connectivity, neurologists might be interested in questions such as "which brain regions play the central role in conducting a functional task?", "in what patterns are cognitive functions segregated and integrated among brain regions?" or "how does this brain connectivity network react to the presence of a disease?" Simply reporting a vast and plain network without any highlights does not answer these questions. Graphical models notably have visualized network structures, so it is natural to analyze their structures as an important post-processing in their applications in brain connectivity, as discussed in (Bullmore & Sporns, 2009; Stam & Reijneveld, 2007).

The history of graph theory can be traced back to nearly three hundred years ago, marked by preeminent Swiss mathematician Euler's paper on the Seven Bridges of Königsberg. Its application to real-world complex networks was boosted at the end of last century by a series of discoveries on the architecture of world-wide-web, social networks, cellular networks, etc. These systems, despite their tremendous variety, share certain common properties, such as the "small world" (Watts & Strogatz, 1998), the "scale free" (Barabasi & Albert, 1999) and the "self-similarity" (Song et al., 2005) properties. These properties might hint how these networks evolve and grow, and are also related to their functions and interactions with the environment (Watts & Strogatz, 1998).

Some well-know properties such as the "scale-free" or "self-similarity" properties are more suitable for large networks, than for networks of moderate size (with dozens of nodes), because their statistics need large scale observations. However, the number of time points of an fMRI scan is relatively small, approximately several hundred, and cannot support reliably discovery of large scale networks. Therefore, in this section, we focus on network analysis suitable for brain connectivity networks of moderate size.

4.1 Network measures

Graphs can be studied at different levels from basically nodes and edges, to paths, or more intricately, sub-graphs. According to the object of interest, network measures can be broadly classified into two categories: (1) local measures that focus on local objects in the network, for example, a node, an edge, or a sub-graph, and (2) global measures that feature the pattern of the overall architecture. Local measures usually, yet not necessarily, put a local object in the global view. For example, the importance of a node could be defined as the proportion of communication in the whole network that must go through it. Vice versa, global measures are usually built on local features. For example, the "scale-free" property is about the distribution of node degrees. Fig. 9 illustrates those network measures listed below. Most network measures are ultimately linked to fundamental concepts such as node degree and path length.

- **Centrality and local contribution to network communication.** A local object, for instance a node or an edge, that plays an important role in network communication is considered to be central in the network. The centrality of a node can be measured by its relay of the communication between other nodes. For example, betweenness centrality (Freeman, 1977) is based on the number of shortest paths between other nodes passing through a node. It can also be assessed by the geodesic distance to other nodes, as closeness centrality (Beauchamp, 1965) does, or by deleting a node and then comparing the connectivity loss of the "impaired" network, as Shapley ratings (Kötter et al., 2007) do. Similar ideas can be applied to define the centrality of an edge or a sub-graph. Some measures are not as intuitive as the aforementioned ones: for instance, eigenvector centrality (Bonacich, 1972) and sub-graph centrality (Estrada & Rodrguez-Velzquez, 2005) are also implemented for the same concept.

- **Modularity and brain function organization.** It is believed that various cognitive functions are localized in different brain regions, and that these distributed functions are integrated together for complicated information processing. Such a perspective on brain function organization naturally leads to a network structure where some nodes are densely clustered and form function modules. The "small-world" property, at the global level,

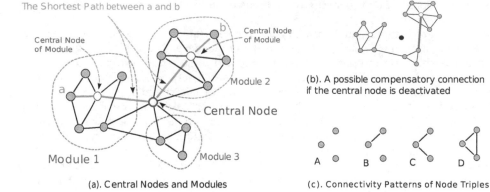

(a). Central Nodes and Modules

(b). A possible compensatory connection if the central node is deactivated

(c). Connectivity Patterns of Node Triples

Fig. 9. Network measures suitable for graphs of moderate size. A central node, as the red nodes in sub-figure (a), plays an important role in network communication. Nodes densely clustered form modules, as those circled by dotted lines in sub-figure (a). The blue edge in sub-figure (b) is a possible compensatory edge to restore the connectivity impaired by deactivation of the central node (thick black). Sub-figure (c) shows the possible connectivity patterns of node triples. Connectivity patterns appear significantly more frequently than those in random graphs are called "network motif".

features systems that are highly locally clustered, like regular lattices, but still have small geodesic diameter, like random graphs (Watts & Strogatz, 1998). Modules can be detected by hierarchical clustering algorithms that groups node from the most linked pairs to the least pairs, or by community detection algorithms (Girvan & Newman, 2002) that draw module boundaries by breaking unimportant edges one by one.

- **Perturbation and compensation mechanisms.** It is believed that as a dynamic system, the brain will respond to impairment such as that induced by disease, by recruiting other neural resources to compensate the partially disabled function. This compensation mechanism is an important hypothesis of neuro-rehabilitation, and also related to many neurological diseases. Network analysis for the compensation mechanism can take a perturbation-and-recovery approach: deleting a connection or deactivating a node, and then searching for the most efficient changes that are needed to restore the impaired connectivity. Such mechanism could be developing a new connection other than the deleted one, or increasing the functionality of the most central node of the "lesioned" network (Kötter et al., 2007).

- **Motif and connectivity pattern.** Inter-connected nodes are building blocks of a big network, and the connectivity patterns among neighboring nodes characterize how information is processed at the local level. It has been found that in real-world networks certain patterns of inter-connections occur much more frequently than in random networks, and these "signature" local patterns are called network "motif" (Milo et al., 2002; Sporns & Kötter, 2004). Another network measure related to the "small-world" property is clustering coefficient, which is a function of the counts of pattern C and pattern D in Fig. 9-(c).

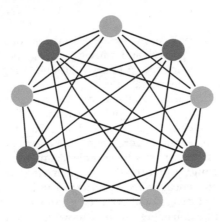

Fig. 10. An example of the discriminability of different centrality measures. With the betweenness, the closeness and the eigenvector centrality, all the nodes are identical, while with the sub-graph centrality, the nodes are distinguishable, with score 45.696 for blue nodes, and 45.651 for green nodes. This example is from (Estrada & Rodrguez-Velzquez, 2005).

4.2 Discriminability of network measures

When using network measures to quantitatively reveal the differences with respect to a certain network concept, we naturally expect that the measure could sensitively detect even subtle differences. As various calculation methods could be proposed to quantify the same network concept, this raises the concern of the discriminability of these calculation methods. For example, to measure the centrality of a node, there are options such as the betweenness (Freeman, 1977), the closeness (Beauchamp, 1965), the sub-graph (Estrada & Rodrguez-Velzquez, 2005), and the eigenvector centrality (Bonacich, 1972). As Fig. 10 shows, certain difference can only be detected by some measures.

This situation motivates the future development of theoretical criteria for rigorously comparing network measures and guiding their design, besides just evaluating them empirically. Theoretically, it is possible to use just a real number to uniquely represent a binary graph, achieving perfect discriminability. For instance, the adjacency matrix can be lined straight as the binary coding of a rational number. Though this simple mapping may not be meaningfully related to any network concept, it at least shows that with a single index all graphs can be distinguished.

For network measures of a graph, an available criterion is the mutual information between the measure and the "isomorphic" class of graphs (Corneil & Gotlieb, 1970). Two graphs G_1 and G_2 are isomorphic if and only if there is a one-to-one mapping f between the nodes of G_1 and G_2 such that for every adjacent node pair a and b in G_1, their mirrors in G_2, ie. $f(a)$ and $f(b)$, are also adjacent, and vice versa. Similarly, for network measures about a node in a graph, their discriminability can quantified with the mutual information between the measure and the "isomorphic" class of the nodes. Two nodes a and b in a graph G are isomorphic if and only if there a permutation p of the nodes of G such that $p(a) = b$ and $p(b) = a$ and that for every adjacent node pair c and d (which can be a or b), $p(c)$ and $p(d)$ are also adjacent. It is of great theoretic and practical importance to further pursue criteria for rigorously comparing the discriminability of network measures.

5. Concluding remarks

In this article, we reviewed the application of graphical models for inferring brain connectivity from fMRI data. We have described and provided signal processing solutions for the challenges raised in this highly interdisciplinary and innovating research field related to model reliability, generality and interpretability.

The importance of error control during brain network structure learning has been increasingly recognized, with a series of papers being published since 2005. These papers proposed solutions from the perspective of both classical and Bayesian statistics, and provided some theoretical conclusions. Because brain regions are not just algebraically isolated variables, but rather located in a three-dimension space with complex geometric structure, a desirable future direction is to exploit this geometric information for improving the error control.

Group analysis is a frequently encountered requirement in biomedical research. Graphical models introduce inter-subject diversity at both the parameter level and the structure level. Most existing methods can be considered to take a two-level framework: a lower level of models for each individual subject, and a group level integrating individual models and describing inter-subject commonality and diversity. Being modular, incrementally updatable, and scalable is highly desirable, yet not well implemented features for current group analysis. Network analysis is an important post-processing for extracting interpretable and human-understandable information from graphical models. Network concepts such as centrality, modularity, connection patterns, the "small-world", "scale-free" property have been actively explored in the analysis of brain connectivity. As various calculation methods could be proposed to quantify the same network concept, it is of great theoretic and practical importance to further pursue criteria for rigorously comparing the discriminability of network measures.

6. Appendix

Software and databases

The interest on modeling brain connectivity using fMRI has been experiencing an increasing, important growth in the signal processing community during the last decade. One of the factors of this success is the availability of public-available software and databases. As a reference for interested readers, here we provide an overview of several widely used computer programs related to fMRI brain connectivity analysis. This list is by no means complete.

- **Statistical Parametric Mapping (SPM)**: Developed by the Wellcome Trust Centre for Neuroimaging.
  Website: http://www.fil.ion.ucl.ac.uk/spm
  Brief description: The SPM software package, probably the most popular one, has been designed for the analysis of brain imaging data sequences. The sequences can be a series of images from different cohorts, or time-series from the same subject. The current release is designed for the analysis of fMRI, PET, SPECT, EEG and MEG.

- **LONI Software**: Developed by the Laboratory of Neuro Imaging at the University of California, Los Angeles.
  Website: http://www.loni.ucla.edu/Software
  Brief description: The popular LONI Software is a comprehensive library for neuroimaging analysis, including pipelines for automated processing, web-based applications, tools for image processing and visualization, etc.

- **FMRIB Software Library (FSL)**: Developed mainly by the FMRIB Analysis Group at the University of Oxford.
  Website: http://www.fmrib.ox.ac.uk/fsl
  Brief description: FSL is a comprehensive library of analysis tools for fMRI, MRI and DTI brain imaging data.

- **MRIcro**: Developed by Professor Chris Rorden's group at the University of South Carolina.
  Website: http://www.sph.sc.edu/comd/rorden
  Brief description: MRIcro allows efficient viewing and exporting of brain images. It can create Analyze format headers for exporting brain images to other platforms, such as SPM. In addition, it allows neuropsychologists to identify regions of interest (ROIs).

- **FreeSurfer**: Developed by the Athinoula A. Martinos Center for Biomedical Imaging.
  Website: http://surfer.nmr.mgh.harvard.edu
  Brief description: FreeSurfer is a set of automated tools for reconstruction of the brain cortical surface from structural MRI data, and overlay of functional MRI data onto the reconstructed surface.

- **Brain Connectivity Toolbox (BCT)**: Developed mainly by the Computational Cognitive Neuroscience Laboratory at Indiana University.
  Website: http://www.brain-connectivity-toolbox.net
  Brief description: This toolbox provides an access to a large selection of complex network measures in Matlab. Such measures aim to characterize brain connectivity by neuro-biologically meaningful statistics, and are used in the description of structural and functional connectivity datasets.

There are normally fMRI datasets associated with the above software. Here we also briefly mention a few publicly-available fMRI databases. Details related with the experiment, design and data content are available in the associated website links.

- **fMRI Data Center (fMRIDC)**: Funded by the National Science Foundation, the W. M. Keck Foundation.
  Website: http://www.fmridc.org

- **Biomedical Informatics Research Network (BIRN) Data Repository**
  Website: http://nbirn.net/bdr

- **The Neuroimaging Informatics Tools and Resources Clearinghouse (NITRC)**: Funded by the National Institutes of Health Blueprint for Neuroscience Research.
  Website: http://www.nitrc.org

7. References

Akaike, H. (1974). A new look at the statistical model identification, *Automatic Control, IEEE Transactions on* 19(6): 716–723.

Ali, R., Richardson, T. & Spirtes, P. (2009). Markov equivalence for ancestral graphs, *The Annals of Statistics* 37(5B): 2808–2837.

Barabasi, A.-L. & Albert, R. (1999). Emergence of Scaling in Random Networks, *Science* 286(5439): 509–512.

Bassett, D. S. & Bullmore, E. (2006). Small-World Brain Networks, *Neuroscientist* 12(6): 512–523.

Beauchamp, M. A. (1965). An improved index of centrality, *Behavioral Science* 10(2): 161–163.

Benjamini, Y. & Yekutieli, D. (2001). The control of the false discovery rate in multiple testing under dependency, *Ann. Stat.* 29(4): 1165–1188.

Bollen, K. A. (1989). *Structural Equations With Latent Variables*, John Wiley.

Bonacich, P. (1972). Factoring and weighting approaches to status scores and clique identification, *Journal of Mathematical Sociology* 2(1): 113–120.

Bullmore, E., Fadili, J., Maxim, V., Sendur, L., Whitcher, B., Suckling, J., Brammer, M. & Breakspear, M. (2004). Wavelets and functional magnetic resonance imaging of the human brain., *Neuroimage* 23 Suppl 1: S234–S249.

Bullmore, E. & Sporns, O. (2009). Complex brain networks: graph theoretical analysis of structural and functional systems., *Nat Rev Neurosci* 10(3): 186–198.

Calhoun, V., Adali, T., Pearlson, G. & Pekar, J. (2001). A method for making group inferences from functional mri data using independent component analysis, *Human Brain Mapping* 14(3): 140–151.

Cao, J. & Worsley, K. (1999). The geometry of correlation fields with an application to functional connectivity of the brain, *The Annals of Applied Probability* 9(4): 1021–1057.

Catani, M. & ffytche, D. H. (2005). The rises and falls of disconnection syndromes., *Brain* 128: 2224–2239.

Corneil, D. & Gotlieb, C. (1970). An efficient algorithm for graph isomorphism, *Journal of the ACM (JACM)* 17(1): 51–64.

Edelman, G. M. & Gally, J. A. (2001). Degeneracy and complexity in biological systems, *PNAS* 98(24): 13763–13768.

Estrada, E. & Rodrguez-Velzquez, J. A. (2005). Subgraph centrality in complex networks, *Phys. Rev. E* 71(5): 056103.

Freeman, L. C. (1977). A set of measures of centrality based on betweenness, *Sociometry* 40(1): 35–41.

Friedman, N. & Koller, D. (2003). Being Bayesian about network structure. A Bayesian approach to structure discovery in Bayesian networks, *MACH LEARN* 50(1): 95–125.

Friston, K. J., Harrison, L. & Penny, W. (2003). Dynamic causal modelling, *NeuroImage* 19(4): 1273–1302.

Girvan, M. & Newman, M. E. J. (2002). Community structure in social and biological networks., *Proc Natl Acad Sci U S A* 99(12): 7821–7826.

Granger, C. W. J. (Aug., 1969). Investigating causal relations by econometric models and cross-spectral methods, *Econometrica* 37(3): 424–438.

Harville, D. A. (1977). Maximum likelihood approaches to variance component estimation and to related problems, *Journal of the American Statistical Association* 72(358): 320–338.

Heckerman, D., Geiger, D. & Chickering, D. M. (1995). Learning Bayesian networks: The combination of knowledge and statistical data, *Machine Learning* 20(3): 197–243.

Heller, R., Stanley, D., Yekutieli, D., Rubin, N. & Benjamini, Y. (2006). Cluster-based analysis of fMRI data, *NeuroImage* 33(2): 599–608.

Kalisch, M. & Bühlmann, P. (2007). Estimating high-dimensional directed acyclic graphs with the PC-algorithm, *Journal of Machine Learning Research* 8: 613–636.

Kaminski, M. (2005). Determination of transmission patterns in multichannel data, *Phil. Trans. R. Soc. B* 360(1457): 947–952.

Kasess, C. H., Stephan, K. E., Weissenbacher, A., Pezawas, L., Moser, E. & Windischberger, C. (2010). Multi-subject analyses with dynamic causal modeling, *NeuroImage* 49(4): 3065–3074.

Koivisto, M. & Sood, K. (2004). Exact Bayesian structure discovery in Bayesian networks, *J MACH LEARN RES* 5: 549–573.

Kötter, R., Reid, A. T., Krumnack, A., Wanke, E. & Sporns, O. (2007). Shapley ratings in brain networks., *Front Neuroinformatics* 1: 2.

Lauritzen, S. L. (1996). *Graphical Models*, Clarendon Press, Oxford University Press, Oxford, New York.

Li, J. & Wang, Z. J. (2009). Controlling the false discovery rate of the association/causality structure learned with the PC algorithm, *J MACH LEARN RES* pp. 475–514.

Li, J., Wang, Z. J., Palmer, S. J. & McKeown, M. J. (2008). Dynamic bayesian network modeling of fMRI: A comparison of group-analysis methods, *NeuroImage* 41(2): 398 – 407.

Listgarten, J. & Heckerman, D. (2007). Determining the number of non-spurious arcs in a learned DAG model: Investigation of a Bayesian and a frequentist approach, *Proceedings of the 23rd Conference on Uncertainty in Artificial Intelligence*.

Madigan, D., York, J. & Allard, D. (1995). Bayesian graphical models for discrete data, *INT STAT REV* 63(2): 215–232.

McKeown, M. J. (2000). Cortical activation related to arm-movement combinations, *Muscle & Nerve* 23(S9): S19–S25.

Mechelli, A., Penny, W. D., Price, C. J., Gitelman, D. R. & Friston, K. J. (2002). Effective connectivity and intersubject variability: Using a multisubject network to test differences and commonalities, *NeuroImage* 17(3): 1459–1469.

Milo, R., Shen-Orr, S., Itzkovitz, S., Kashtan, N., Chklovskii, D. & Alon, U. (2002). Network motifs: Simple building blocks of complex networks, *Science* 298(5594): 824–827.

Mumford, J. A. & Nichols, T. (2006). Modeling and inference of multisubject fMRI data, *IEEE Eng Med Biol* 25(2): 42–51.

Neumann, J. & Lohmann, G. (2003). Bayesian second-level analysis of functional magnetic resonance images., *Neuroimage* 20(2): 1346–1355.

Niculescu-Mizil, A. & Caruana, R. (2007). Inductive transfer for Bayesian network structure learning, *Proceedings of the 11th International Conference on AI and Statistics (AISTATS '07)*.

Palmer, S. J., Eigenraam, L., Hoque, T., McCaig, R. G., Troiano, A. & McKeown, M. J. (2009). Levodopa-sensitive, dynamic changes in effective connectivity during simultaneous movements in Parkinson's disease., *Neuroscience* 158(2): 693–704.

Price, C. J. & Friston, K. J. (2002). Degeneracy and cognitive anatomy, *Trends in Cognitive Sciences* 6(10): 416–421.

Richardson, T. (2003). Markov properties for acyclic directed mixed graphs, *Scandinavian Journal of Statistics* 30(1): 145–157.

Roweis, S. & Ghahramani, Z. (1999). A unifying review of linear Gaussian models, *Neural Computation* 11(2): 305–345.

Schlösser, R. G. M., Wagner, G., Koch, K., Dahnke, R., Reichenbach, J. R. & Sauer, H. (2008). Fronto-cingulate effective connectivity in major depression: a study with fMRI and dynamic causal modeling., *Neuroimage* 43(3): 645–655.

Schwarz, G. (1978). Estimating the dimension of a model, *The Annals of Statistics* 6(2): 461–464. Short Communications.

Song, C., Havlin, S. & Makse, H. A. (2005). Self-similarity of complex networks, *Nature* 433(7024): 392–395.

Spirtes, P., Glymour, C. & Scheines, R. (2001). *Causation, Prediction, and Search*, The MIT Press.

Spirtes, P., Richardson, T., Meek, C., Scheines, R. & Glymour, C. (1998). Using path diagrams as a structural equation modeling tool, *Sociological Methods Research* 27(2): 182–225.

Sporns, O. & Kötter, R. (2004). Motifs in brain networks, *PLoS Biol* 2(11): e369.

Stam, C. J. & Reijneveld, J. C. (2007). Graph theoretical analysis of complex networks in the brain., *Nonlinear Biomed Phys* 1(1): 3.

Steinsky, B. (2003). Enumeration of labelled chain graphs and labelled essential directed acyclic graphs, *Discrete Mathematics* 270(1-3): 267–278.

Stephan, K. E., Penny, W. D., Daunizeau, J., Moran, R. J. & Friston, K. J. (2009). Bayesian model selection for group studies, *NeuroImage* 46(4): 1004–1017.

Storey, J. D. (2002). A direct approach to false discovery rates, *Journal of the Royal Statistical Society. Series B (Statistical Methodology)* 64(3): 479–498.

Supekar, K., Menon, V., Rubin, D., Musen, M. & Greicius, M. D. (2008). Network analysis of intrinsic functional brain connectivity in Alzheimer's disease., *PLoS Comput Biol* 4(6): e1000100.

Tsamardinos, I. & Brown, L. E. (July, 2008). Bounding the false discovery rate in local Bayesian network learning, *Proceedings of the Twenty-Third AAAI Conference on Artificial Intelligence*.

Valdes-Sosa, P., Sanchez-Bornot, J., Lage-Castellanos, A., Vega-Hernandez, M., Bosch-Bayard, J., Melie-Garcia, L. & Canales-Rodriguez, E. (2005). Estimating brain functional connectivity with sparse multivariate autoregression, *Phil. Trans. R. Soc. B* 360(1457): 969–981.

Watts, D. J. & Strogatz, S. H. (1998). Collective dynamics of "small-world" networks, *Nature* 393(6684): 440–442.

Woolrich, M. W., Behrens, T. E. J., Beckmann, C. F., Jenkinson, M. & Smith, S. M. (2004). Multilevel linear modelling for fMRI group analysis using Bayesian inference, *NeuroImage* 21(4): 1732–1747.

Worsley, K. J., Liao, C. H., Aston, J., Petre, V., Duncan, G. H., Morales, F. & Evans, A. C. (2002). A general statistical analysis for fMRI data., *Neuroimage* 15(1): 1–15.

Zheng, X. & Rajapakse, J. C. (2006). Learning functional structure from fMR images, *NeuroImage* 31(4): 1601–1613.

8

Neuroimaging Studies in Carbon Monoxide Intoxication

Ya-Ting Chang[1], Wen-Neng Chang[1], Shu-Hua Huang[2], Chun-Chung Lui[3],
Chen-Chang Lee[3], Nai-Ching Chen[1] and Chiung-Chih Chang[1,4]

[1]Department of Neurology,
[2]Nuclear Medicine,
[3]Radiology,
Chang Gung Memorial Hospital, Kaohsiung Medical Center
and Chang Gung University College of Medicine,
[4]Department of Biological Science, National Sun Yet-sen University
Taiwan

1. Introduction

CO is a tasteless, odorless and colorless gas. The existence of endogenous CO in the human body arises from heme catabolism (Meredith and Vale 1988; Ernst and Zibrak 1998) and oxidation of organic molecules (Marilena 1997). Endogenous CO acts as a neurotransmitter for long-term potentiation, consequently playing a key role in memory and learning (Marilena 1997). It also plays a role in modulating inflammation, apoptosis, cell proliferation, mitochondrial biogenesis (Weaver 2009) and vascular relaxation (Marilena 1997).

Exogenous sources of CO intoxication include smoking, forest fires, pollutants, and improper usage of heaters or furnaces (Weaver 2009; Kumar, Prakash et al. 2010). CO intoxication usually indicates exposure to exogenous sources and is considered one of the most common causes of poisoning worldwide (Prockop and Chichkova 2007; Weaver 2009), with 1000 deaths annually in Britain (Meredith and Vale 1988), and 4000-6000 deaths annually in the United States (Tibbles and Perrotta 1994; Ernst and Zibrak 1998; Weaver 1999). In Asia, the exact epidemiology remains unclear. In Japan, Hong Kong and Taiwan, a common CO etiology of intoxication is charcoal burning suicide (Lee, Chan et al. 2002). In Japan, poisoning by charcoal burning is the most lethal form of suicide and is a highly prevalent method among men aged 25-64 years of age (Kamizato, Yoshitome et al. 2009), in contrast to a high rate of drug poisoning as a method of suicide in women. In Hong Kong, the risk factors of suicide by charcoal burning are male and living alone with financial stress (Lee and Leung 2009). In Taiwan, charcoal burning was not a common method of suicide before 1998, with a rate of only 0.14 per 10^5 people per year (Lin and Lu 2008). With the dissemination of media and the internet, the rate of charcoal burning suicides dramatically increased by 40-fold, reaching a rate of 5.38 per 10^5 people per year in 2005 (Lin and Lu 2008).

2. Mechanisms of CO intoxication

2.1 Tissue hypoxia

CO competes with oxygen in binding with hemoglobin to form carboxyhemoglobin. The affinity between CO and hemoglobin is 200 times higher than that of oxygen (Ernst and Zibrak 1998; Piantadosi 2002; Weaver 2009). The production of carboxyhemoglobin shifts the oxygen-hemoglobin curve to the left and dissociates oxygen from hemoglobin (Ernst and Zibrak 1998). These reactions consequently reduce oxygen delivery to tissues and result in a hypoxic microenvironment.

2.2 Oxidative stress

In brief, CO intoxication leads to oxidative stress through the following mechanisms:
1. CO increases cytosolic heme levels leading to increased heme oxygenase-1 protein, causing intracellular oxidative stress and direct cellular injury (Ernst and Zibrak 1998; Weaver 2009).
2. CO binds to cytochrome c oxidase and impairs mitochondrial function. Cytochrome c oxidase is one of the mitochondrial complexes involved in electric chain transport and is essential for energy production. Binding of CO to cytochrome c oxidase can lead to activation of hypoxia-inducible factor 1α or production of reactive oxygen species with direct cellular injury. Related downstream reactions include apoptosis, lipid peroxidation, lymphocyte proliferation, inflammation and necrosis (Weaver 2009).
3. CO binds to platelet heme protein and induces biogenesis of nitric oxide peroxynitrite, consequently leading to enhanced adhesion of neutrophils to the vascular lining, neutrophil aggregation and release of myeloperoxidase. All of these reactions not only trigger inflammatory processes but also produce more reactive oxygen species (Ernst and Zibrak 1998; Weaver 2009).

2.3 Reoxygenation injury

H_2O_2 production has been noted to increase extensively in brain tissues during reoxygenation after CO intoxication (Zhang and Piantadosi 1992). Salicylate hydroxylation products and 2,3- and 2,5-dihydroxybenzoic acid are also significantly increased during reoxygenation. During this period, CO still binds to cytochrome c oxidase and inhibits the mitochondrial electron transport chain. If the reaction exists in iron-rich regions such as the basal ganglia, it causes persistent acidosis and active iron, which can further damage cells (Zhang and Piantadosi 1992).

2.4 Mechanisms related to central nervous system (CNS) injury
2.4.1 Acute CNS injury

In animal models, an initial cerebral blood flow increment after CO exposure is thought to maintain the baseline energy state (MacMillan 1975). A change of blood flow depends on both the reaction of the cerebrovasculature and cardiac function in CO intoxication. In either failure of cerebrovasculature dilatation or impairment of cardiac pumping function, there is no compensatory blood supply increase in the status of acute carboxyhemoglobin elevation and oxyhemoglobin reduction. (Raub and Benignus 2002). After initially compensated hyperperfusion, focal hypoperfusion has been noted in several studies (Choi, Lee et al. 1992; Choi and Lee 1993) which might be related to clinical manifestation (Sesay, Bidabe et al. 1996). Hypoperfusion over the basal ganglion (Sesay, Bidabe et al. 1996; Kao, Hung et al.

1998), cerebral cortical (Choi, Lee et al. 1992; Kao, Hung et al. 1998), and white matter (WM) (Sesay, Bidabe et al. 1996) areas have been noticed. Cerebral WM and the globus pallidum (GPi) were noted to have relatively low cerebral blood flow after acute CO intoxication in one animal study (Okeda, Matsuo et al. 1987).

Hypoxia in the CNS induces decreased adenosine-5′-triphosphate, influx of Ca2+ and Na+, release of glutamate, noradrenaline and acetylcholine and causes cell swelling and death (Weinachter, Blavet et al. 1990; Kluge 1991). Increased glutamate with both neuronal necrosis and apoptosis was noted immediately after CO intoxication in one animal study (Piantadosi, Zhang et al. 1997). However, how hypoxia affects the CNS in the acute stage of CO intoxication has not been well established (Piantadosi, Zhang et al. 1997; Gorman, Drewry et al. 2003). Aside from changes of cerebral blood flow and hypoxia, increasing intracranial pressure and brain tissue necrosis have been noted in animals and humans after acute CO intoxication (Jiang and Tyssebotn 1997; Piantadosi, Zhang et al. 1997; Uemura, Harada et al. 2001; Lo, Chen et al. 2007).

2.4.2 Chronic CNS injury
The pathogenesis of delayed CNS injury in CO intoxication is complicated. Hypoperfusion (Sesay, Bidabe et al. 1996; Watanabe, Nohara et al. 2002; Chu, Jung et al. 2004) and hypoxia (Opeskin and Drummer 1994) still play an important role. Demyelination (Murata, Kimura et al. 2001; Kamijo, Soma et al. 2007; Ide and Kamijo 2008), cytotoxic edema (Kim, Chang et al. 2003; Chu, Jung et al. 2004; Kwon, Chung et al. 2004), hemorrhage (Ramsey 2001) and infarction (Schwartz, Hennerici et al. 1985; Sung, Yu et al. 2010) have also been associated with delayed neurological deficits. Hypoperfusion and cytotoxic edema in delayed CNS injury have been noted in WM areas and the cerebral cortex (Chu, Jung et al. 2004), and ischemia and necrosis have been noted in the globus pallidus (Chang, Han et al. 1992). Although demyelination and axonal damage might co-exist in CO intoxication, demyelination more than axonal damage is suggested in the literature (Chang, Han et al. 1992; Murata, Kimura et al. 2001; Kamijo, Soma et al. 2007; Ide and Kamijo 2008).

2.5 Other mechanisms
CO also inhibits a number of proteins essential for cells. Myoglobin in the heart and skeletal muscle systems, neuroglobin in the brain, cytochrome P450 (Weiner 1986), dopamine and tryptophan oxygenase (Raub and Benignus 2002) have all been reported to be affected. A high CO concentration transforms xanthine dehydrogenase to xanthine oxidase and produces more free radicals in tissues (Piantadosi, Tatro et al. 1995). Inhibiting the normal function of these intracellular proteins causes further damage or systemic injury in CO intoxication.

3. Clinical manifestation

3.1 The diagnosis of CO intoxication
The diagnosis of CO intoxication is based on the clinical history of exposure or elevated carboxyhemoglobin level (> 10%) (Handa and Tai 2005; Chang, Lee et al. 2009). There is currently no definition of clinical staging in CO intoxication in the literature, although the pathophysiology follows that of hypoxic–ischemic encephalopathy (Gutierrez, Rovira et al.).

3.2 Symptoms in the acute phase

Tightness across the forehead, headache, throbbing in the temples, nausea, vomiting, dimness of vision, dizziness, general weakness, syncope, convulsion, and coma are commonly found in patients with CO exposure within one day (Choi 2001). Cortical blindness with initially normal visual evoked potentials has also been reported in a case (Katafuchi, Nishimi et al. 1985). The pathogenesis contributing to the clinical manifestations includes change of blood flow (Penney 1990; Lo, Chen et al. 2007), hypoxia (Lo, Chen et al. 2007), and neurochemistry abnormalities (Penney 1990).

3.3 Symptoms in the late phase

Following initial neurological deficits after acute CO intoxication, some patients experience progressive neurological deterioration, while others nearly complete recovery of symptoms. Some patients have a delayed onset of neurological deficits after an initial symptom-free period (Lee and Marsden 1994). The latter is often termed as delayed neuropsychiatric sequela in CO intoxication. The lucid interval after acute CO poisoning, on average, is around 20 days, varying from one to 240 days (Choi 1983; Lee and Marsden 1994; Ernst and Zibrak 1998; Pavese, Napolitano et al. 1999; Hsiao, Kuo et al. 2004), with a prevalence of 0.2-40% (Hsiao, Kuo et al. 2004; Otubo, Shirakawa et al. 2007). Delayed neuropsychiatric sequelae include parkinsonism (Lee and Marsden 1994), chorea (Park and Choi 2004), akinetic mutism (Lee and Marsden 1994), increased irritability, verbal aggressiveness, violence, impulsiveness (Meredith and Vale 1988), mood disorders (Weaver 2009), dementia (Meredith and Vale 1988; Ernst and Zibrak 1998; Weaver 2009), psychosis (Ernst and Zibrak 1998), sleep disturbances (Weaver 2009), cortical blindness (Quattrocolo, Leotta et al. 1987; Senol, Yildiz et al. 2009) and incontinence (Ernst and Zibrak 1998).

The cognitive deficits are often very diverse (Hurley, Hopkins et al. 2001; Parkinson, Hopkins et al. 2002; Raub and Benignus 2002) including impairment in verbal or visual episodic memory, language, visuospatial ability, executive function and calculation (Chang, Chang et al. 2010). No specific neuropsychiatric battery has been designed for the cognitive deficits in CO intoxication. For general cognitive performance, most researchers apply the mini-mental state examination (Folstein, Folstein et al. 1975) or Wechsler Adult Intelligence Scale (Dorken and Greenbloom 1953) for evaluation. Chang *et al.* (Chang, Lee et al. 2009) used the clinical dementia rating scale (Morris 1997) to evaluate the functional capability of these patients since they may have physical disabilities. Tasks that have been used for evaluation are as follows: Alzheimer's Disease Assessment Scale-Cognitive word-recognition test (Rosen, Mohs et al. 1984) for verbal episodic memory; recollection of Rey-Osterrieth complex figures for visuospatial ability (Boone 2000); Boston naming test for language ability (Boone 2000); digit span, digit-symbol, digit backward (Cronholm and Viding 1956; Sherman and Blatt 1968; Rudel and Denckla 1974); Trail Making Part A and Part B, block design, and design fluency (Gieseking, Lubin et al. 1956; Arbuthnott and Frank 2000) for executive function; and neuropsychiatric inventory for behavioral changes (Cummings, Mega et al. 1994).

4. Neuroimaging study results of CO intoxication by anatomical classification

4.1 Basal ganglion lesions emphasized on the globus pallidus (GP)

The basal ganglion includes the putamen, caudate nucleus, and GP. GP lesions are often considered as pathognomonic signs for patients with CO intoxication, however the prevalence differs among studies (Silver, Cross et al. 1996; O'Donnell, Buxton et al. 2000). One study showed 63% of abnormal lesions in the GP with 26% in the rest of the basal ganglia (O'Donnell, Buxton et al. 2000). Another study with 73 patients revealed only one patient (1.4%) with basal ganglia lesions scanned two weeks after CO poisoning (Parkinson, Hopkins et al. 2002).

4.1.1 Imaging features suggesting edematous change in the acute phase

Low density GP lesions, commonly seen in computed tomography (CT), are considered as characteristic findings in patients with CO intoxication (Kanaya, Imaizumi et al. 1992; Gotoh, Kuyama et al. 1993; Uchino, Hasuo et al. 1994; Chu, Jung et al. 2004; Kinoshita, Sugihara et al. 2005; Hopkins, Fearing et al. 2006). Low density lesions of the putamen and caudate nucleus, in contrast, have only been reported in one case (Ferrier, Wallace et al. 1994). The nature of GP lesions has been studied further by diffusion-weighted imaging (DWI) and apparent diffusion coefficient (ADC) mapping (Chu, Jung et al. 2004; Kinoshita, Sugihara et al. 2005). One case report interpreted low ADC values and high intensity GP lesions on DWI as restriction of water diffusion (i.e. cytotoxic edema) (Kinoshita, Sugihara et al. 2005). Vasogenic edema can also be visualized on ADC and DWI as increased signal intensity lesions (Chalela, Wolf et al. 2001). The high signal on DWI is due to the T2 shine-through effect.

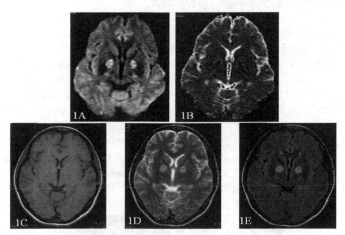

Fig. 1. Magnetic resonance imaging study in the acute stage of carbon monoxide intoxication.

Six days after CO intoxication, a 42-year-old woman with a globus pallidus interna lesion with hyperintensity in diffusion weighted imaging (1A), hypointensity in apparent diffusion coefficient (1B), hypointensity in T1 weighted image (WI) (1C), hyperintensity in T2WI (1D), and hyperintensity in fluid-attenuated inversion recovery (1E).

4.1.2 Imaging features suggesting necrosis

Imaging studies showing cavity-changes by T1 or T2WI often suggest necrosis of the GP (Mendelsohn and Hertzanu 1983; Pulst, Walshe et al. 1983; Ko, Ahn et al. 2004). Autopsies of patients with CO intoxication have confirmed the histology of necrosis and/or neuronal degeneration of the GP (Jones, Lagasse et al. 1994). The pathogenesis of necrosis is believed to be due to edema-induced ischemia or hemorrhage transformation (Chang, Han et al.

1992). Follow-up GP images often show volume shrinkage (Vieregge, Klostermann et al. 1989; Kanaya, Imaizumi et al. 1992).

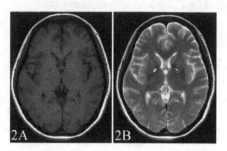

Fig. 2. Magnetic resonance imaging in the delayed stage of carbon monoxide intoxication.

Four years after CO intoxication, a 41-year-old woman with a globus pallidus lesion showed hypointensity in T1 weighted image (T1WI) (2A) and cavity changes with hyperintensity in T2WI (2B).

4.1.3 Imaging features suggesting hemorrhage

Hemorrhage of the GP is seen both in the acute and delayed stages after CO intoxication (Silverman, Brenner et al. 1993; Bianco and Floris 1996), while only one case report has demonstrated putaminal hemorrhage by CT (Schils, Cabay et al. 1999). Temporal sequences in conventional MRI have been noted to be similar to intracranial hemorrhage (Bradley 1993). Hemorrhage may occur within days after CO intoxication with high signal intensity in T1-weighted imaging (T1WI) and T2-weighted imaging (T2WI) (Bianco and Floris 1996). High T1WI and low T2WI signals have been observed up to two months after intoxication, suggesting delayed hemorrhage (Yoshii, Kozuma et al. 1998). One case report described abnormal signals in the GP, with shorter T1 characteristics and longer T2 characteristics suggesting a prior focal hemorrhage three years after CO intoxication (Silverman, Brenner et al. 1993). In one study, widespread multiple pin point hemorrhages in the thalamus and GP were found in 40% of postpartum autopsies (Mehta, Niyogi et al. 2001).

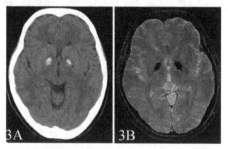

Fig. 3. Computed tomography and gradient echo T2WI after carbon monoxide intoxication.

Two days after CO intoxication, a 57-year-old woman with hemorrhage in the globus pallidus showed hyperdensity in CT (3A) and a follow-up one month later with low signal intensity on gradient echo (3B).

4.1.4 Imaging features suggesting calcification

Calcification of the GP has also been reported in the literature (Illum 1980; Lugaresi, Montagna et al. 1990; Adam, Baulac et al. 2008). The clinical presentations included acute neurological deficits with loss of initiative and slowness of thinking and acting (Adam, Baulac et al. 2008), and delayed neurological deficits with personality changes and akinesia (Lugaresi, Montagna et al. 1990). However one case was free of any neurological sequelae after 48 years of follow-up (Illum 1980).

4.1.5 Functional imaging features suggesting hypometabolism

[18F]fluorodeoxyglucose (FDG) PET has been used to evaluate glucose metabolism activity. Decreased metabolism in the basal ganglion and frontal lobe has been frequently reported (Tengvar, Johansson et al. 2004; Hon, Yeung et al. 2006). The largest series on PET and CO intoxication with basal ganglion lesions included eight patients with their behavioral and MRI patterns (Laplane, Levasseur et al. 1989). Seven patients revealed hypometabolism of the prefrontal cortex in relation to other parts of the brain, leading to a concept of prefrontal-pallidum circuit dysfunction. A functional study using [18F] F-DOPA showed presynaptic dopaminergic deficits in one case with parkinsonism symptoms after CO intoxication (Rissanen, Paavilainen et al. 2010). In this case, normal uptake of [11C] raclopride implicated normal postsynaptic dopaminergic function (Rissanen, Paavilainen et al. 2010).

Single photon emission computed tomography (SPECT) provides perfusion patterns of GM and the basal ganglion (Chang, Liu et al. 2008) with tracers such as 99mTc-ethylcysteinate dimer and 99mTc-Hexamethylpropyleneamine oxime. (99mTc-ECD) brain SPECT is considered to be more sensitive than brain CT for the early detection of hypoperfusion status (Wu, Changlai et al. 2003). In the acute stage, 50% to 85% of the patients with CO intoxication have been reported to have basal ganglion hypoperfusion (Wu, Changlai et al. 2003; Pach, Hubalewska et al. 2004).

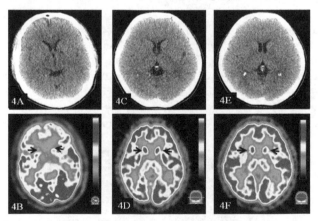

Fig. 4. [18F]fluorodeoxyglucose positron emission tomography (PET) of two patients after CO poisoning.

Two and a half months after CO intoxication, a 33-year-old patient's CT showed low intensity of the globus pallidus (4A) on brain computed tomography (CT) while PET revealed a remarkably reduced uptake of FDG in bilateral striatum (arrows) and thalamus (4B). Five months after CO intoxication, another 36-year-old patient's CT showed no obvious lesions (4C, 4E) while PET revealed normal FDG uptake in bilateral striatum (4D, 4F arrows) and normal thalamic uptake.

4.1.6 Imaging features suggesting pallidoreticular damage

In CO intoxication, pallidoreticular damage specifically targeting the fiber tract along the pallidum and substantia nigra pars reticulata was first described by Auer and Benveniste (Auer and Benveniste 1996). One case report revealed cytotoxic edema of bilateral GP with concurrent substantia nigra pars reticulata involvement in a patient scanned 12 days after CO intoxication (Kinoshita, Sugihara et al. 2005). Two case reports revealed pallidoreticular distribution after one year showing hyperintensities on T2WI and hypointensities on T1WI (Kawanami, Kato et al. 1998; Gandini, Prockop et al. 2002). The authors suggested that these two iron rich regions had selective tissue vulnerability due to the high affinity of CO to heme molecules (Kawanami, Kato et al. 1998; Gandini, Prockop et al. 2002; Kinoshita, Sugihara et al. 2005).

4.2 WM lesions

An increasing number of studies have established that WM lesions are the most common findings in CO intoxication patients, either in the acute phase or in those with delayed neuropsychiatric sequelae (Miura, Mitomo et al. 1985; Chang, Han et al. 1992; Choi, Kim et al. 1993; Lee and Marsden 1994). The largest study included 129 patients, and 33% of them had WM lesions on brain CT (Choi, Kim et al. 1993). In patients with improvements of neurological deficits, resolution of WM changes have also been noted (Klostermann, Vieregge et al. 1993; Matsushita, Takahashi et al. 1996; Pavese, Napolitano et al. 1999). Lesions of the WM area are believed to be associated with clinical outcomes (Miura, Mitomo et al. 1985; Vieregge, Klostermann et al. 1989; Choi, Kim et al. 1993).

4.2.1 Imaging features suggesting WM cytotoxic/vasogenic edema

In a pathological series, cytotoxic and vasogenic edema after CO intoxication were often mixed within three months, and the presence of cytotoxic edema was often noted to be in the acute phase (Ginsberg, Myers et al. 1974; Ginsberg 1985; Thom, Bhopale et al. 2004). The presence of cytotoxic edema lesions can be detected as early as the first day of CO intoxication (Sener 2003) or during the delayed phase (Murata, Kimura et al. 2001; Kim, Chang et al. 2003; Chu, Jung et al. 2004). Imaging features suggesting cytotoxic edema of the

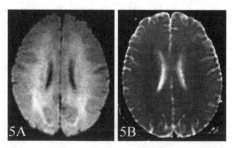

Fig. 5. Diffusion weighted image (5A) and apparent diffusion coefficient (5B) in one case presenting as delayed neuropsychiatric sequelae after carbon monoxide intoxication.

WM area show low ADC values with high DWI intensities, while vasogenic edema shows high signals on both sequences.

One month after CO intoxication, a 41-year-old woman with white matter hyperintensity in DWI (6A) and iso- to low-signal intensity in ADC (6B) indicating cytotoxic edema.

4.2.2 Imaging features suggesting WM demyelination or axonopathy

The prevalence of imaging features suggesting WM demyelination or axonopathy range from 12% to 100% in CO intoxication (Chang, Han et al. 1992; Parkinson, Hopkins et al. 2002). The largest MRI study focusing on WM included 73 patients scanned on day 1, 2 weeks and 6 months after CO intoxication (Parkinson, Hopkins et al. 2002). Semiquantitative scores were rated on bilateral periventricular and centrum semiovale areas (Parkinson, Hopkins et al. 2002). Twelve percent of the patients had WM hyperintensities on T2WI on day 1 (Parkinson, Hopkins et al. 2002) with significantly more periventricular, but not centrum semiovale distributions as compared with age-matched controls. The WM lesions in the CO group did not change from day 1 to 6 months follow-up, however the hyperintensities in the centrum semiovale were related to worse cognitive performance. The study revealed no correlation between WM hyperintensities and carboxyhemoglobin level, or duration of CO exposure at any of the three scan times (Parkinson, Hopkins et al. 2002).

Hyperintensities in T2WI and fluid-attenuated inversion recovery (FLAIR) and hypointensities in T1WI often suggest WM demyelination or axonopathy (Chang, Han et al. 1992; Pavese, Napolitano et al. 1999; Parkinson, Hopkins et al. 2002). From a pathological perspective, myelin damage is constant and can vary from discrete perivascular lesions to extensive periventricular demyelination and/or axonal destruction (Funata, Okeda et al. 1982; Prockop and Chichkova 2007). An autopsy study after CO intoxication showed that diffuse WM hyperintensities reflected apoptosis of oligodendrocytes (Akaiwa, Hozumi et al. 2002). Another autopsy study of brains three days after CO intoxication revealed a normal cortex and injured WM with disrupted myelin and pyknotic oligodendroglia, whilst the axons, astrocytes and capillaries were normal (Foncin and Le Beau 1978).

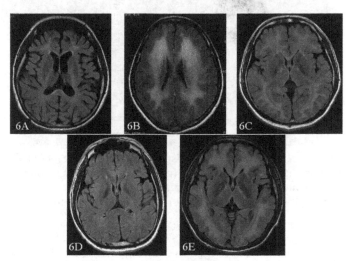

Fig. 6. A wide spectrum of white matter hyperintensities in fluid-attenuated inversion recovery after carbon monoxide intoxication with cognitive deficits.

Focal white matter hyperintensities (WMHs) over bilateral frontal horns in a 29-year-old woman, two years after CO exposure (6A). Diffuse and confluent WMHs in a 42-year-old woman, one and a half months after CO exposure (6B). Prominent subcortical U fiber hyperintensity with globus pallidus hyperintensity in a 35-year-old man, one and a half months after CO exposure (6C). A 31-year-old woman presented in a confused state without obvious WMHs four days after CO intoxication (6D). Extensive subcortical WMHs with globus pallidus hypointensity two years later (6E).

A study by Weaver (Weaver, Valentine et al. 2007) suggested that cognitive sequelae at six weeks benefited from hyperbaric oxygen (HBO) in patients aged 36 years and older, or who were exposed to CO for a duration of 24 hours or more. Two studies explored changes of fractional anisotropy (FA) in CO intoxication after HBO. Both studies revealed lower FA values in the patient group compared to that of controls three months after HBO (Lo, Chen et al. 2007; Chang, Lee et al. 2009). The mini-mental state examination scores completely recovered after three months of follow-up in all evaluated patients in one study (Lo, Chen et al. 2007), while another study showed that HBO treatment may not reverse the damage caused by CO intoxication (Chang, Lee et al. 2009). A longitudinal study used diffusion tensor imaging (DTI) and compared the changes of diffusion measurements in CO intoxication patients including mean diffusivity, axial diffusivity and radial diffusivity with follow-up scans three months and 10 months later. Extensive changes found in the FA maps at both three and 10 months in the CO group were attributed to initial increments of radial diffusivities, while a decrement of axial diffusivities were found at 10 months follow-up (Chang, Chang et al. 2010). The study suggested that changes in diffusion parameters might reflect WM demyelination at three months followed by subsequent axonopathy.

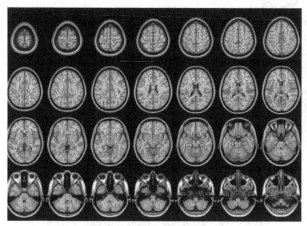

Fig. 7. An example of Tract Based Spatial Statistics with decreased Fractional Anisotropy (FA) (blue) overlaid on the mean FA skeleton (green) in a sample of carbon monoxide intoxication (n=30) as compared with age-matched controls. Diffuse white matter damage was detected including the subcortical areas, brain stem and cerebellum.

White matter insults after CO intoxication lead to transient or permanent injuries, which consequently lead to decreased WM volumes. Diffusion indices including mean diffusivity, axial diffusivity and radial diffusivity reflect WM injuries earlier than volume reduction, while the major regions of WM atrophy in one study were in the periventricular WM areas (Chang, Chang et al. 2010).

4.2.3 Imaging features suggesting WM hemorrhage

In the acute phase, petechial hemorrhages of the WM, particularly the corpus callosum, are common (Funata, Okeda et al. 1982; Finelli and DiMario 2004; Weaver and Hopkins 2005). Gradient echo T2WI uses a shorter repetition time than spin-echo T2WI and can detect metal material such as ferritin and ferritin-containing substances such as hemosiderin, thus detecting hemorrhages and microbleeds (Atlas, Grossman et al. 1988; Bradley 1993). Susceptibility-weighted imaging (SWI) is a heavy T2*-weighted gradient-recalled 3-D fast low-angle shot sequence with full flow compensation in all three directions (Sehgal, Delproposto et al. 2005). Microhemorrhages have been reported in patients with CO intoxication with the complimentary information provided by gradient echo T2WI and SWI (Finelli and DiMario 2004; Weaver and Hopkins 2005). In gradient echo T2WI, hemorrhages along the nerve fibers are distributed predominantly over the posterior WM (Finelli and DiMario 2004).

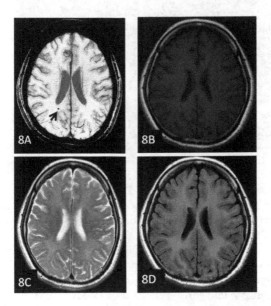

Fig. 8. Microhemorrhage shown on susceptibility-weighted imaging.

Four months after carbon monoxide intoxication, a 53-year-old woman with a low signal intensity lesion on susceptibility-weighted imaging (8A, arrow) suggesting microhemorrhage of white matter which was invisible on T1 (8B), T2 (8C), and fluid-attenuated inversion recovery (8D).

4.3 Cortex
4.3.1 Imaging features suggesting cortical injury and atrophy

Pure cortical involvement without concurrent WM lesions in CO intoxication is not common (Choi, Kim et al. 1993). Using DWI, imaging features suggesting cortical cytotoxic edema were described in bilateral posterior temporal lobes and bilateral occipital lobes in one patient, bilateral posterior temporal lobes and left parietal lobe in another patient, and right frontal, temporal and parietal lobes in another (Hon, Yeung et al. 2006). Hippocampal involvement has been linked with anterograde amnesia, with pathological findings of necrosis and apoptosis (Uemura, Harada et al. 2001; Mahmoud, Mestour et al. 2009).

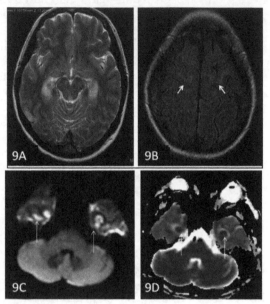

Fig. 9. Cortical injuries after CO intoxication.

Four days after CO intoxication, a 37-year-old woman with hyperintensities in bilateral hippocampi in a T2-weighted image (9A). Six days after CO intoxication, a 42-year-old woman with hyperintensities in bilateral superior frontal gyrus in fluid-attenuated inversion recovery (9B). Another 28-year-old female five days after CO intoxication showed bilateral medial temporal region high signal intensity lesions (9C, diffusion weighted image, arrows) with corresponding low intensity lesions on apparent diffusion coefficient map (9D, arrows) suggesting cytotoxic edema.

Cortical volume reduction is a late consequence of CO intoxication. Significant ventricle and sulcus dilatation in comparison with the controls were found in all 34 patients evaluated during the chronic phase of CO intoxication in a study by Kono et al. (Kono, Kono et al. 1983), with a 19-year interval from CO intoxication. In a case report several months after CO intoxication, brain MRI revealed bilateral atrophy of lateral temporal lobes and the clinical deficits included severe cognitive impairment and a transient Klüver-Bucy-like behavior (Muller and Gruber 2001). Voxel based morphometry (Ashburner and Friston 2001) enables the quantification of grey and WM volume changes between groups. In one study using voxel based morphometry, no significant differences in the GM were found in the patient group compared to age-matched controls ten months after CO intoxication (Chang, Chang et al. 2010), while atrophy of WM was evident in the periventricular areas. In another study of 13 patients with brain MRI studies 25 years after CO poisoning, the parieto-occipital region was most frequently involved, and six of the 13 patients had dilated temporal horns (Uchino, Hasuo et al. 1994).

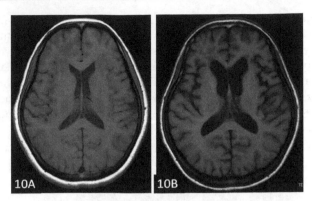

Fig. 10. Cortical atrophy after carbon monoxide intoxication revealed in T1-weighted image.

A 47-year-old woman with rapid cortical atrophy after CO intoxication as revealed in T1WI three months (9A) and 20 months (9B) after CO exposure.

4.3.2 Imaging features suggesting cortical hemorrhage

Hemorrhage in the cortical areas has also been reported in CO intoxication. One 28-year-old man had achromatopsia five months after CO intoxication (Fine and Parker 1996). Brain MRI revealed hemorrhage in the bilateral temporal and occipital lobes (Fine and Parker 1996). Another case demonstrated a 7-year-old boy who had generalized convulsions, coma and right hemiparesis on the day of CO intoxication (El Khashab and Nejat 2009). Brain CT on the same day revealed a left temporal hemorrhage (El Khashab and Nejat 2009). Micro-vascular impairment and brain reperfusion injury were the suspected pathogenetic mechanisms causing the damage (El Khashab and Nejat 2009).

4.3.3 Imaging features suggesting cortical hypoperfusion and hypometabolism

Six studies have reported SPECT findings in the evaluation of cortical blood flow after CO intoxication (Choi, Lee et al. 1992; Choi, Kim et al. 1995; Watanabe, Nohara et al. 2002; Pach, Hubalewska et al. 2004; Huang SH, Chang Chiung Chih2 et al. 2005; Pach, Urbanik et al. 2005). The largest one included 20 cases with 85% of the patients showing hypoperfusion over the frontal-parietal cortex (Pach, Hubalewska et al. 2004). In a study on follow-up SPECT in patients with CO intoxication, six of seven patients had improvement of hypoperfusion throughout the cortex, while their clinical conditions also improved concomitantly (Choi, Kim et al. 1995). In a comparison between those with delayed neuropsychiatric sequelae and those without sequelae, significant hypoperfusion was noted over bilateral frontal lobes, bilateral insula and right temporal lobe in patients with delayed neuropsychiatric sequelae, whilst only bilateral frontal lobe hypoperfusion was noted in those without neuropsychiatric sequelae (Watanabe, Nohara et al. 2002).

To date, there have only been a limited number of reports on [18F] FDG-PET in the evaluation of metabolic dysfunction in the cortical areas of patients with CO intoxication (Tengvar, Johansson et al. 2004; Senol, Yildiz et al. 2009). One case report of a middle-aged man revealed hypometabolism of bilateral frontal lobes and anterior cingulate cortices (Tengvar, Johansson et al. 2004), and his neurological deficit of akinetic mutism was regarded as the consequence of the hypometabolism state of the involved regions (Tengvar, Johansson et al. 2004). In a study of serial [18F] FDG-PET follow-up scans, persistent hypometabolism of bilateral frontal lobes was found in a 29-year-old woman who demonstrated impaired responsiveness to stimuli for one year after CO poisoning (Shimosegawa, Hatazawa et al. 1992). In another case report on a 21-year-old woman who had coma, seizure and cortical blindness within three days after CO poisoning, the neurological deficit of cortical blindness remained. A subsequent [18F] FDG-PET four years later still showed hypometabolism of bilateral posterior temporal and occipital lobes (Senol, Yildiz et al. 2009).

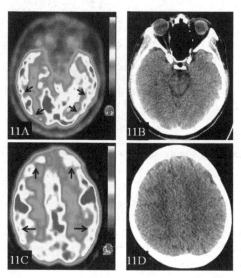

Fig. 11. [18F]fluorodeoxyglucose positron emission tomography of two patients after carbon monoxide intoxication.

One month after CO intoxication, a patient's (age: 30) PET revealed reduced uptake of FDG in bilateral temporal and occipital lobes (11A, arrows), while the brain CT (11B) did not detect any hypodense lesions over the corresponding areas. One month after CO intoxication, another patient's (age: 58) PET revealed reduced uptake of FDG in bilateral frontal and parietal lobes (11C, arrows) with negative findings on the CT scan (11D).

5. Nerves and muscles

Although peripheral neuropathy has been reported in CO intoxication (Choi 1982), only electrophysiological studies but not neuroimaging studies are available (Choi 1982).
Skeletal muscle injuries have been reported in CO intoxication. In one case report, skeletal muscle MRI was performed showing hyperintensity lesions in T2WI of the thigh muscles three months after CO intoxication (Chen, Huang et al. 2010). The muscle biopsy in this patient proved the diagnosis of heterotopic ossification selectively involving the iliopsoas, the tensor fascia lata, rectus femoris, sartorius and quadriceps muscles. Another study using Tc99m-sestamibi SPECT to evaluate the skeletal muscular injuries in 25 patients after CO intoxication showed decreased uptake in the patient group as compared with the controls (Huang, Chang et al. 2011). The low uptake was related to mitochondrial dysfunction.

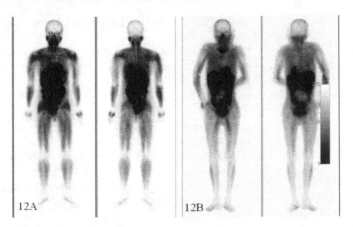

Fig. 12. Planar view of technetium-99m-sestamibi (^{99m}Tc-MIBI) in the evaluation of muscle injury in a patient with carbon monoxide intoxication.

Compared with muscle ^{99m}Tc-MIBI of a normal control (12A), a 59-year-old man showed decreased ^{99m}Tc-MIBI uptake in the thigh muscles two months after CO intoxication (12B).

6. Conclusion

Damage to the neurological system after CO intoxication includes the basal ganglia, cerebral WM, cortex and muscles. The mechanisms of damage can be identified by MRI and correlated with clinical features. Apart from MRI, functional imaging can provide information about brain perfusion and metabolism in CO intoxication. With muscle MIBI, mitochondrial function can be assessed in patients with CO intoxication.

7. Acknowledgments

The study was supported by grants CMRPG 880951, 890871 and 860171 from Kaohsiung Chang Gung Memorial Hospital.

8. References

Adam, J., M. Baulac, et al. (2008). Behavioral symptoms after pallido-nigral lesions: a clinico-pathological case. *Neurocase* 14, 2: pp. 125-130.

Akaiwa, Y., I. Hozumi, et al. (2002). [A case suspected of acute gas poisoning by carbon monoxide (CO), presenting with progressive diffuse leukoencephalopathy associated with marked brain edema]. *No To Shinkei* 54, 6: pp. 493-497.

Arbuthnott, K. and J. Frank (2000). Trail making test, part B as a measure of executive control: validation using a set-switching paradigm. *J Clin Exp Neuropsychol* 22, 4: pp. 518-528.

Ashburner, J. and K. J. Friston (2001). Why voxel-based morphometry should be used. *Neuroimage* 14, 6: pp. 1238-1243.

Atlas, S. W., R. I. Grossman, et al. (1988). Calcified intracranial lesions: detection with gradient-echo-acquisition rapid MR imaging. *AJR Am J Roentgenol* 150, 6: pp. 1383-1389.

Auer, R. N. and H. Benveniste (1996). Carbon monoxide poisoning *Greenfield's neuropathology* 1: pp. 275-276.

Bianco, F. and R. Floris (1996). MRI appearances consistent with haemorrhagic infarction as an early manifestation of carbon monoxide poisoning. *Neuroradiology* 38 Suppl 1: pp. S70-72.

Boone, K. B. (2000). The Boston Qualitative Scoring System for the Rey-Osterrieth Complex Figure. *J Clin Exp Neuropsychol* 22, 3: pp. 430-434.

Bradley, W. G., Jr. (1993). MR appearance of hemorrhage in the brain. *Radiology* 189, 1: pp. 15-26.

Chalela, J. A., R. L. Wolf, et al. (2001). MRI identification of early white matter injury in anoxic-ischemic encephalopathy. *Neurology* 56, 4: pp. 481-485.

Chang, C. C., W. N. Chang, et al. (2010). Longitudinal study of carbon monoxide intoxication by diffusion tensor imaging with neuropsychiatric correlation. *J Psychiatry Neurosci* 35, 2: pp. 115-125.

Chang, C. C., Y. C. Lee, et al. (2009). Damage of white matter tract correlated with neuropsychological deficits in carbon monoxide intoxication after hyperbaric oxygen therapy. *J Neurotrauma* 26, 8: pp. 1263-1270.

Chang, C. C., J. S. Liu, et al. (2008). (99m)Tc-ethyl cysteinate dimer brain SPECT findings in early stage of dementia with Lewy bodies and Parkinson's disease patients: a correlation with neuropsychological tests. *Eur J Neurol* 15, 1: pp. 61-65.

Chang, K. H., M. H. Han, et al. (1992). Delayed encephalopathy after acute carbon monoxide intoxication: MR imaging features and distribution of cerebral white matter lesions. *Radiology* 184, 1: pp. 117-122.

Chen, S. H., S. H. Huang, et al. (2010). Heterotopic ossification as a complication of carbon monoxide intoxication. *Acta Neurol Taiwan* 19, 2: pp. 120-124.

Choi, I. S. (1982). A clinical study of peripheral neuropathy in carbon monoxide intoxication. *Yonsei Med J* 23, 2: pp. 174-177.

Choi, I. S. (1983). Delayed neurologic sequelae in carbon monoxide intoxication. *Arch Neurol* 40, 7: pp. 433-435.

Choi, I. S. (2001). Carbon monoxide poisoning: systemic manifestations and complications. *J Korean Med Sci* 16, 3: pp. 253-261.

Choi, I. S., S. K. Kim, et al. (1993). Evaluation of outcome after acute carbon monoxide poisoning by brain CT. *J Korean Med Sci* 8, 1: pp. 78-83.

Choi, I. S., S. K. Kim, et al. (1995). Evaluation of outcome of delayed neurologic sequelae after carbon monoxide poisoning by technetium-99m hexamethylpropylene amine oxime brain single photon emission computed tomography. *Eur Neurol* 35, 3: pp. 137-142.

Choi, I. S. and M. S. Lee (1993). Early hypoperfusion of technetium-99m hexamethylprophylene amine oxime brain single photon emission computed tomography in a patient with carbon monoxide poisoning. *Eur Neurol* 33, 6: pp. 461-464.

Choi, I. S., M. S. Lee, et al. (1992). Technetium-99m HM-PAO SPECT in patients with delayed neurologic sequelae after carbon monoxide poisoning. *J Korean Med Sci* 7, 1: pp. 11-18.

Chu, K., K. H. Jung, et al. (2004). Diffusion-weighted MRI and 99mTc-HMPAO SPECT in delayed relapsing type of carbon monoxide poisoning: evidence of delayed cytotoxic edema. *Eur Neurol* 51, 2: pp. 98-103.

Cronholm, B. and G. Viding (1956). [Digit span as a test of immediate memory]. *Nord Med* 56, 45: pp. 1612-1614.

Cummings, J. L., M. Mega, et al. (1994). The Neuropsychiatric Inventory: comprehensive assessment of psychopathology in dementia. *Neurology* 44, 12: pp. 2308-2314.

Dorken, H., Jr. and G. C. Greenbloom (1953). Psychological investigation of senile dementia. II. The Wechsler-Bellevue adult intelligence scale. *Geriatrics* 8, 6: pp. 324-333.

El Khashab, M. and F. Nejat (2009). Hemorrhagic cerebral infarction in carbon monoxide poisoning: a case report. *Cases J* 2: pp. 96.

Ernst, A. and J. D. Zibrak (1998). Carbon monoxide poisoning. *N Engl J Med* 339, 22: pp. 1603-1608.

Ferrier, D., C. J. Wallace, et al. (1994). Magnetic resonance features in carbon monoxide poisoning. *Can Assoc Radiol J* 45, 6: pp. 466-468.

Fine, R. D. and G. D. Parker (1996). Disturbance of central vision after carbon monoxide poisoning. *Aust N Z J Ophthalmol* 24, 2: pp. 137-141.

Finelli, P. F. and F. J. DiMario, Jr. (2004). Hemorrhagic infarction in white matter following acute carbon monoxide poisoning. *Neurology* 63, 6: pp. 1102-1104.

Folstein, M. F., S. E. Folstein, et al. (1975). "Mini-mental state". A practical method for grading the cognitive state of patients for the clinician. *J Psychiatr Res* 12, 3: pp. 189-198.

Foncin, J. F. and J. Le Beau (1978). [Myelinopathy due to carbon monoxyde poisoning. A study in ultrastructural neuropathology (author's transl)]. *Acta Neuropathol* 43, 1-2: pp. 153-159.

Funata, N., R. Okeda, et al. (1982). Electron microscopic observations of experimental carbon monoxide encephalopathy in the acute phase. *Acta Pathol Jpn* 32, 2: pp. 219-229.

Gandini, C., L. D. Prockop, et al. (2002). Pallidoreticular-rubral brain damage on magnetic resonance imaging after carbon monoxide poisoning. *J Neuroimaging* 12, 2: pp. 102-103.

Gieseking, C., A. Lubin, et al. (1956). The relation of brain injury and visual perception to block design rotation. *J Consult Psychol* 20, 4: pp. 275-280.

Ginsberg, M. D. (1985). Carbon monoxide intoxication: clinical features, neuropathology and mechanisms of injury. *J Toxicol Clin Toxicol* 23, 4-6: pp. 281-288.

Ginsberg, M. D., R. E. Myers, et al. (1974). Experimental carbon monoxide encephalopathy in the primate. II. Clinical aspects, neuropathology, and physiologic correlation. *Arch Neurol* 30, 3: pp. 209-216.

Gorman, D., A. Drewry, et al. (2003). The clinical toxicology of carbon monoxide. *Toxicology* 187, 1: pp. 25-38.

Gotoh, M., H. Kuyama, et al. (1993). Sequential changes in MR images of the brain in acute carbon monoxide poisoning. *Comput Med Imaging Graph* 17, 1: pp. 55-59.

Gutierrez, L. G., A. Rovira, et al. CT and MR in non-neonatal hypoxic-ischemic encephalopathy: radiological findings with pathophysiological correlations. *Neuroradiology* 52, 11: pp. 949-976.

Handa, P. K. and D. Y. Tai (2005). Carbon monoxide poisoning: a five year review at Tan Tock Seng Hospital, Singapore. *Ann Acad Med Singapore* 34, 10: pp. 611-614.

Hon, K. L., W. L. Yeung, et al. (2006). Neurologic and radiologic manifestations of three girls surviving acute carbon monoxide poisoning. *J Child Neurol* 21, 9: pp. 737-741.

Hopkins, R. O., M. A. Fearing, et al. (2006). Basal ganglia lesions following carbon monoxide poisoning. *Brain Inj* 20, 3: pp. 273-281.

Hsiao, C. L., H. C. Kuo, et al. (2004). Delayed encephalopathy after carbon monoxide intoxication--long-term prognosis and correlation of clinical manifestations and neuroimages. *Acta Neurol Taiwan* 13, 2: pp. 64-70.

Huang SH, Chang Chiung Chih2, et al. (2005). Technetium-99m ECD Brain Single Photon Emission Computed Tomography in a Patient with Delayed Neurological Sequelae after Carbon Monoxide Poisoning. *Ann Nucl Med Sci* 18: pp. 57-61.

Huang, S. H., W. N. Chang, et al. (2011). Tc99m-sestamibi thigh SPECT/CT images for noninvasive assessment of skeletal muscle injury in carbon monoxide intoxication with clinical and pathological correlation. *Clin Nucl Med* 36, 3: pp. 199-205.

Hurley, R. A., R. O. Hopkins, et al. (2001). Applications of functional imaging to carbon monoxide poisoning. *J Neuropsychiatry Clin Neurosci* 13, 2: pp. 157-160.

Ide, T. and Y. Kamijo (2008). Myelin basic protein in cerebrospinal fluid: a predictive marker of delayed encephalopathy from carbon monoxide poisoning. *Am J Emerg Med* 26, 8: pp. 908-912.

Illum, F. (1980). Calcification of the basal ganglia following carbon monoxide poisoning. *Neuroradiology* 19, 4: pp. 213-214.

Jiang, J. and I. Tyssebotn (1997). Cerebrospinal fluid pressure changes after acute carbon monoxide poisoning and therapeutic effects of normobaric and hyperbaric oxygen in conscious rats. *Undersea Hyperb Med* 24, 4: pp. 245-254.

Jones, J. S., J. Lagasse, et al. (1994). Computed tomographic findings after acute carbon monoxide poisoning. *Am J Emerg Med* 12, 4: pp. 448-451.

Kamijo, Y., K. Soma, et al. (2007). Recurrent myelin basic protein elevation in cerebrospinal fluid as a predictive marker of delayed encephalopathy after carbon monoxide poisoning. *Am J Emerg Med* 25, 4: pp. 483-485.

Kamizato, E., K. Yoshitome, et al. (2009). Factors affecting the choice of suicide method in Okayama: a database analysis from a forensic perspective. *Acta Med Okayama* 63, 4: pp. 177-186.

Kanaya, N., H. Imaizumi, et al. (1992). The utility of MRI in acute stage of carbon monoxide poisoning. *Intensive Care Med* 18, 6: pp. 371-372.

Kao, C. H., D. Z. Hung, et al. (1998). HMPAO brain SPECT in acute carbon monoxide poisoning. *J Nucl Med* 39, 5: pp. 769-772.

Katafuchi, Y., T. Nishimi, et al. (1985). Cortical blindness in acute carbon monoxide poisoning. *Brain Dev* 7, 5: pp. 516-519.

Kawanami, T., T. Kato, et al. (1998). The pallidoreticular pattern of brain damage on MRI in a patient with carbon monoxide poisoning. *J Neurol Neurosurg Psychiatry* 64, 2: pp. 282.

Kim, J. H., K. H. Chang, et al. (2003). Delayed encephalopathy of acute carbon monoxide intoxication: diffusivity of cerebral white matter lesions. *AJNR Am J Neuroradiol* 24, 8: pp. 1592-1597.

Kinoshita, T., S. Sugihara, et al. (2005). Pallidoreticular damage in acute carbon monoxide poisoning: diffusion-weighted MR imaging findings. *AJNR Am J Neuroradiol* 26, 7: pp. 1845-1848.

Klostermann, W., P. Vieregge, et al. (1993). [Carbon monoxide poisoning: the importance of computed and magnetic resonance tomographic cranial findings for the clinical picture and follow-up]. *Rofo* 159, 4: pp. 361-367.

Kluge, H. (1991). Calcium and hypoxic/ischemic brain damage--some critical and conceptual remarks. *Exp Pathol* 42, 4: pp. 239-244.

Ko, S. B., T. B. Ahn, et al. (2004). A case of adult onset tic disorder following carbon monoxide intoxication. *Can J Neurol Sci* 31, 2: pp. 268-270.

Kono, E., R. Kono, et al. (1983). Computerized tomographies of 34 patients at the chronic stage of acute carbon monoxide poisoning. *Arch Psychiatr Nervenkr* 233, 4: pp. 271-278.

Kumar, R., S. Prakash, et al. (2010). Breath carbon monoxide concentration in cigarette and bidi smokers in India. *Indian J Chest Dis Allied Sci* 52, 1: pp. 19-24.

Kwon, O. Y., S. P. Chung, et al. (2004). Delayed postanoxic encephalopathy after carbon monoxide poisoning. *Emerg Med J* 21, 2: pp. 250-251.

Laplane, D., M. Levasseur, et al. (1989). Obsessive-compulsive and other behavioural changes with bilateral basal ganglia lesions. A neuropsychological, magnetic resonance imaging and positron tomography study. *Brain* 112 (Pt 3): pp. 699-725.

Lee, D. T., K. P. Chan, et al. (2002). Burning charcoal: a novel and contagious method of suicide in Asia. *Arch Gen Psychiatry* 59, 3: pp. 293-294.

Lee, E. and C. M. Leung (2009). High-risk groups for charcoal-burning suicide attempt in Hong Kong, China, 2004. *J Clin Psychiatry* 70, 3: pp. 431.

Lee, M. S. and C. D. Marsden (1994). Neurological sequelae following carbon monoxide poisoning clinical course and outcome according to the clinical types and brain computed tomography scan findings. *Mov Disord* 9, 5: pp. 550-558.

Lin, J. J. and T. H. Lu (2008). High-risk groups for charcoal-burning suicide in Taiwan, 2001-2005. *J Clin Psychiatry* 69, 9: pp. 1499-1501.

Lo, C. P., S. Y. Chen, et al. (2007). Diffusion-tensor MR imaging for evaluation of the efficacy of hyperbaric oxygen therapy in patients with delayed neuropsychiatric syndrome caused by carbon monoxide inhalation. *Eur J Neurol* 14, 7: pp. 777-782.

Lo, C. P., S. Y. Chen, et al. (2007). Brain injury after acute carbon monoxide poisoning: early and late complications. *AJR Am J Roentgenol* 189, 4: pp. W205-211.

Lugaresi, A., P. Montagna, et al. (1990). 'Psychic akinesia' following carbon monoxide poisoning. *Eur Neurol* 30, 3: pp. 167-169.

MacMillan, V. (1975). Regional cerebral blood flow of the rat in acute carbon monoxide intoxication. *Can J Physiol Pharmacol* 53, 4: pp. 644-650.

Mahmoud, O., M. Mestour, et al. (2009). [Carbon monoxide intoxication and anterograde amnesia]. *Encephale* 35, 3: pp. 281-285.

Marilena, G. (1997). New physiological importance of two classic residual products: carbon monoxide and bilirubin. *Biochem Mol Med* 61, 2: pp. 136-142.

Matsushita, H., S. Takahashi, et al. (1996). [MR imaging of carbon monoxide intoxication: evaluation of 13 cases to discuss the relation between MR findings and clinical course]. *Nippon Igaku Hoshasen Gakkai Zasshi* 56, 13: pp. 948-954.

Mehta, S. R., M. Niyogi, et al. (2001). Carbon monoxide poisoning. *J Assoc Physicians India* 49: pp. 622-625.

Mendelsohn, D. B. and Y. Hertzanu (1983). Carbon monoxide poisoning. Report of a case with 1-year computed tomographic follow-up. *S Afr Med J* 64, 19: pp. 751-752.

Meredith, T. and A. Vale (1988). Carbon monoxide poisoning. *Br Med J (Clin Res Ed)* 296, 6615: pp. 77-79.

Miura, T., M. Mitomo, et al. (1985). CT of the brain in acute carbon monoxide intoxication: characteristic features and prognosis. *AJNR Am J Neuroradiol* 6, 5: pp. 739-742.

Morris, J. C. (1997). Clinical dementia rating: a reliable and valid diagnostic and staging measure for dementia of the Alzheimer type. *Int Psychogeriatr* 9 Suppl 1: pp. 173-176; discussion 177-178.

Muller, N. G. and O. Gruber (2001). High-resolution magnetic resonance imaging reveals symmetric bitemporal cortical necrosis after carbon monoxide intoxication. *J Neuroimaging* 11, 3: pp. 322-325.

Murata, T., H. Kimura, et al. (2001). Neuronal damage in the interval form of CO poisoning determined by serial diffusion weighted magnetic resonance imaging plus 1H-magnetic resonance spectroscopy. *J Neurol Neurosurg Psychiatry* 71, 2: pp. 250-253.

O'Donnell, P., P. J. Buxton, et al. (2000). The magnetic resonance imaging appearances of the brain in acute carbon monoxide poisoning. *Clin Radiol* 55, 4: pp. 273-280.

Okeda, R., T. Matsuo, et al. (1987). Regional cerebral blood flow of acute carbon monoxide poisoning in cats. *Acta Neuropathol* 72, 4: pp. 389-393.

Opeskin, K. and O. H. Drummer (1994). Delayed death following carbon monoxide poisoning. A case report. *Am J Forensic Med Pathol* 15, 1: pp. 36-39.

Otubo, S., Y. Shirakawa, et al. (2007). [Magnetic resonance imaging could predict delayed encephalopathy after acute carbon monoxide intoxication]. *Chudoku Kenkyu* 20, 3: pp. 253-261.

Pach, D., A. Hubalewska, et al. (2004). Evaluation of regional cerebral perfusion using 99mTc-HmPAO single photon emission tomography (SPET) in carbon monoxide acutely poisoned patients. *Przegl Lek* 61, 4: pp. 217-221.

Pach, D., A. Urbanik, et al. (2005). (99m)Tc-HmPAO single photon emission tomography, magnetic resonance proton spectroscopy and neuropsychological testing in evaluation of carbon monoxide neurotoxicity. *Przegl Lek* 62, 6: pp. 441-445.

Park, S. and I. S. Choi (2004). Chorea following acute carbon monoxide poisoning. *Yonsei Med J* 45, 3: pp. 363-366.

Parkinson, R. B., R. O. Hopkins, et al. (2002). White matter hyperintensities and neuropsychological outcome following carbon monoxide poisoning. *Neurology* 58, 10: pp. 1525-1532.

Pavese, N., A. Napolitano, et al. (1999). Clinical outcome and magnetic resonance imaging of carbon monoxide intoxication. A long-term follow-up study. *Ital J Neurol Sci* 20, 3: pp. 171-178.

Penney, D. G. (1990). Acute carbon monoxide poisoning: animal models: a review. *Toxicology* 62, 2: pp. 123-160.

Piantadosi, C. A. (2002). Carbon monoxide poisoning. *N Engl J Med* 347, 14: pp. 1054-1055.

Piantadosi, C. A., L. Tatro, et al. (1995). Hydroxyl radical production in the brain after CO hypoxia in rats. *Free Radic Biol Med* 18, 3: pp. 603-609.

Piantadosi, C. A., J. Zhang, et al. (1997). Production of hydroxyl radical in the hippocampus after CO hypoxia or hypoxic hypoxia in the rat. *Free Radic Biol Med* 22, 4: pp. 725-732.

Piantadosi, C. A., J. Zhang, et al. (1997). Apoptosis and delayed neuronal damage after carbon monoxide poisoning in the rat. *Exp Neurol* 147, 1: pp. 103-114.

Prockop, L. D. and R. I. Chichkova (2007). Carbon monoxide intoxication: an updated review. *J Neurol Sci* 262, 1-2: pp. 122-130.

Pulst, S. M., T. M. Walshe, et al. (1983). Carbon monoxide poisoning with features of Gilles de la Tourette's syndrome. *Arch Neurol* 40, 7: pp. 443-444.

Quattrocolo, G., D. Leotta, et al. (1987). A case of cortical blindness due to carbon monoxide poisoning. *Ital J Neurol Sci* 8, 1: pp. 57-58.

Ramsey, P. (2001). Delayed postpartum hemorrhage: a rare presentation of carbon monoxide poisoning. *Am J Obstet Gynecol. 2001 Jan;* 184, 2: pp. 2.

Raub, J. A. and V. A. Benignus (2002). Carbon monoxide and the nervous system. *Neurosci Biobehav Rev* 26, 8: pp. 925-940.

Rissanen, E., T. Paavilainen, et al. (2010). Carbon monoxide poisoning-induced nigrostriatal dopaminergic dysfunction detected using positron emission tomography (PET). *Neurotoxicology* 31, 4: pp. 403-407.

Rosen, W. G., R. C. Mohs, et al. (1984). A new rating scale for Alzheimer's disease. *Am J Psychiatry* 141, 11: pp. 1356-1364.

Rudel, R. G. and M. B. Denckla (1974). Relation of forward and backward digit repetition to neurological impairment in children with learning disabilities. *Neuropsychologia* 12, 1: pp. 109-118.

Schils, F., J. E. Cabay, et al. (1999). Unusual CT and MRI appearance of carbon monoxide poisoning. *JBR-BTR* 82, 1: pp. 13-15.

Schwartz, A., M. Hennerici, et al. (1985). Delayed choreoathetosis following acute carbon monoxide poisoning. *Neurology* 35, 1: pp. 98-99.

Sehgal, V., Z. Delproposto, et al. (2005). Clinical applications of neuroimaging with susceptibility-weighted imaging. *J Magn Reson Imaging* 22, 4: pp. 439-450.

Sener, R. N. (2003). Acute carbon monoxide poisoning: diffusion MR imaging findings. *AJNR Am J Neuroradiol* 24, 7: pp. 1475-1477.

Senol, M. G., S. Yildiz, et al. (2009). Carbon monoxide-induced cortical visual loss: treatment with hyperbaric oxygen four years later. *Med Princ Pract* 18, 1: pp. 67-69.

Sesay, M., A. M. Bidabe, et al. (1996). Regional cerebral blood flow measurements with Xenon-CT in the prediction of delayed encephalopathy after carbon monoxide intoxication. *Acta Neurol Scand Suppl* 166: pp. 22-27.

Sherman, A. R. and S. J. Blatt (1968). WAIS digit span, digit symbol, and vocabulary performance as a function of prior experiences of success and failure. *J Consult Clin Psychol* 32, 4: pp. 407-412.

Shimosegawa, E., J. Hatazawa, et al. (1992). Cerebral blood flow and glucose metabolism measurements in a patient surviving one year after carbon monoxide intoxication. *J Nucl Med* 33, 9: pp. 1696-1698.

Silver, D. A., M. Cross, et al. (1996). Computed tomography of the brain in acute carbon monoxide poisoning. *Clin Radiol* 51, 7: pp. 480-483.

Silverman, C. S., J. Brenner, et al. (1993). Hemorrhagic necrosis and vascular injury in carbon monoxide poisoning: MR demonstration. *AJNR Am J Neuroradiol* 14, 1: pp. 168-170.

Sung, P. S., C. Y. Yu, et al. (2010). Asymmetrical delayed encephalopathy after acute CO intoxication: a case report. *Neurotoxicology* 31, 1: pp. 161-163.

Tengvar, C., B. Johansson, et al. (2004). Frontal lobe and cingulate cortical metabolic dysfunction in acquired akinetic mutism: a PET study of the interval form of carbon monoxide poisoning. *Brain Inj* 18, 6: pp. 615-625.

Thom, S. R., V. M. Bhopale, et al. (2004). Delayed neuropathology after carbon monoxide poisoning is immune-mediated. *Proc Natl Acad Sci U S A* 101, 37: pp. 13660-13665.

Tibbles, P. M. and P. L. Perrotta (1994). Treatment of carbon monoxide poisoning: a critical review of human outcome studies comparing normobaric oxygen with hyperbaric oxygen. *Ann Emerg Med* 24, 2: pp. 269-276.

Uchino, A., K. Hasuo, et al. (1994). MRI of the brain in chronic carbon monoxide poisoning. *Neuroradiology* 36, 5: pp. 399-401.

Uemura, K., K. Harada, et al. (2001). Apoptotic and necrotic brain lesions in a fatal case of carbon monoxide poisoning. *Forensic Sci Int* 116, 2-3: pp. 213-219.

Vieregge, P., W. Klostermann, et al. (1989). Carbon monoxide poisoning: clinical, neurophysiological, and brain imaging observations in acute disease and follow-up. *J Neurol* 236, 8: pp. 478-481.

Watanabe, N., S. Nohara, et al. (2002). Statistical parametric mapping in brain single photon computed emission tomography after carbon monoxide intoxication. *Nucl Med Commun* 23, 4: pp. 355-366.

Weaver, L. K. (1999). Carbon monoxide poisoning. *Crit Care Clin* 15, 2: pp. 297-317, viii.

Weaver, L. K. (2009). Clinical practice. Carbon monoxide poisoning. *N Engl J Med* 360, 12: pp. 1217-1225.

Weaver, L. K. and R. O. Hopkins (2005). Hemorrhagic infarction in white matter following acute carbon monoxide poisoning. *Neurology* 64, 6: pp. 1101; author reply 1101.

Weaver, L. K., K. J. Valentine, et al. (2007). Carbon monoxide poisoning: risk factors for cognitive sequelae and the role of hyperbaric oxygen. *Am J Respir Crit Care Med* 176, 5: pp. 491-497.

Weinachter, S. N., N. Blavet, et al. (1990). Models of hypoxia and cerebral ischemia. *Pharmacopsychiatry* 23 Suppl 2: pp. 94-97; discussion 98.

Weiner, L. M. (1986). Magnetic resonance study of the structure and functions of cytochrome P450. *CRC Crit Rev Biochem* 20, 2: pp. 139-200.

Wu, C. I., S. P. Changlai, et al. (2003). Usefulness of 99mTc ethyl cysteinate dimer brain SPECT to detect abnormal regional cerebral blood flow in patients with acute carbon monoxide poisoning. *Nucl Med Commun* 24, 11: pp. 1185-1188.

Yoshii, F., R. Kozuma, et al. (1998). Magnetic resonance imaging and 11C-N-methylspiperone/positron emission tomography studies in a patient with the interval form of carbon monoxide poisoning. *J Neurol Sci* 160, 1: pp. 87-91.

Zhang, J. and C. A. Piantadosi (1992). Mitochondrial oxidative stress after carbon monoxide hypoxia in the rat brain. *J Clin Invest* 90, 4: pp. 1193-1199.

9

Neuroimaging Outcomes of Brain Training Trials

Chao Suo and Michael J. Valenzuela
Regenerative Neuroscience Group, School of Psychiatry & Brain and
Ageing Research Program, University of New South Wales
Australia

1. Introduction

The brain remains plastic throughout the human lifespan. This unique property holds great promise for the better treatment of cognitive disorders, and forms the basis for behavioural interventions aimed at promoting mental function that may help delay and prevent the onset of dementia. Brain training (BT) is a direct method for targeting brain plasticity that employs repetitive cognitive exercises. Over the past decade increasing evidence has accumulated that BT can lead to clinical and cognitive benefits in psychiatric samples (McGurk et al., 2005, 2007), as well as in healthy older individuals (Valenzuela & Sachdev, 2009). However, the neurobiological mechanisms underlying these clinical benefits are not well understood. Advances in neuroimaging therefore has potential for revealing the complex *in vivo* structural, functional and metabolic brain changes that accompany BT. The aim of this systematic review was to compare and integrate results of several recent clinical trials of BT that have employed Magnetic Resonance Imaging (MRI), with a particular emphasis on design and technical issues. These studies are beginning to provide fascinating insights into the nature of BT effects on the human brain.

2. Definition of brain training

The wider cognitive intervention field abounds with multiple ill-defined terms that have hampered their development and validation, and can also explain mixed findings to date (Gates & Valenzuela, 2010). Clare and Woods divide this general area into 'cognitive rehabilitation', 'cognitive stimulation', or 'cognitive training' (CT) (Clare & Woods, 2004). We have proposed a specific operational definition for cognitive training (CT) to include cognitive interventions that meet the following four criteria: 1) involves repeated practice, 2) on tasks with an inherent problem, 3) using standardized exercises, and 4) that specifically target a cognitive domain (Gates & Valenzuela, 2010) . Here, the terms BT and CT are identical and are used interchangeably.

3. Method

3.1 Search strategy

The Medline (1996 – 04/2011) database was searched for original research articles in English that met the following criteria. (a) 'brain training', 'cognitive training', 'cognitive intervention', 'cognitive exercise', 'mental exercise', 'cognitive activity' or 'cognitive stimulation', and (b) 'individuals', 'adults', 'persons', 'subjects', but no 'children' or 'teenagers', and (c) 'Magnetic Resonance Image', 'MRI' or 'brain scans'. Combined intervention, subject, and method terms were searched across all fields and produced 144 studies. The title and abstract of these studies were reviewed to identify potentially relevant trials, and these were supplemented by manual checking through reference lists of published reports.

3.2 Inclusion criteria & study quality

Studies were selected for review if they met the following criteria: i) comprised a longitudinal clinical trial with either a randomized controlled trial (RCT) design or uncontrolled clinical trial design (UCT), ii) sample included only healthy individuals not selected against clinical psychiatric criteria, iii) had MRI assessment at least at baseline (before training) and at post-training, and iv) the nature of the intervention met our definition for cognitive training (described above). The qualities of included studies were assessed against CONSORT 2001 criteria for clinical trials (www.consort-statement.org).

4. Results

4.1 Search results

After reviewing the 144 abstracts returned by our search, nine studies containing ten trials met our criteria. These included 7 RCT and 3 UCT. Details are provided in **Table 1**.

4.2 Study quality

Quality of studies varied between 13.5 and 19.5 (out of a maximum of 24). The main limiting factors were unspecified sample size calculations, or details about method of randomizing and blinding. CONSORT criteria scores for RCTs are provided in **Table 1** (maximum = 25).

4.3 Subjects

There were a total of 309 subjects included in the ten identified trials, split between training (N=168) and control groups (N=138). Sample size varied from 10 (Dahlin et al., 2008; Takeuchi et al., 2010) to 58 (Mozolic et al., 2010). Studies divided into three main groups based on age of participants: five studies of young adults with average age of 20-30 years (Dahlin et al., 2008; Erickson et al., 2007a; Olesen et al., 2004; Takeuchi et al., 2010), three studies of elderly subjects with mean age over 60 years (Engvig et al., 2010; Mozolic et al., 2010; Valenzuela et al., 2003), and two studies that combined both elderly and young adult age groups (Erickson et al., 2007b; Lovden et al., 2010). Recruitment source was also variable: young adult subjects were mainly university students, while elderly subjects were from the community based on newspaper advertisements (Dahlin et al., 2008; Engvig et al., 2010; Lovden et al., 2010). All subjects were cognitively-intact.

4.4 Nature of brain training

Because two studies used the same BT protocols (Erickson et al., 2007a, 2007b), a total of nine protocols were reviewed. These could be distinguished on the basis of implementation, either computer-based exercises (Dahlin et al., 2008; Erickson et al., 2007a, 2007b; Lovden et al., 2010; Olesen et al., 2004; Takeuchi et al., 2010), or non-computerized 'paper-and-pencil' exercises (Engvig et al., 2010; Valenzuela et al., 2003). Computerized BT most commonly

Citation	Intervention Summary	Targeted Cognitive Domain	Difficulty Level	Delivery	Time per Session	Frequency	Training Period	CONSORT Scores
Erickson 2007a / Erickson 2007b	Pure or combined colour discrimination or letter discrimination tasks	Memory and decision	RT feedback	Computer	60 mins	Five sessions in total across 2-3 weeks		17.5 / 17.5
Lovden 2010	Three working memory tasks, three episodic memory tasks, and six perceptual speed tasks	Memory and perceptual speed	Adjusted automatically by performance	Computer	60 mins	Average of 101 sessions in 6 months		18
Olesen 2004 (Experiment I)	Three working memory tasks: visuo-spatial working memory task, a backwards digit span task and a letter span task	Memory	adjusted automatically by performance	Computer	35-45mins	Daily	5 weeks	N/A
Olesen 2004 (Experiment II)	Three spatial memory tasks only: Grid, Grid rotation and 3D Grid (Cogmed cognitive medical systems)	Memory	adjusted automatically by performance	Computer	35-45mins	Daily	5 weeks	N/A
Takeuchi 2010	Computer based working memory training	Memory	adjusted automatically by performance	Computer	25 mins	Daily	2 months	N/A
Mozolic 2010	Visual and auditory tasks with visual and auditory distracters	Detecting classifying and sequencing	adjusted automatically by performance	Computer	60 mins	Once per week	2 months	15.5
Dahlin 2008	One letter memory criterion task and five other updating tasks	Memory and updating	adjusted automatically by performance	Computer	45 mins	3 sessions per week	5 weeks	13.5
Engvig 2010	MOL(method of loci) verbal recollection memory task	Memory strategy	lengthen the word list	Group session +homework	60 mins	5 sessions per week	2 months	19.5
Valenzuela 2003	MOL, remember a list of unrelated concrete nouns	Memory strategy	lengthen the word list	Group session	15-20 mins	Once per week	5 weeks	16

Table 1. Summary of brain training interventions with MRI outcomes.

consisted of different memory-based exercises (i.e., unidomain) (Dahlin et al., 2008; Erickson et al., 2007a, 2007b; Lovden et al., 2010; Olesen et al., 2004; Takeuchi et al., 2010). BT exercises were generally custom-designed by the research group, although one study investigated a multi-domain commercial program which included detecting, classifying, and/or sequencing with audio and visual distracters (Mozolic et al., 2010). Non-computerized BT studies used a specific mnemonic strategy known as the Method of Loci (MoL) (Engvig et al., 2010; Valenzuela et al., 2003). Further BT details are available in **Table 1**.

For most of the computerized BT interventions, difficulty level was automatically adjusted based on performance on previous tasks, whereas the Erickson group utilized continuous real-time feedback (response time) to help motivate and challenge subjects (Erickson et al., 2007a). Across all studies, training was session-based, varying form 20 minutes to 60 minutes per session. Frequencies of BT also varied from one session per week to daily. The duration of interventions were generally around two months) (Dahlin et al., 2008; Engvig et al., 2010; Mozolic et al., 2010; Olesen et al., 2004; Takeuchi et al., 2010; Valenzuela et al., 2003), except for one 6 month training study (Lovden et al., 2010) and two 2-week training studies (Erickson et al., 2007a, 2007b).

Definition of control training in RCTs was predominantly a no-intervention wait-and-see condition in 6 studies, whilst one study used an active control training condition, which comprised an educational lecture program and quizzes (Mozolic et al., 2010).

4.5 Types of MRI

Five studies used an event-related fMRI approach, employing in-scanner tasks either identical or highly similar to the offline training exercises (Erickson et al., 2007a, 2007b; Olesen et al., 2004). One fMRI study is unique for investigating functional BT-related changes related to both the trained task as well as to non-trained tasks within the scanner (Dahlin et al., 2008). Two studies investigated BT-induced changes to white matter fractional anisotropy (FA) and mean diffusivity (MD) using DTI (Lovden et al., 2010; Takeuchi et al., 2010). Another study used perfusion MRI (pMRI) to investigate BT effects on whole-brain cerebral blood flow (Mozolic et al., 2010). Finally, one study employed MR spectroscopy (MRS) to explore biochemical change before and after BT in several cortical and subcortical areas (Valenzuela et al., 2003).

Whilst all studies were selected for employing a baseline and post-training scan, one study conducted dual baseline scans in one experiment, and 5 serial scans over 5 weeks during BT in another experiment (Olesen et al., 2004). T1 structural MRI (sMRI) were common to all studies, however only two studies have specifically reported structural BT outcomes (Engvig et al., 2010; Lovden et al., 2010). Three out of ten studies used a 3 Tesla scanner, remaining studies used 1.5 Tesla field strength. No study specifically reported the presence or absence of hardware scanner changes or upgrades during the follow-up period.

4.6 Approaches to MRI pre-processing

Three main software platforms were used to perform MRI preprocessing: Four papers used different versions (SPM99, SPM2, SPM5) of Statistical Parametric Mapping (SPM, http://www.fil.ion.ucl.ac.uk/spm/) (Dahlin et al., 2008; Mozolic et al., 2010; Olesen et al., 2004; Takeuchi et al., 2010), two studies used FSL (FMRIB Software Library http://www.fmrib.ox.ac.uk/fsl/) (Erickson et al., 2007a, 2007b), and one study was based on Freesurfer (http://surfer.nmr.mgh.harvard.edu/) (Engvig et al., 2010). Further MRI pre-processing information is summarized in **Table 2**.

Citation	MRI	MRI assessment point	Main MRI protocol	Scanner info	Pre-processing platform	Pre-processing steps
Erickson 2007a	2	Pre- and Post training	fMRI (training tasks)	3T	FSL	Slice timing, motion-corrected, temporally filtered (1.5s-50s) and smoothing (7mm)
Erickson 2007 b	2	Pre- and Post training				
Lovden 2010	2	Pre- and Post training	DTI	1.5T	Semi-auto algorithm	Motion correction, generating MD and FA maps and semi-auto corpus callosum (CC) segmentation
Olesen 2004 (Experiment I)	3	twice at Pre- and once at Post training	fMRI (lowload working memory task and control task)	1.5T	SPM99	Motion correction, normalized by using T1 localizer and smoothing (6mm)
Olesen 2004 (Experiment II)	5	5 scans during 5 weeks (day 0, 2,4,8 23)	fMRI(highload and lowload memory tasks and control tasks)			
Takeuchi 2010	2	Pre- and Post training	DTI	3T	SPM5	Optimised VBM, intra-subject coregistration and smoothing (10mm)
Mozolic 2010	2	Pre- and Post training	perfusion MRI and structural MRI	1.5T	SPM5	Optimised VBM and smoothing (8mm)
Dahlin 2008	2	Pre- and Post training	fMRI (letter memory, n-back and Stroop)	1.5T	SPM2	Slice timing, realigned and unwarped, normalized and smoothing (8mm)
Engvig 2010	2	Pre- and Post training	Structural MRI	1.5T	Freesufer	Tissue segmentation, cortical thickness measures, subtraction of pre BT from post BT after coregistration to mid point and smoothing (30mm)
Valenzuela 2003	2	Pre- and Post training	MRS at right hippocampus, left frontal lobe and occipital-parietal	1.5T	Not applicable	N-acetylaspartate, choline and phosphocreatine relative to internal water peak corrected by cerebral spinal fluid percentage using voxel segmentation and white matter hyper-intensity volume

Table 2. Hardware and preprocessing information of reviewed studies.

Irrespective of MRI modality or research interest, the goal of preprocessing should be to prepare data so that further analytical assumptions are valid (Klein et al., 2009). For example, motion correction and spatial normalization maximizes the likelihood that a particular voxel property comes from same location across subjects. In the ten studies reviewed, fMRI preprocessing procedures were similar, including slice timing, motion correction, normalization, and smoothing. pMRI, DTI and sMRI studies created sample-specific template for coregistration and normalization purpose. Two studies (Mozolic et al., 2010; Takeuchi et al., 2010) followed the Optimized VBM (Good et al., 2001) approach, and one study created subject-specific templates by averaging image pairs across pre- and post-sessions (Engvig et al., 2010). Finally, the Lovden group used a semi-automatic algorithm for analysis of the corpus callosum (Niogi et al., 2007).

MRS studies require no geometric preprocessing. Rather, quantitative MRS assessment of neurometabolites may be influenced by scanning parameters such as shimming and receiver gain. MRS studies generally report relative metabolic signal intensity against a reference signal, and creatine is by far the most common reference signal. However, because subclinical degenerative disease and the intervention itself could hypothetically alter resting state phosphocreatine-creatine turnover (Valenzuela & Sachdev, 2001), we have used tissue-water as a more reliable reference signal in studies of ageing and BT (Valenzuela et al., 2003).

4.7 Approaches to MRI statistical inference

The General Linear Model (GLM) assumes an individual's MRI signal of interest is a function of a 'ground truth' signal modified by one or more experimental conditions and affected by error. The strengths (Friston et al., 2007) and weaknesses (Haynes, 2011) of the GLM approach therefore apply generally to the present set of fMRI, sMRI and DTI studies. In the context of longitudinal BT studies, statistical inference was mainly geared at testing Group (BT vs control) × Time (Pre vs Post-BT) interactions. In addition, one study carried out a regression analysis when analyzing DTI, using total BT amount (completed sessions) as the covariate of interest (Takeuchi et al., 2010).

When testing the null hypothesis, BT MRI studies have generally adopted a 'mass univariate' voxel-by-voxel test, either across the whole-brain or restricted to some ROI defined by prior knowledge. This approach assumes each voxel (or larger cluster of voxels) is necessarily an independent observation, an assumption that contradicts brain biology and introduces a significant multiple-comparison problem (Nichols & Hayasaka, 2003). Four studies used cluster-level correction (Dahlin et al., 2008; Erickson et al., 2007a, 2007b; Mozolic et al., 2010; Olesen et al., 2004), and one study voxel-level correction (Engvig et al., 2010). Some studies designed an initial experiment, and such first-level results were consequently used as an explicit mask for the next experiment (Dahlin et al., 2008; Erickson et al., 2007a, 2007b; Mozolic et al., 2010; Olesen et al., 2004). In this case, close attention is required to avoid non-independence errors (Kriegeskorte et al., 2009; Vul et al., 2009). Interestingly, one study used a split-half validation approach that uses a more relaxed multiple-correction threshold in one half of the sample to generate hypotheses for rigorous (but more constrained) testing in the other half of the sample (Engvig et al., 2010). Notably, alternative network approaches that consider covariance patterns across and between ensembles of brain locations (Haynes 2011), including Partial Least Squares analysis (Krishnan et al., 2011), Independent Components Analysis (Biswal & Ulmer, 1999; Calhoun et al., 2001), or graph-based analysis (Bullmore & Sporns, 2009), have not yet been applied to BT studies. Further details are available in **Table 3**.

Citation	Post-processing steps	Multiple Correction Approach
Erickson 2007a	1. Extract the mean signal from first level task-contrast activation and test interaction with time × group 2. Whole brain voxel wise interaction analysis 3. Test correlation between activity change and performance improvement.	1. Threshold cluster at z<2.33 (p<0.01) uncorrected, then use p(corrected)<0.01 to define ROI 2. Threshold cluster at z<3.1 (p<0.001) uncorrected, then p(corrected)<0.01
Erickson 2007 b	1. Extract the mean signal from first level task-contrast activation and test interaction with time × group 2. Whole brain time × group analysis 3. Test other interaction (time × group × condition × age) on these regions from step2	To define ROI: z>3.1(p<0.001)uncorrected=>cluster level correction at p=0.01
Lovden 2010	1. Time × Group × Age interaction test of the FA and MD of 5 segments of Corpus Callosum (CC) 2. Test correlation of performances and DTI result 3. Structure change of voxel for each segmented CC	Not involved
Olesen 2004 (Experiment I)	Whole brain time × group analysis	Threshold at z<2.33(p<0.01) uncorrected, then threshold at p<0.01 cluster level correction
Olesen 2004 (Experiment II)	1. First level analysis (task-control task) 2. Regression analysis on the level one contrast with individual working memory capacities	Threshold at t>2.44 (p<0.022) uncorrected, then threshold at p<0.01 cluster level correction
Takeuchi 2010	1. Pre- and post-training groups paired-t analysis 2. Regression analysis between different fractional anisotropy (FA) map and the total amount of BT within step 1 regions 3. Test correlation between total BT and mean FA changes within step 1 regions	Threshold at p<0.005 uncorrected, then threshold at p<0.05 cluster level correction
Mozolic 2010	1. Whole brain time × group interaction test on cerebral blood flow (CBF) map 2. GM time × group interaction test within ROI from step1 3. Test correlation on changes of CBF and performance improvements	1. p(uncorrected)<0.001, then extent p(corrected)<0.05; 2. Biological Parametric Mapping toolbox to correct
Dahlin 2008	1. First level pre-training scans for three tasks 2. Second level time × group interaction analysis for each tasks 3. A conjunction analysis of letter memory task and 3-back tasks	1. p(FDR)<0.01 for two tasks, p(uncorrected)<0.005 for Stroop task; 2, p(uncorrected)>0.05
Engvig 2010	1. Time × group interaction whole brain 2. Split-half validation 3. Memory improvement correlates with the mean ROI GM thickness change	1. p(FWE)<0.05 peak level; 2. p(uncorrected)<0.05 and overlap the two split-half results
Valenzuela 2003	Regression analysis in SPSS	Not involved

Table 3. Post-processing and statistical correction details.

	Citation	Regions	Main Results
MRI	Erickson 2007a	Bilateral dorsolateral prefrontal cortex (DLPFC)	↑ activation
		Right inferior frontal gyrus, right superior parietal lobule, right dorsal inferior frontal gyrus and left superior parietal lobule (trend)	↓ activation
	Erickson2007 b	Left ventral prefrontal cortex, bilateral DLPFC	↑ activation
		Right ventral prefrontal cortex	↓ activation
fMRI	Olesen 2004 (Experiment I)	Right middle frontal gyrus, right inferior parietal cortex, and bilateral intraparietal cortex	↑ activation
		Cingulate sulcus	↓ activation
	Olesen 2004 (Experiment II)	Left middle frontal gyrus; bilateral superior parietal cortex, bilateral inferior parietal cortex, left intraparietal cortex, thalamus, and right caudate head	↑ activation
		Cingulate suclus; right inferior frontal sulcus and left postcentral gyrus	↓ activation
	Dahlin 2008	Bilateral putamen, right temporal lobe, and right occipital lobe	↑ activation
		Right frontal lobe, right parietal lobe	↓ activation
		Left frontal lobe, left parietal lobe, left temporal lobe and left putamen	↑ activation
DTI	Takeuchi 2010	WM adjacent to the inferior parietal sulcus; the border between the frontal lobe and parietal lob; adjacent to the intraparietal suclus; anterior part of the corpus callosum	↑ fractional anisotropy
	Lovden 2010	Segment 1 (anterior) of corpus callosum	↑ fractional anisotropy and voxels
pMRI	Mozolic 2010	Right inferior prefrontal cortex	↑ cerebral blood flow
sMRI	Engvig 2010	Right insular, right lateral orbitofrontal cortex, right fusiform cortex, and left lateral orbitofrontal cortex	↑cortical thickness
		Global	↑ right hemisphere thickness
MRS	Valenzuela 2003	Hippocampus (right)	↑ creatine and choline

Table 4. Summary of MRI results of brain training in healthy adults.

4.8 Neuroimaging outcomes in BT trials

All MRI studies have to date revealed significant training-induced brain changes. Moreover, there is some overlap between studies in terms of topographical distribution. Training-related adaptation in the frontal lobe is most common. In fact, frontal lobe functional changes were reported in all fMRI studies, although the direction of changes was not consistent, and the precise localization of differences also varied (see **Table 4**). Even in the same experiments, there was evidence of both increased and reduced activation in distinct frontal lobe areas (Erickson et al., 2007a, 2007b). These functional changes are also supported by BT-related increments to cerebral blood flow (Mozolic et al., 2010), and in one study, increased cortical thickness (Engvig et al., 2010). Since all BT (either explicitly or implicitly) requires repetitive high-load engagement of working memory, it is not altogether surprising that frontal lobe plasticity is consistently implicated. Differences in BT design may help explain regional heterogeneity in these fMRI studies.

Another working-memory related area is the parietal lobe (Osaka et al., 2007), also implicated in multimodal integration (Fogassi et al., 2005), and hence potentially relevant to BT. Greater superior or inferior parietal lobe activity was detected in five fMRi studies after training compared with the untrained groups (Dahlin et al., 2008; Erickson et al., 2007a, 2007b; Olesen et al., 2004), with the exception of one study which found reduced activation in the right superior parietal lobe (Dahlin et al., 2008). Furthermore, a DTI study found increased fractional anisotropy (FA) in white matter regions adjacent to the inferior parietal sulcus, as well as at the border between the frontal and parietal lobe (Takeuchi et al., 2010).

Two studies have investigated the corpus callosum (CC) using DTI, and both revealed increased FA of the anterior CC after BT (Lovden et al., 2010; Takeuchi et al., 2010). Finally, only one study has focused on BT-related changes in the hippocampus, arguably the brain's most plastic area (Burke & Barnes, 2006; Gage et al., 2008), using MRS after a five-week Method of Loci trial (Valenzuela et al., 2003). Increased phosphocreatine was found in the hippocampus, but not other grey and white matter areas, suggestive of an activity-dependent upregulation of cellular-energy resting state, potentially of neuroprotective benefit (Brustovetky et al., 2001) in an area highly susceptible to degeneration.

There were also several differences in outcomes between studies, and so it is important to consider possible moderating factors. Session number or frequencies are unlikely to have had a major impact as they were relatively consistent between studies. Age, however, may be salient to BT outcomes. For example, in Erickson and colleagues' study (Erickson et al., 2007b), whilst a significant group × time interaction was for both elderly and young subjects at the dorsal prefrontal cortex bilaterally, the direction of the effects were opposite: in the older subjects there was reduced activation after BT, and increased activation amongst young subjects. Age differences have also been observed in a DTI study, whereby FA increased after BT only in the older group (Lovden et al., 2010).

5. Discussion

5.1 A biological insight into the trained brain

One of the major unresolved challenges for the BT field is to adequately demonstrate transfer or generalizability of outcomes (Gates & Valenzuela, 2010; Valenzuela & Sachdev, 2009). Individuals will predictably improve on almost any trained task – in clinical terms this is rather trivial unless gains can also be demonstrated in non-trained tasks. Neuroimaging studies are only beginning to address this issue. For example, one study found that the effect of training in one task translates to functional brain changes in non-trained tasks (Dahlin et al., 2008). Brain imaging studies can therefore provide independent biological evidence about the impact of BT on brain structure, function and biochemistry.

So far, BT studies have been universally positive, each study reporting at least one significant brain imaging outcome. It is of course impossible to assess the role of publication bias, as null studies may have been self-censored by authors, or rejected by editors and reviewers. The field is also manifestly young, only 10 studies were found following a systematic search, across a mix of BT designs, approaches, MRI modalities and subjects. Nevertheless, a number of studies point to the key role of frontal lobe plasticity in potentially mediating BT benefits. All fMRI studies have so far found changes in this region, and as mentioned, this may reflect the heavy working memory demands of BT itself. Interestingly, repetitive practice of working memory problems does not necessarily lead to straightforward increases (in terms of signal change or spread of suprathreshold voxels) in task-related functional activity. Rather, a complex series of increases and decreases in brain activity have been observed. BT may therefore lead to two major types of functional adaptations including (Lustig et al., 2009): i) task-related hyperactivation, where the network of brain regions that normally subserves a given task becomes primed to activate, and ii) efficiency gains, where for a less extensive brain response, the same (or increased) cognitive proficiency is possible.

The cellular and molecular mechanisms that underlie BT-related frontal lobe plasticity are currently not known. Environmental enrichment, (in part) a model for BT in animals, is known to produce a wide range of neurobiological changes, including enhanced synaptic plasticity, neurogenesis and angiogenesis, as well as macroscopic structural changes including increased brain volume (Nithianantharajah & Hannan, 2006; Valenzuela et al., 2007). Interestingly, one sMRI has found that extensive memory training (2 months, 5 days a week) can translate into increased cortical thickness in the frontal lobe (Engvig et al., 2010), and two DTI studies further suggest frontal lobe structural plasticity in the form of increased FA in the anterior corpus callosum (Lovden et al., 2010; Takeuchi et al., 2010). The temporal dynamics of such structural BT changes are not understood, but studies of mental activity outside of our BT definition do provide some clues. Knowledge acquisition amongst college students led to persistent hippocampal volumetric increases even 3 month after the end of study (Draganski et al., 2006), whilst motor training studies suggest gray matter volume reaches a zenith after just 7 days of training and gains are reversed three months later (Boyke et al,. 2008; Driemeyer et al., 2008). With sufficient practice, functional BT effects may transform into detectable structural brain changes. From a practical viewpoint, sMRI plasticity may take longer to develop, or simply produce subtle changes, and hence studies with this outcome in mind need to pay attention to adequate BT dosage, power and sample size.

5.2 Limitations and challenges for the field

Whilst BT research has so far employed the full range of MR modalities, the field conspicuously lacks multi-modal studies. Each modality has its strengths and weaknesses, and so combining MR approaches will allow the clearest insight into putative neurobiological mechanisms. Use of network-based analyses will also help integrate findings across modalities, as well as recognize the interconnected and dynamic nature of human brain plasticity (Bullmore & Sporns, 2009). However, of more fundamental concern is the absence of any active control group in almost all reviewed RCTs. Since BT typically involves participants coming into a centre for some level of person-to-person instruction, as well as often undertaking training in group sessions, receiving personalized feedback, and a host of other non-specific stimulatory factors, it is altogether unclear whether results so far reflect the benefits of BT specifically, or the neural manifestation of social contact, motivation, generic mental activity, and other Hawthorne effects. Future studies must employ active control conditions to ensure that valid neurobiological inferences are possible. Similarly, whilst BT often implicates working memory-related brain regions such as the prefrontal lobe, few studies have demonstrated a clear correlation between MRI-changes and BT-induced cognitive benefits (Engvig et al., 2010; Erickson et al., 2007a, 2007b). Of course, when testing for such links there are numerous technical MR processing pitfalls that could lead to spurious results. This has been graphically illustrated by Thomas et al., 2009, who found that a period of mirror-reading training led, alternatively, to either nil, modest, or widespread structural brain changes depending on which Voxel-Base-Morphometry assumptions were made, or even which software package was chosen. Recently, a systematic comparison of different sMRI software platforms found each had strengths and weaknesses, depending on the nature of the question (de Bresser et al., 2011). Clearly, for the field to advance on solid ground, claims of BT-related plasticity should not be pipeline-dependent (Valenzuela, et al., *in press*), and the strongest results will be those with some level of cross-validation, either though the use of multiple imaging modalities, verification by manual methods, or parameter-based sensitivity testing.

Finally, a technical factor that is often overlooked is the role of hardware MRI upgrades during the intervention period (Ridgway et al., 2008). These routinely occur, often outside the control of the investigator, and become increasingly relevant in longitudinal studies. Reporting of any hardware changes during a BT trial should be standard, and if this change selectively affects some subjects but not others, at a bare minimum this information should be added to analyses as a nuisance covariate.

6. Conclusions

Neuroimaging studies of BT emphasize the brain's potential to adapt and change during the whole of life. Functional BT changes are most frequently implicated, with consistent findings of altered activity patterns in frontal and parietal lobe areas. Cross-validation of these results is also emerging with MR studies reporting BT-induced structural, blood flow and biochemical adaptation. Multimodal imaging investigation of BT is needed, recognizing that structural BT-related plasticity may be subtle and have a different time course to functional BT-related plasticity. A major challenge for the field is to start to draw connections between BT-related changes in brain structure and function to the cognitive benefits increasingly evident in clinical studies. Future studies should also take care to design active control conditions, as well as ensure that results are not overly influenced by arbitrary processing decisions.

7. References

Biswal, B. B., & Ulmer, J. L. (1999). Blind source separation of multiple signal sources of fMRI data sets using independent component analysis. *J Comput Assist Tomogr*, Vol.23, No.2, (1999/03/30), pp. 265-271, ISSN 0363-8715

Boyke, J., Driemeyer, J., Gaser, C., Buchel, C., & May, A. (2008). Training-induced brain structure changes in the elderly. *J Neurosci*, Vol.28, No.28, (2008/07/11), pp. 7031-7035, ISSN 1529-2401

Brustovetsky, N., Brustovetsky, T., & Dubinsky, J. M. (2001). On the mechanisms of neuroprotection by creatine and phosphocreatine. *J Neurochem*, Vol.76, No.2, (2001/02/24), pp. 425-434, ISSN 0022-3042

Bullmore, E., & Sporns, O. (2009). Complex brain networks: graph theoretical analysis of structural and functional systems. *Nat Rev Neurosci*, Vol.10, No.3, (2009/02/05), pp. 186-198, ISSN 1471-0048

Burke, S. N., & Barnes, C. A. (2006). Neural plasticity in the ageing brain. *Nat Rev Neurosci*, Vol.7, No.1, (2005/12/24), pp. 30-40, ISSN 1471-003X

Calhoun, V. D., Adali, T., McGinty, V. B., Pekar, J. J., Watson, T. D., & Pearlson, G. D. (2001). fMRI activation in a visual-perception task: network of areas detected using the general linear model and independent components analysis. *Neuroimage*, Vol.14, No.5, 1080-1088, ISSN 1053-8119

Clare, L., & Woods, R. T. (2004). Cognitive training and cognitive rehabilitation for people with early-stage Alzheimer's disease: A review. *Neuropsychological Rehabilitation: An International Journal*, Vol.14, No.4, 385 - 401, ISSN 0960-2011

Dahlin, E., Neely, A. S., Larsson, A., Backman, L., & Nyberg, L. (2008). Transfer of learning after updating training mediated by the striatum. *Science*, Vol.320, No.5882, (2008/06/17), pp. 1510-1512, ISSN 1095-9203

de Bresser, J., Portegies, M. P., Leemans, A., Biessels, G. J., Kappelle, L. J., & Viergever, M. A. (2011). A comparison of MR based segmentation methods for measuring brain atrophy progression. *Neuroimage*, Vol.54, No.2, (2010/10/05), pp. 760-768, ISSN 1095-9572

Draganski, B., Gaser, C., Kempermann, G., Kuhn, H. G., Winkler, J., Buchel, C., et al. (2006). Temporal and spatial dynamics of brain structure changes during extensive learning. *J Neurosci*, Vol.26, No.23, (2006/06/10), pp. 6314-6317, ISSN 1529-2401

Driemeyer, J., Boyke, J., Gaser, C., Buchel, C., & May, A. (2008). Changes in gray matter induced by learning--revisited. *PLoS One*, Vol.3, No.7, (2008/07/24), pp. e2669, ISSN 1932-6203

Engvig, A., Fjell, A. M., Westlye, L. T., Moberget, T., Sundseth, O., Larsen, V. A., et al. (2010). Effects of memory training on cortical thickness in the elderly. *Neuroimage*, Vol.52, No.4, (2010/06/29), pp. 1667-1676, ISSN 1095-9572

Erickson, K. I., Colcombe, S. J., Wadhwa, R., Bherer, L., Peterson, M. S., Scalf, P. E., et al. (2007a). Training-induced functional activation changes in dual-task processing: an FMRI study. *Cereb Cortex*, Vol.17, No.1, (2006/02/10), pp. 192-204, ISSN 1047-3211

Erickson, K. I., Colcombe, S. J., Wadhwa, R., Bherer, L., Peterson, M. S., Scalf, P. E., et al. (2007b). Training-induced plasticity in older adults: effects of training on hemispheric asymmetry. *Neurobiol Aging*, Vol.28, No.2, (2006/02/17), pp. 272-283, ISSN 1558-1497

Fogassi, L., Ferrari, P. F., Gesierich, B., Rozzi, S., Chersi, F., & Rizzolatti, G. (2005). Parietal lobe: from action organization to intention understanding. *Science*, Vol.308, No.5722, (2005/04/30), pp. 662-667, ISSN 1095-9203

Friston, K., Ashburner, J., Penny, W., Keibel, S., & Nicholas, M. (2007). *Statistical parametric mapping : the analysis of functional brain images.* London : Academic, ISBN 0123725607, London

Gage, F. H., Kempermann, G., & Song, H. (Eds.). (2008). *Adult neurogenesis.* Cold Spring Harbor, N.Y. : Cold Spring Harbor Laboratory Press, ISBN 9780879697846, N.Y.

Gates, N., & Valenzuela, M. (2010). Cognitive exercise and its role in cognitive function in older adults. *Curr Psychiatry Rep,* Vol.12, No.1, (2010/04/29), pp. 20-27, ISSN 1535-1645

Haynes, J. D. (2011). Multivariate decoding and brain reading: Introduction to the special issue. *Neuroimage,* Vol.56, No.2, (2011/03/31), pp. 385-386, ISSN 1095-9572

Klein, A., Andersson, J., Ardekani, B. A., Ashburner, J., Avants, B., Chiang, M. C., et al. (2009). Evaluation of 14 nonlinear deformation algorithms applied to human brain MRI registration. *Neuroimage,* Vol.46, No.3, (2009/02/07), pp. 786-802, ISSN 1095-9572

Kriegeskorte, N., Simmons, W. K., Bellgowan, P. S., & Baker, C. I. (2009). Circular analysis in systems neuroscience: the dangers of double dipping. *Nat Neurosci,* Vol.12, No.5, (2009/04/28), pp. 535-540, ISSN 1546-1726

Krishnan, A., Williams, L. J., McIntosh, A. R., & Abdi, H. (2011). Partial Least Squares (PLS) methods for neuroimaging: A tutorial and review. *Neuroimage,* Vol.56, No.2, (2010/07/27), pp. 455-475, ISSN 1095-9572

Lovden, M., Bodammer, N. C., Kuhn, S., Kaufmann, J., Schutze, H., Tempelmann, C., et al. (2010). Experience-dependent plasticity of white-matter microstructure extends into old age. *Neuropsychologia,* Vol.48, No.13, (2010/09/08), pp. 3878-3883, ISSN 1873-3514

Lustig, C., Shah, P., Seidler, R., & Reuter-Lorenz, P. A. (2009). Aging, training, and the brain: a review and future directions. *Neuropsychol Rev,* Vol.19, No.4, (2009/10/31), pp. 504-522, ISSN 1573-6660

McGurk, S. R., Mueser, K. T., & Pascaris, A. (2005). Cognitive training and supported employment for persons with severe mental illness: one-year results from a randomized controlled trial. *Schizophr Bull,* Vol.31, No.4, (2005/08/05), pp. 898-909, ISSN 0586-7614

McGurk, S. R., Twamley, E. W., Sitzer, D. I., McHugo, G. J., & Mueser, K. T. (2007). A meta-analysis of cognitive remediation in schizophrenia. *Am J Psychiatry,* Vol.164, No.12, (2007/12/07), pp. 1791-1802, ISSN 0002-953X

Mozolic, J. L., Hayasaka, S., & Laurienti, P. J. (2010). A cognitive training intervention increases resting cerebral blood flow in healthy older adults. *Front Hum Neurosci,* Vol.4, (2010/03/20), pp. 16, ISSN 1662-5161

Nichols, T., & Hayasaka, S. (2003). Controlling the familywise error rate in functional neuroimaging: a comparative review. *Stat Methods Med Res,* Vol.12, No.5, (2003/11/06), pp. 419-446, ISSN 0962-2802

Niogi, S. N., Mukherjee, P., & McCandliss, B. D. (2007). Diffusion tensor imaging segmentation of white matter structures using a Reproducible Objective Quantification Scheme (ROQS). *Neuroimage,* Vol.35, No.1, (2007/01/09), pp. 166-174, ISSN 1053-8119

Nithiananatharajah, J., & Hannan, A. J. (2006). Enriched environments, experience-dependent plasticity and disorders of the nervous system. *Nat Rev Neurosci,* Vol.7, No.9, (2006/08/23), pp. 697-709, ISSN 1471-003X

Osaka, N., Logie, R. H., & D'Esposito, M. (2007). The cognitive neuroscience of working memory. Oxford ; New York : Oxford University Press, ISBN 978-0-19-857039-4, Oxford ; New York

Takeuchi, H., Sekiguchi, A., Taki, Y., Yokoyama, S., Yomogida, Y., Komuro, N., et al. (2010). Training of working memory impacts structural connectivity. *J Neurosci*, Vol.30, No.9, (2010/03/06), pp. 3297-3303, ISSN 1529-2401

Thomas, A. G., Marrett, S., Saad, Z. S., Ruff, D. A., Martin, A., & Bandettini, P. A. (2009). Functional but not structural changes associated with learning: an exploration of longitudinal voxel-based morphometry (VBM). *Neuroimage*, Vol.48, No.1, (2009/06/13), pp. 117-125, ISSN 1095-9572

Valenzuela, M., Bartres-Faz, D., Beg, F., Fornito, A., Merlo-Pich, E., Muller, U., et al. (in press). Neuroimaging as Endpoints in Clinical Trials: Are We There Yet? Perspective from the first Provence Workshop. *Molecular Psychiatry*.

Valenzuela, M., & Sachdev, P. (2009). Can cognitive exercise prevent the onset of dementia? Systematic review of randomized clinical trials with longitudinal follow-up. *Am J Geriatr Psychiatry*, Vol.17, No.3, (2009/02/20), pp. 179-187, ISSN 1545-7214

Valenzuela, M. J., Jones, M., Wen, W., Rae, C., Graham, S., Shnier, R., et al. (2003). Memory training alters hippocampal neurochemistry in healthy elderly. *Neuroreport*, Vol.14, No.10, (2003/07/24), pp. 1333-1337, ISSN 0959-4965

Valenzuela, M. J., & Sachdev, P. (2001). Magnetic resonance spectroscopy in AD. *Neurology*, Vol.56, No.5, (2001/03/23), pp. 592-598, ISSN 0028-3878

Valenzuela, M. J., Sachdev, P. S., Wen, W., Shnier, R., Brodaty, H., & Gillies, D. (2000). Dual voxel proton magnetic resonance spectroscopy in the healthy elderly: subcortical-frontal axonal N-acetylaspartate levels are correlated with fluid cognitive abilities independent of structural brain changes. *Neuroimage*, Vol.12, No.6, (2000/12/09), pp. 747-756, ISSN 1053-8119

Vul, E., Harris, C., Winkielman, P., & Pashler, H. (2009). Voodoo correlations in social neuroscience. *Perspectives on Psychological Science*, Vol.4, No.3, 274-290, ISSN 1745-6916

10

Event-Related Potential Studies of Cognitive and Social Neuroscience

Agustin Ibanez[1,2,3,4], Phil Baker[1] and Alvaro Moya[1]
[1]Laboratory of Experimental Psychology and Neuroscience (LPEN),
Institute of Cognitive Neurology (INECO), Buenos Aires
[2]National Scientific and Technical Research Council (CONICET), Buenos Aires,
[3]Laboratory of Cognitive Neuroscience, Universidad Diego Portales, Santiago,
[4]Institute of Neuroscience, Favaloro University, Buenos Aires,
[1,2,4]Argentina
[3]Chile

1. Introduction

In this chapter, we assess the role of Event-Related Potentials (ERP) in the field of cognitive neuroscience, particularly in the emergent area of social neuroscience. This is new ground that combines approaches from cognitive neuroscience and social psychology, highlighting the multilevel approach to emotional, social and cognitive phenomena, and representing one of the most promising fields of cognitive neuroscience (Adolphs, 2003, 2010; Blakemore, Winston and Frith, 2004; Cunningham and Zelazo, 2007; Decety and Sommerville, 2003; Frith and Frith, 2010; Insel, 2010; Lieberman and Eisenberger, 2009; Miller, 2006; Ochsner, 2004; Rilling and Sanfey, 2011; Sanfey, 2007; Singer and Lamm, 2009; Zaki and Ochsner, 2009).

The technique of ERPs is a precise tool regarding time resolution (on the order of milliseconds). ERPs are useful not only for their excellent temporal resolution but because recent advances (e.g., dense arrays, single trial analysis, source localization algorithms, connectivity and frequency measures, among others) provide multiples sources of brain activity in response to cognitive events.

First, a definition of ERPs and an explanation about the recordings and features of main components (P1, N1, N170, VPP, EPN, N2, P2, P3, N400, N400-like LPC, LPP, P600, ERN, fERN, CNV, RP; LRP, MP, RAP) are detailed (including a description of their generating sources when available). We then introduce some representative examples of cognitive and social neuroscience: contextual approaches to language, emotions and emotional body language; empathy; and decision-making cognition. All these areas are reviewed, highlighting their relevance for cognitive neuroscience and clinical research (neuropsychiatry and pathophysiology). Finally, important issues, such as sleep research, intracranial ERPs recordings, source location in dense arrays and co-recordings with fMRI, are discussed.

2. Event-Related Potentials (ERPs)

The technique of ERPs is a precise tool regarding time resolution (on the order of milliseconds) that incorporates the recording of ongoing electrophysiological activity using electroencephalography (EEG). ERPs result from the synchronous activation of neural subpopulations that occur in response to events (sensory, motor or cognitive). ERPs are useful not only for their excellent temporal resolution but because recent advances (e.g., dense arrays, single-trial analysis, source localization algorithms, connectivity and frequency measures, among others) provide multiples sources of brain activity in response to cognitive events.

To measure the brain activity, the ERP quantifies electrical fields through the skull and scalp. This last procedure is named electroencephalography (EEG). ERPs are the ongoing electrophysiological activity resulting from the synchronous activation of several neural subpopulations that occur in response to sensory, motor or cognitive events (Hillyard and Picton, 1987). ERPs are the summed activity of excitatory postsynaptic potential (EPSP) and inhibitory postsynaptic potential (IPSP) activated in response to each new stimulus or subject response. The ERPs are less precise for the anatomical localization of the neural generators than the neuroimaging techniques. Nonetheless, this technique has an exceptional temporal resolution of milliseconds (Kutas and Federmeier, 2000). An ERP's spatial distribution on the scalp is not indicative of its brain-source generators (although some mathematical tools for source algorithm localization can enhance the spatial precision).

Electrodes are attached to diverse points on the scalp relative to bony landmarks. Using a standardized EEG-measurement technique to determine the correct spots, the entire head is measured. Normally, the participants are placed in front of a computer screen with electrodes fixed onto the scalp and connected to electric amplifiers and auditory headsets displaying a pattern of stimuli. One computer records and amplifies the electrical peaks elicited by each stimulus onset (or the participant response).

The EEG activity is time-locked to several presentations of similar events (stimuli or participants responses), and the averaging of these segmented EEG traced together is the usual procedure. The average decreases the influence of noisy activity (i.e., EEG not related to experimental events or background noise) while maintaining the event-related activity. Several signal processing steps, such as filtering (e.g., 0.5 to 30 hz), segmentation, artifact detection and correction, bad channel replacements, re-referencing, baseline correction and averaging, are usually required to obtain a suitable signal-to-noise ratio (see Figure 1). After these processing steps, positive or negative changes of voltage constitute ERPs that appear at specific latencies after the stimulus presentation. Most ERP components are referred to by a preceding letter (e.g., "N"), indicating polarity followed by the typical peak latency in milliseconds (e.g., the "N400" ERP component is described as a negative voltage deflection occurring approximately 400 ms after the stimulus onset). The timing of the brain processing is measured by the timing of these cortical responses.

The simplest ERP parameters are latency (how long after the event they appear), direction (positive or negative), amplitude (the strength of the voltage change) and topological distribution of the component on the surface of the head (frontal, parietal, occipital, etc.). The standard procedure to visualize and measure the ERP activity consists of quantifying the amplitude and latency (measured in microvolts and milliseconds, respectively) of the waveform associated with a specific stimulus or response. By means of this procedure, different stimuli or conditions can be contrasted in terms of amplitude or latency. It is usually stated that a given ERP "is modulated by," "is sensitive to" or "discriminates" a given condition when statistically significant differences are found in latency, amplitude or morphology, respectively, as a function of such condition manipulation.

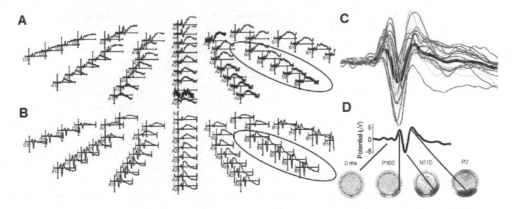

Fig. 1. ERP signal-to-noise ratio. A) ERPs at temporo-occipital scalp in response to face stimuli without preprocessing and (B) with preprocessing. Note how the N170 can be clearly observed after preprocessing over the right occipito-temporal sites (comparing both ellipses). C) N170 estimation over a representative electrode (T8) demonstrating the signal-to-noise ratio reduction in between the subject's average waveform (black line). D). Voltage map reconstruction by interpolation showing the scalp activity at 0, P100, N170, 200 and P2 after the presentation of face stimuli.

A continuous reconstruction of electrical activity on the scalp, normally based on spatial interpolation of the electrode sites, is termed a topographical map (or a voltage map or topomap). Each component usually has a relatively specific topographic distribution. The so-called long latency components (cognitive components or endogenous components) occur after 100 ms and are sensitive to changes in cognitive processing, as the meaning of the stimulus, or resources of processing required in the task performed (Hillyard, 2000). In the following section, we provide a succinct description of several components.

3. A selective description of main components

3.1 P100 and N100 (P1 and N1)
Eason et al. (1969) found that visual stimuli situated in visual fields with focused attention elicited components with larger amplitude (approximately 100 ms after stimulus onset, P1 and N1), compared with ignored or unnoticed stimuli. This amplitude enhancement is at its maximum in the temporal-occipital region, contralateral to the localization of the stimuli and is sensitive to the specific localization of the stimuli in the visual field (Mangun et al., 1993). Comparable results were obtained in the auditory modality by a dichotic listening paradigm (Hillyard et al., 1973). This auditory early-attention effect reflects a response increase of the auditory primary cortex (Woldorff et al., 1993). The P1 and N1 components are also modulated by several factors in the attentional task, such as emotional saliency, relevance or familiarity.

3.2 P200 (or P2)
Is a positive deflection occurring approximately 200 ms after the onset of the stimulus? P200 has been interpreted as reflecting selective attention (Hackley, Woldorff and Hillyard, 1990) and visual-feature detection processes (Luck and Hillyard, 1994). Similarly, P2 has been

shown to be sensitive to orthographic/phonological tasks, semantic categorization tasks, reward-punishment discrimination and lexical decision tasks.

3.3 N200 (or N2)

Is a negative deflection resulting from a deviation in form or context of a prevailing stimulus? Normally, N2 is evoked 180 to 235 ms following the presentation of a specific visual or auditory stimulus. Additionally, the N2 is considered to be a family of different components, but its classic consideration can be elicited through an experimental oddball paradigm and is sensitive to perceptual features (Bentin et al., 1999). This component is also associated with conflict detection during the regulation of successful behavior (Nieuwenhuis, Yeung, Van Den Wildenberg and Ridderinkhof, 2003). The source of N2 modulation compromises the anterior cingulate cortex (ACC hereafter, a brain area susceptible to social monitoring of conflict) and other prefrontal cortex areas (Nieuwenhuis et al., 2003).

3.4 N170/Vertex Positive Potential (N170/VPP)

The N170/VPP complex is a negative peak around 170 ms in the temporal-occipital regions and simultaneously one central-frontal positivity (VPP), functionally equivalent (Joyce and Rossion, 2005). The source of N170 compromises the inferior temporal gyrus and the fusiform gyrus (two neural areas associated with specific face processing). Its amplitude is greater for human faces, compared with objects or other stimuli (Bentin, Allison, Puce, Perez and McCarthy, 1996; Jeffreys, 1989). During the face-processing task, N170 is sometimes followed by a P2, a N250 and an LPP component modulated by other variables. The N170 component has shown amplitude/latency modulation based on race cues (Ibanez et al., 2010c; Ito and Ulrand, 2005; Gonzales et al., 2008), emotional variables (Ashley, Vuilleunier and Swick, 2004) and contextual effects (Ibanez et al. 2011d).

3.5 Early Posterior Negativity (EPN)

The EPN is a middle-latency component that has been associated with different stages of valence information processing and affective discrimination (Schupp et al., 2004a, 2004b). Di Russo, Taddei, Apnile and Spinelli (2006) suggested that EPN would reflect early valence discrimination and response selection processes. Additionally, Schupp et al. (2004a) have stated that the processing indexed by the EPN is modulated by perceptual features that facilitate further evaluation of arousing stimuli. Different studies have found a modulation differing from the neutral for both emotional (pleasant, unpleasant) categories of pictures (e.g., Dufey et al., 2010; Cuthbert, Schupp, Bradley, Birbaumer and Lang (2000). Nevertheless, specific effects (task or stimuli-dependent) on EPN in relation to valence and the influence of arousal should be further assessed.

3.6 P300 (or P3)

This component has been described as engaging higher-order cognitive operations related to selective attention and resource allocation (Donchin and Coles, 1988). The P3 amplitude may serve as a covert measure of attention that arises independently of behavioral responding (Gray et al., 2004). The component has also been related to a post-decisional "cognitive closure" mechanism (Desmedt, 1980; Verleger, 1998); and to the access of information for consciousness (Picton, 1992). Its amplitude generally varies as a function of the temporal distance between a target and a preceding outgoing stimulus (e.g., Cornejo et al., 2007). There are two sub-components (P3a and P3b). The P3a has a more frontal distribution and is observed after an unexpected event, regardless of the relevance of the stimulus. Usually, it is associated with automatic attentional modulation. The P3b is related to attention, working memory and superior cognitive functions and is observed at centro-parietal sites. This ERP is affected by several psychological processes, the most important of which are motivation and sustained attention.

3.7 Late Positive Components (LPP, PPC, P600)

The late positive potential (LPP) is considered to be a family of components (although initially was described by Sutton in 1965 as a unique, frontal bilateral positivity). This late component (300 to 700 ms) is sensitive to stimuli valence and to the previous emotional context (Cacioppo et al., 1994, Schupp et al., 2000). Its amplitude, according to several studies, increases in response to motivationally relevant stimuli (i.e., pleasant or unpleasant images; Cuthbert et al., 2000; Schupp et al., 2000; Schupp, Junghofer, Weike and Hamm, 2004). The amplitude, latency and topography of LPP are modulated by the semantic emotional valence of stimuli (Cunningham et al., 2007) and contextual information (Cornejo et al., 2009; Hurtado et al., 2009). The late positive complex (LPC) is a component similar to LPP and has been related to the process of re-analysis of the incongruent situation produced by inconsistent meaning (Ibanez et al., 2010a, 2011b; Sitnikova, Kuperberg and Holcomb, 2003). The P600 is considered to be an index for second pass-parsing processes of information processing, having much in common with working memory operations. It is associated with superior frontal, temporal and parietal regions, which are believed to contribute to some aspects of information processing during recognition memory.

3.8 N400 and N400-like

The N400 is a negative component that appears around 400 ms after the presentation of semantically unrelated information between two words or between a context and a word. Although this component was first studied in the linguistic field, recent studies have extended previous results to richer action sequences and pictorial stimuli (sometimes called N350 or N400-like), such as congruent-incongruent pictures or videos of gestures, actions and motor events (Aravena et al., 2010; Cornejo et al., 2009; Proverbio et al., 2010; Ibañez et al., 2010b, 2011; Guerra et al., 2009; Sitnikova et al., 2003). Although spatial resolution provided by ERP does not allow a precise localization of N400 neural generators, evidence from lesion studies, MEG and intracranial recordings converge to implicate temporal areas (left superior/middle temporal gyrus, the anterior-medial temporal lobe, the PHC and anterior fusiform gyrus) as the possible sources of N400 (Van Petten and Luka, 2006). This N400 points to a distributed and multimodal system that is simultaneously open to verbal and nonverbal meanings (Kutas and Federmeier, 2000).

3.9 Contingent Negative Variation (CNV)

CNV is an extended and prolonged negative potential recorded during simple, warned reaction time paradigms from central and parietal scalp fields. Its scalp distribution always begins bilaterally and symmetrically at the midline of the precentral-parietal regions, approximately 1.000 to 1.500 ms before response movement. CNV is a correlate of anticipation of the latter presentation of a stimulus target (Picton and Hillyard, 1988; Walter, Cooper, Aldridge, McCallum and Winter, 1964).

3.10 Error-Related Negativity (ERN) and Feedback Error-Related Negativity (fERN)

The ERN is a component observed 50 to 100 ms after a response characterized as being of high conflict in which a dominant response is inconsistent with respect to the correct response (Hohnsbein, Falkenstein and Hoormann, 1995 and others). The ERN is an index for the general sensitivity of the conflict monitoring system, which can be used to predict successful patterns of control (Yeung, Botvinick, and Cohen, 2004). Feedback error-related negativity (fERN) has been referred to as a negative deflection in the event-related potential (ERP), which distinguishes between wins/losses or correct/error trials in terms of expected and unexpected outcomes (e.g., San Martin et al., 2010). In correct (ERN) or win trials (fERN), similar components have been named Correct Related Negativity (CRN) and

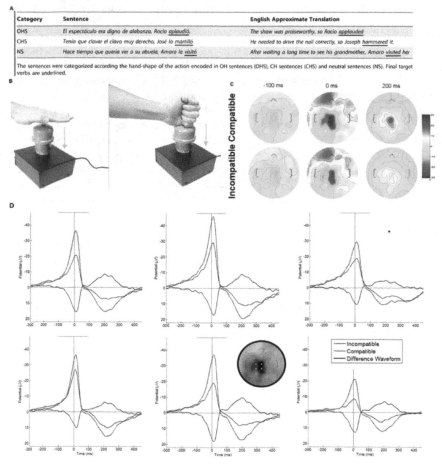

Fig. 2. Motor potential (MP and RAP) modulated by compatibility with semantic stimuli. A) Verbal stimuli used in an action-sentence compatibility paradigm. B) Participants' open- and close-hand responses. C) Scalp topography of the motor response at baseline, zero-time response and 200 ms after the response. D) Motor potential (MP and RAP) modulated by the compatibility between the participant motor responses (open or close) and the semantic stimuli (sentences containing open- or close-hand actions). Modified from Aravena et al., 2010.

feedback correct-related positivity (fCRP), respectively. According to an extended theory called the "reinforcement learning theory of ERN," both forms of ERN/fERN reflect the function of a generic, high-level error-processing system in humans (Holroyd and Coles, 2002). Both the ERN and fERN have a main source on the cingulate cortex, the anterior and the posterior division.

3.11 Motor components (RP, LRP, MP, RAP)

The movement-related cortical potentials (MRCP) associated with self-paced movements are considered to be a measure of motor cortex excitability and allow the exploration of cortical changes related to motor preparation and execution. The readiness potential (RP, or in its original German name, Bereitschaftspotential) precedes voluntary muscle movement and represents the cortical contribution to the pre-motor planning of volitional movement. The RP was first described in 1964 by Hans Helmut Kornhuber and Lüder Deecke. The lateralized readiness potential (LRP) is a particular form of RP in response to certain movements of one side (left or right) of the body. Being related to RP, another negativity measured over Cz beginning shortly before the response onset (-90 ms) has been named the motor potential (MP) or late motor-related potential (late MRP; Aravena et al., 2010). The MP is likely to represent pyramidal neuron activity in the primary cortex (M1) at motor execution. MP amplitude modulation has been associated with the rapidness and precision of movement and also with short-term training effects. Finally, another component with a peak over Cz after movement onset (200-300 ms) has been named the re-afferent potential (RAP). RAP is an index of movement-related sensory feedback to the primary sensory-motor cortex and is considered an indicator of attention (Aravena et al., 2010, see Figure 2).

4. Representative areas of social cognitive neuroscience

4.1 Contextual approaches to language

Context-dependence effects are pervasive in everyday cognition (Barutta et al., 2011; Cosmelli and Ibañez, 2008; Ibanez and Cosmelli, 2008; Ibanez et al., 2010a), especially in the case of language (Ledoux, Camblin, Swaab and Gordon, 2006; Rodriguez-Fornells, Cunillera, Mestres-Misse and de Diego-Balaguer, 2009). We listen and say words within other streams of words. We perceive the emotion of a face altogether with the emotional body language, the semantics, the prosody and other cues from the situation. Language use can be tracked by assessing the influence of context parameters (such as intonation, lexical choice, prosody, and paralinguistic clues) in a current communicative situation. ERPs studies of early (N170 and ELAN) and late components (N400, LPC, LPP) have provided important insights about the temporal brain dynamics of contextual effects in language. For instance, important issues, such as automaticity of contextual effects, multimodal blending of meanings, action-sentence coupling, language-like gesture processing, language and social information coupling, and early emotional word processing have been demonstrated within ERP research (Aravena et al., 2010; Cornejo et al., 2009; Hagoort, 2008; Ibanez et al., 2006, 2009, 2010b, 2010c, 2011b; 2011c, 2011d, 2011e, Van Petten and Luka, 2006). Contextual effects in language assessed with ERPs is a relevant topic in diverse areas of neuropsychiatric research, such as schizophrenia (Guerra et al., 2009; Ibanez et al., 2011c), Alzheimer's disease and mild cognitive impairment (Schwartz et al., 2003; Taylor and Olichney, 2007), focal basal ganglia lesions (Paulmann, Pell and Kotz, 2008) alcoholism (Roopesh et al., 2009) and aphasia (Wassenaar and Hagoort, 2005), among other conditions.

4.2 Emotion and emotional body language

Today, it is well known that complex social skills depend on basic emotional processing and inference (Grossmann, 2010). Moreover, facial emotional expressions can provide an automatic and rapid shortcut to alarm signals, mentalizing and inter-subjective communication. Important issues in emotion research, such as face emotional processing (Eimer and Holmes, 2007), emotion regulation (Hajcak, MacNamara and Olvet, 2010) and the intertwining of attention and emotion (Schupp, Flaisch, Stockburger & Junghofer, 2006) have a long tradition in ERP research.

Early, automatic and unaware processing of emotion in faces, words and pictures have been demonstrated within ERP research (Guex et al., 2011; Ibanez et al., 2010c, 2011d, In press, Submitted b, see Figure 3.A). Theoretical models of emotion perception (Vuilleumier and Pourtois, 2007) propose a parallel and interactive system indexing object recognition (e.g., triggered by the fusiform gyrus) and emotional discrimination (e.g., triggered by the amygdala). Emotional signs that can denote confidence or danger may occur before and parallel to the process of object codification. In other words, emotional significance can be processed before a stimulus is completely identified. At the same time, processing of complex social stimuli intermixed with emotional processing has been reported at late stages, indexed with the LPP and LPC (Dufey et al., 2010; Hurtado et al., 2009; Ibanez et al.,

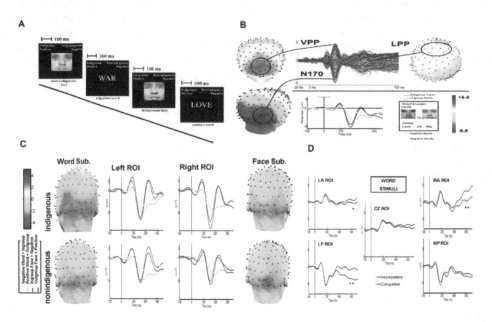

Fig. 3. Early and late emotional-cognitive processing. A) Implicit association test (IAT) schematic representation. Both ingroup and outgroup faces, along with words of positive and negative valence, are presented. The subject is required to classify each stimulus to the left or to the right according to labels displayed on top of the screen. B) Early (N170) and late (LPP) effects of IAT. C) N170 contextual modulation based on valence and membership stimuli. D) Late processing (LPP) of semantic stimuli compatibility. Modified from Hurtado et al. 2009 and Ibanez et al 2010c.

2009, 2010b, 2011b, see Figure 3.B). Emotional body language (EBL) is another emergent area in neuroscience research (de Gelder, 2006). Neuroimaging studies have shown that the EBL activates similar areas of emotional face processing, such as amygdala and fusiform gyrus. EBL signals are automatically perceived and influence emotional communication and decision making. ERP research has demonstrated that EMB (a) is automatic and processed early in the brain; (b) influences the emotional recognition of face processing; and (c) is processed in an integrated way with face processing (de Gelder et al., 2006; Meeren, van Heijnsbergen and de Gelder, 2005).

4.3 Empathy

A large number of studies using functional MRI, and more recently electrophysiology, have used the presentation of stimuli depicting people in pain (i.e., people suffering from physical injuries or expressing facial expressions of pain) to characterize the neural underpinnings of empathic processing (Botvinick et al., 2005; Jackson et al., 2006; Cheng et al., 2008a; Fan et al., 2008; Han et al., 2008; Akitsuki and Decety, 2009, Decety et al., 2010c). The results from these studies suggest that empathy for pain involves a somatosensory resonance mechanism between other and self that draws on the affective and sensory dimensions of pain processing (Jackson et al., 2006). This mechanism provides crucial and rapid information to help us understand the affective states of others and respond to them (Decety and Lamm, 2006).

ERP studies of empathy for pain showed an N1 differentiation (neutral pictures eliciting greater negative amplitudes) over the frontal area, as well as a late P3 over the centro-parietal region (pain pictures producing greater positive amplitudes; Fan et al., 2008; Han et al., 2008; Decety et al., 2010). These ERPs studies have shown early modulation by contextual reality of stimuli and late modulation based on cognitive regulatory and task demands (Fan and Han, 2008; Han et al., 2008; Decety et al., 2010c; Li and Han, 2010), as well as 'other-related' information, such as priming for treat signaling (Ibanez et al. 2011e). ERP studies have provided important insights regarding the context-dependent processing and differences in automatic-controlled processing on empathy for pain research.

4.4 Decision making and reward

The current neuroscience of decision making has assessed multiple processes engaged in this complex cognitive ability. Evidence from animals, healthy human volunteers and neuropsychiatric patients (e.g., Bechara and van Der Linden, 2005; Brand et al., 2006; Camerer et al. 2008; Gleichgerrcht et al. 2010; Kable and Glimcher, 2009; Glimcher and Rustichini, 2004; Rangel 2008; Rangel, Rushworth et al., 2007) highlights the role of frontostriatal and limbic loops in decision making. Despite some discrepancies between different models, three main systems are thought to be involved in frontostriatal and limbic loop: a stimulus-encoding system (orbitofrontal cortex), a reward-based action-selection and monitoring system (cingulate cortex) and an expected-reward system (basal ganglia and amygdala). We have shown (Gleichgerrcht et al., 2010) that these systems are crucial in the decision-making process in normal voluntaries, as well as in neuropsychiatric disorders, such as neurodegenerative diseases (Figure 4). The action-selection and monitoring system can be tracked directly with the P2, the ERN and the fERN, opening a new branch of research (Nieuwenhuis et al., 2004, 2005). Gambling and decision-making tasks can be assessed with ERPs (e.g., San martin et al., 2010). Behavioral measures of affective and risky decision-making tasks would be not so sensitive as to assess subtle deficits in decision making in disorders such as adult attention deficit hyperactivity disorder and bipolar disorders. Conversely, ERP abnormal neural processing of valence and magnitude of rewards in a gambling task in those disorders may help to integrate reward, action-selection and monitoring systems, providing an excellent shortcut to goal-directed action (Ibanez et al., Submitted a). ERP research on gambling tasks provides both a clinical and a theoretical branch of research linking decision making, soft frontal diseases, monitoring-reward systems and psychiatry.

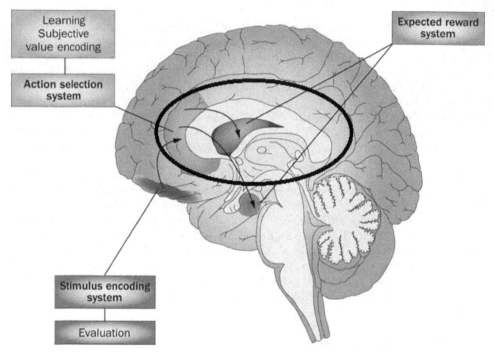

Fig. 4. A neuroanatomical model of decision making. Three main systems are thought to be involved in decision making: a stimulus-encoding system (orbitofrontal cortex shown in red), an action-selection system (anterior cingulate cortex shown in green) and an expected-reward system (basal ganglia and amygdala shown in blue). The anterior, medial and posterior cingulate cortex, together with basal ganglia (ellipse), seem to modulate the ERN and fERN in gambling and error-monitoring tasks. Modified from Gleichgerrcht et al., 2010.

5. Complementary issues

We have described several ERP components involved in studies of social and cognitive neuroscience. Now, in this section we review some methodological approaches of ERP research that complement and improve the advances in traditional ERP assessment: sleep research, intracranial recordings, source location analysis and co-recordings with fMRI.

5.1 Sleep research

The study of cognitive processing during sleep is a topic of great interest because ERPs allow the study of stimulation with passive paradigms (without conscious or behavioral response), opening multiple research possibilities during different sleep phases (Ibanez et al., 2008a). Different cognitive discriminations during sleep related to the learning, frequency, intensity, duration, saliency, novelty, proportion of appearance, meaning and even sentential integration of stimuli are topics of intense research (e.g., Ibanez et al., 2006). Methodological control of ERP sleep research, such the use of qualitative and quantitative measures of sleep stages (see Figure 5), the control of the so-called first night effect and the assessment of sleep disturbances are important factors for improving this research area (Ibanez et al., 2008b). Better control of experimental paradigms is relevant for the growth of the neuroscience of sleep.

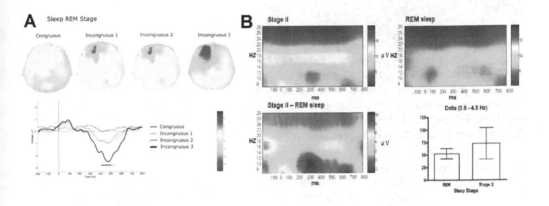

Fig. 5. Quantitative assessment of sleep stages during ERP recordings. A) The voltage maps and N400 waveform modulation of contextual semantic discrimination during REM sleep. B).Comparison of frequency bands between sleep stages (time-frequency charts for stage II sleep, REM sleep and stage II-minus-REM subtraction). Microvolt differences (mean and standard deviations) of delta band activity during stage II and REM (right bottom). Modified from Ibanez et al., 2006, 2008b.

5.2 Intracraneal recordings

The use of local field potentials (LFP) and electrocorticography (ECoG) in patients with surgically implanted electrodes (Figure 6) have provided a recent, new pathway to study the spatiotemporal brain dynamics of cognition. Intracraneal recordings help to diagnose and treat neurological conditions, such as epilepsy, Parkinson's disease and tumors. LFP and ECoG are measures of direct brain activity that have better (combined) temporo-spatial resolution than any other human neuroscience method. The ERP assessment, together with evoked oscillatory activity, has provided important insights on working memory, episodic memory, language, face processing, consciousness and spatial cognition (Jacobs and Kahana, 2010; Lachaux et al., 2003).

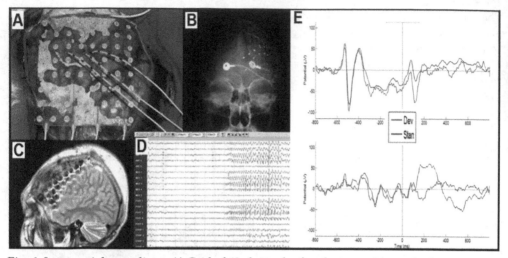

Fig. 6. Intracranial recordings. A) Grid of 63 electrodes for electrocorticography in a patient with refractory epilepsy. B) X-ray computed tomography (CT) and C) MRI showing the electrode grid and deep electrodes for local field potentials. D) Intracranial EEG. E) iERP recordings of deviant (DEV, Blue) and standard (STA, Red) stimuli during a global-local oddball task. Selected electrodes demonstrated an N2 and P3 modulation at the frontal (above) and parieto-temporal sites (below).

5.3 Source location in dense arrays
The current use of dense arrays of electrodes (from 64 to 256 channels) allows a better characterization of field potentials and improves the estimation of cortical brain sources, which generates the ERPs. The source estimation reduces the spatial imprecision of ERPs and links the temporal information with low-resolution anatomical measures. Important advances on parametric and non-parametric methods have been developed recently (Grech et al., 2008). Several engineering solutions of an inverse problem to find ERP sources using parametric and non-parametric approaches are available (e.g., LORETA, sLORETA, VARETA, S-MAP, ST-MAP, Backus-Gilbert, LAURA, SLF, SSLOFO and ALF; BESA, MUSIC and FINES). Methods of distributed sources (Figure 7), including biophysical and psychological constraints (e.g., LAURA), can produce more relevant results. Finally, principal-component analysis (PCA) and independent-component analysis (ICA) are now accessible for ERP source localization. The development of distributed EEG/MEG source analysis using statistical parametric mapping of MRI promises further advances in social-affective neuroscience (e.g., Junghofer, Peyk, Flaisch and Schupp, 2006).

5.4 FMRI-ERP simultaneous recordings
FMRI provides a fine spatial resolution but measures indirect brain signatures (hemodynamic response) and has poor temporal resolution. ERPs are a direct measure of cortical activity but have poor spatial resolution. Combining fMRI and ERPs provides a spatial and temporal fine-ground resolution of cognitive brain activity (Gore, Horovitz, Cannistraci and Skudlarski, 2006). Recently, removal algorithms of fMRI artifacts on ERPs

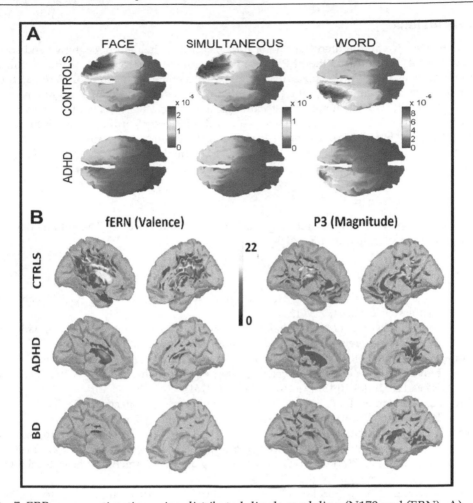

Fig. 7. ERP source estimation using distributed dipole modeling (N170 and fERN). A) N170 source imaging estimation of fusiform gyrus for faces, words and face-word simultaneous stimuli in controls (above) and patients (below) with ADHD. Average values of estimated, standardized current density power at maximum peaks of activation. B) Cortical current density mapping of valence and reward magnitude. The source estimation of distributed valence dipoles (fERN, left) and magnitude effects (P3, right) for controls, patients with ADHD and those with bipolar disorders (BD). Color-map values represent the t-values of comparisons between signal and noise. Modified from Ibanez et al., Accepted, Submitted a.

have been developed, facilitating the combined use of both methods. For instance, ERP/fMRI co-recording allows an enhanced study of origins and locations of ERP neural generators. For example, the spatial (face-processing brain areas) and temporal brain dynamics (N170) of face processing in the human brain have been reported with this methodology (Sadeh et al., 2008)

6. Conclusions

In this chapter, we highlighted the role of ERP research in the field of cognitive and social neuroscience. We introduced the ERP methodology and then a selective description of main components was developed. Subsequently, some representative fields of ERP research on the neural basis of language, emotion, empathy and decision-making cognition were presented. Finally, complementary methodological approaches (sleep research, intracranial recordings, source location in dense arrays and fMRI-ERP co-recordings) were introduced, highlighting the broad horizons of ERP research. By providing the fine, temporal brain dynamics of social and cognitive processes in normal, psychiatric and neurological participants, ERP research constitutes an important branch of human neuroscience.

7. Acknowledgments

This work was partially supported by grants CONICET and FINECO. The authors have no conflicts of interest related to this article.

8. References

Adolphs, R. 2003. Investigating the Cognitive Neuroscience of Social Behavior. *Neuropsychologia*, 41, 119–126.

Akitsuki, Y., & Decety, J. (2009). Social context and perceived agency affects empathy for pain: an event-related fMRI investigation. *Neuroimage*, 47(2), 722-734.

Aravena P, Hurtado E, Riveros R, Cardona F, Manes F, Ibáñez A. Applauding with closed hands: Neural signature of action sentence compatibility effects. (2010), *PLoS ONE* 5(7): e11751. doi:10.1371/journal.pone.0011751

Ashley, V., Vuilleumier, P., & Swick, D. 2004. Time Course and Specificity of Event-Related Potentials to Emotional Expressions. *NeuroReport*, 15, 211–216.

Barutta J, Cornejo C, Ibáñez A. (2011). Theories and theorizers: a contextual approach to theories of cognition. *Integrative Psychological and Behavioral Science*, ;45(2):223-46.

Bechara, A. & van Der Linden, M. Decision making and impulse control after frontal lobe injuries. *Curr. Opin. Neurol.* 18, 734–739 (2005).

Bentin, S., Deouell, L.Y., & Soroker, N. 1999. Selective Visual Streaming in Face Recognition: Evidence from Developmental Prosopagnosia. *Neuroreport*, 10, 823–827.

Bentin, Shlomo, Allison, Truett, Puce, Aina, Perez, Erik, et al. 1996. Electrophysiological Studies of Face Perception in Humans. *Journal of Cognitive Neuroscience*, 8(6):551-565..

Blakemore, S. J., Winston, J., & Frith, U. (2004). Social cognitive neuroscience: where are we heading? *Trends in Cognitive Science*, 8(5), 216-222.

Botvinick, M., Jha, A. P., Bylsma, L. M., Fabian, S. A., Solomon, P. E., & Prkachin, K. M. (2005). Viewing facial expressions of pain engages cortical areas involved in the direct experience of pain. *Neuroimage*, 25(1), 312-319.

Brand, M., Labudda, K. & Markowitsch, H. J. Neuropsychological correlates of decision making in ambiguous and risky situations. *Neural Netw.* 19, 1266–1276 (2006).

Cacioppo, J.T., & Berntson, G. 1994. Relationship between Attitudes and Evaluative Space: A Critical Review, with Enphasis on the Separability of Positive and Negative Subtrates. *Psychological Bulletin*, 115, 401–423.

Cheng, Y., Lee, P. L., Yang, C. Y., Lin, C. P., Hung, D., & Decety, J. (2008). Gender differences in the mu rhythm of the human mirror-neuron system. *PLoS One*, 3(5), e2113.

Cornejo C, Simonetti F, Ibañez, A; Aldunate N, Lopez V, Ceric, F. (2009). Gesture and Metaphor: Electrophysiological evidence of 400 multimodal modulation . *Brain and Cognition*, 70(1):42-52.

Cornejo, C., Simonetti, F., Aldunate, N., Ibáñez, A., López, V., Melloni, L. (2007). Electrophysiological evidence of different interpretive strategies in irony comprehension. *Journal of Psycholinguistic Research*, 36(6):411-30.

Cosmelli, Diego & Ibanez, Agustin. (2008). Human Cognition in Context: On the Biologic, Cognitive and Social reconsideration of Meaning. *Integrative Psychological and Behavioral Sciences*, 42(2):233-44.

Cunningham, W., & Johnson, M. 2007. Attitudes and Evaluation. Toward a Component Process Framework. In E. Harmon-Jones, & P. Winkielman (Eds.), Social Neuroscience. *Integrating Biological and Psychological Explanations of Social Behaviour* (pp. 227–243). NY: The Guilford Press.

Cunningham, W. A., & Zelazo, P. D. (2007). Attitudes and evaluations: a social cognitive neuroscience perspective. *Trends Cognitive Science*, 11(3), 97-104.

Cuthbert, B.N., Schupp, H.T., Bradley, M.M., Birbaumer, N., & y Lang, P.J. 2000. Brain Potentials in Affective Picture Processing: Covariation with Autonomic Arousal and Affective Report. *Biological Psychology*, 52, 95–111.

de Gelder, B. (2006). Towards the neurobiology of emotional body language. *Nat Rev Neurosci*, 7(3), 242-249.

de Gelder, B., Meeren, H. K., Righart, R., van den Stock, J., van de Riet, W. A., & Tamietto, M. (2006). Beyond the face: exploring rapid influences of context on face processing. *Prog Brain Res*, 155, 37-48.

Decety, J., & Sommerville, J. A. (2003). Shared representations between self and other: a social cognitive neuroscience view. *Trends Cognitive Science*, 7(12), 527-533.

Decety, J., & Lamm, C. (2006). Human empathy through the lens of social neuroscience. *ScientificWorldJournal*, 6, 1146-1163.

Decety, J., Yang, C. Y., & Cheng, Y. (2010). Physicians down-regulate their pain empathy response: an event-related brain potential study. *Neuroimage*, 50(4), 1676-1682.

Desmedt, J.E. 1980. P300 in Serial Tasks: An Essential Post-decision Closure Mechanism. *Progressing in Brain Research*, 54, 682–686.

Donchin, E., & Coles, M.G.H. 1988. Is the P300 Component a Manifestation of Cognitive Updating? *The Behavioral and Brain Sciences*, 11, 357–427.

Dufey, M., Hurtado, E. Fernández, A.M. Manes, F, and Ibáñez (2010). Exploring the relationship between vagal tone and event-related potentials in response to an affective picture task. *Social Neuroscience*, 23:1-15.

Di Russo, F., Taddei, F., Apnile, T., & Spinelli, D. (2006). Neural correlates of fast stimulus discrimination and response selection in top-level fencers. *Neurosci Lett*, 408(2), 113-118.

Eimer, M., & Holmes, A. (2007). Event-related brain potential correlates of emotional face processing. *Neuropsychologia*, 45(1), 15-31.

Fan, Y., & Han, S. (2008). Temporal dynamic of neural mechanisms involved in empathy for pain: an event-related brain potential study. *Neuropsychologia*, 46(1), 160-173.

Frith, C., & Frith, U. (2010). Learning from others: introduction to the special review series on social neuroscience. *Neuron*, 65(6), 739-743.

Gleichgerrcht E, Ibanez A, Roca M, Torralva T, Manes F. (2010). Decision Making Cognition in Neurodegenerative Diseases. *Nature Reviews Neurology*, 6, 611–623

Glimcher, P. W. & Rustichini, A. Neuroeconomics: the consilience of brain and decision. *Science* 306, 447–452 (2004).

Gonzalez, R., López, V., Haye, A., Hurtado, E., & Ibañez, A. 2008. N170 and LPP Discrimination of Same Race Versus Other Race Facial Stimuli and Positive and Negative Words in Indigenous and Non-Indigenous Participants. *Clinical Neurophysiology*, 119(9), e155.

Gore, J. C., Horovitz, S. G., Cannistraci, C. J., & Skudlarski, P. (2006). Integration of fMRI, NIROT and ERP for studies of human brain function. *Magn Reson Imaging*, 24(4), 507-513.

Gray, J.R., & Burgess, G.C. 2004. Personality Differences in Cognitive Control? BAS, Processing Efficiency, and the Prefrontal Cortex. *Journal of Research in Personality*, 38, 35– 36.

Grech, R., Cassar, T., Muscat, J., Camilleri, K. P., Fabri, S. G., Zervakis, M., et al. (2008). Review on solving the inverse problem in EEG source analysis. *J Neuroeng Rehabil*, 5, 25.

Grossmann, T. (2010). The development of emotion perception in face and voice during infancy. *Restor Neurol Neurosci*, 28(2), 219-236.

Guerra, S, Ibañez, A, Bobes, A., Martin, M et al. (2009). N400 deficits from semantic matching of pictures in probands and first degrees relatives from multiplex schizophrenia families. *Brain and Cognition*, 70(2):221-30.

Guex, R; Ceric, F; Hurtado, E, Navarro, A, Gonzalez, R; Manes, F, Ibanez, A. Performance errors of ingroup/outgroup stimuli and valence association in the implicit association task: brain bias of ingroup favoritism. *The Open Neuroscience Journal*, Accepted.

Han, S., Fan, Y., & Mao, L. (2008). Gender difference in empathy for pain: an electrophysiological investigation. *Brain Res*, 1196, 85-93.

Hackley, S.A., Woldorff, M., & Hillyard, S.A. 1990. Cross-modal Selective Attention Effects on Retinal, Myogenic, Brainstem and Cerebral Evoked Potentials. *Psychophysiology*, 27, 195–208.

Hagoort, P. (2008). The fractionation of spoken language understanding by measuring electrical and magnetic brain signals. *Philos Trans R Soc Lond B Biol Sci*, 363(1493), 1055-1069.

Hajcak, G., MacNamara, A., & Olvet, D. M. (2010). Event-related potentials, emotion, and emotion regulation: an integrative review. *Dev Neuropsychol*, 35(2), 129-155

Hillyard, S.A. 2000. Electrical and Magnetic Brain Recordings: Contributions to Cognitive Neurosciencies. In Gazzaniga M.S., editor. *Cognitive Neuroscience a Reader* (pp. 25–37). Oxford: Blackwell Publishers Ltd.

Hillyard, S.A., & Picton, T.W. 1987. Electrophysiology of Cognition. *Handbook of Physiology, the Nervous System* (pp. 519-584). New York: Oxford University Press.

Hillyard, S.A., Hink, R.F., Schwent, V.L., & Picton, T.W. 1973. Electrical Signs of Selective Attention in the Human Brain. *Science*, 182, 177–182

Hohnsbein, Joachim, Falkenstein, Michael, & Hoormann, Jörg. 1995. Effects of Attention and Time-Pressure on P300 Subcomponents and Implications for Mental Workload Research. *Biological Psychology*, 40(1–2), 73–81. Special Issue: EEG in Basic and Applied Settings.

Holroyd, C. B., & Coles, M. G. (2002). The neural basis of human error processing: reinforcement learning, dopamine, and the error-related negativity. *Psychol Rev*, 109(4), 679-709.

Hurtado, E, Gonzalez, R; Haye, A; Manes, F., Ibanez, A. (2009). Contextual blending of ingroup/outgroup face stimuli and word valence: LPP modulation and convergence of measures. *BMC Neuroscience*, 26;10:69.

Ibáñez A , Petroni A, Urquina H, Torralva T, Blenkmann A, Beltrachini L, Muravchik C, Baez S, Cetckovih M, Torrente F, Hurtado E, Guex R, Sigman M, Lischinsky A, Manes F. Cortical deficits in emotion processing for faces in adults with ADHD: Its relation to social cognition and executive functioning. *Social Neuroscience* (In press).

Ibáñez A, Gleichgerrcht E, Hurtado E, González R, Haye A, Manes F (2010c). Early Neural Markers of Implicit Attitudes: N170 Modulated by Intergroup and Evaluative Contexts in IAT. *Frontiers in Human Neuroscience*, 4:188. doi:10.3389/fnhum.2010.00188

Ibanez A, Riveros R, Aravena P, Vergara V, Cardona JF, García L, Hurtado E, Martin Reyes M, Barutta J, Manes F. When context is hard to integrate: cortical measures of congruency in schizophrenics and healthy relatives from multiplex families. *Schizophrenia Research 126* (2011c) 303–305

Ibáñez A., Gleichgerrcht, E., Manes, F. (2010a). Clinical Effects of Insular Damage in Humans. *Brain Structure and Function*, 214(5-6):397-410.

Ibanez A; Riveros R; Hurtado E; Gleichgerrcht E; Urquina H; Martin Reyes M; Manes F. (Submitted b) The face and its emotion: *Cortical Deficits in Structural Processing and Early Emotional Discrimination in Schizophrenic and Relatives*

Ibáñez, A, et al., (Submitted a). Neural basis of decision making and reward in euthymic bipolar disorder and adults with ADHD: *A multilevel analysis*

Ibáñez, A, Manes, F; Escobar, J; Trujillo N; Andreucci, P; Hurtado, E. (2010b). Gesture influences the processing of figurative language in non-native speakers. *Neuroscience Letters*, 471, 48–52.

Ibáñez, A, Toro P, Cornejo C, Urquina, H; Manes, F; Weisbrod M, Schröder J. (2011b). High contextual sensitivity of metaphorical expressions and gesture blending: A video ERP design. Psychiatry Research, *Neuroimaging*, 10.1016/j.pscychresns.2010.08.008

Ibáñez, A. Cosmelli D. (2008). Moving Beyond Computational Cognitivism: Understanding Intentionality, Intersubjectivity and Ecology of Mind. *Integrative Psychological and Behavioral Sciences*, 42(2):129-36.

Ibañez, A. San Martin, M. E Hurtado & V. López, (2008b). Methodological considerations related to sleep paradigm using event related potentials. *Biological Research*, 41: 271-275.

Ibáñez, A., Haye, A., González, R., Hurtado, E., Henríquez, R. (2009). Multi-level analysis of cultural phenomena: The role of ERP approach to prejudice. *The Journal for Theory in Social Behavior*, 39, 81-110.

Ibáñez, A., Lopez, V., Cornejo, C. (2006). ERPs and contextual semantic discrimination: Evidence of degrees of congruency in wakefulness and sleep. *Brain and Language*, 98, (3), 264-275.

Ibáñez, A; Hurtado, E., Lobos, A., Trujillo, N., Escobar, J., Baez, S; Huepe D, Manes, F., Decety, J. Subliminal presentation of other faces (but not own face) primes behavioral and evoked cortical processing of empathy for pain. *Brain Research*. (2011e). DOI 10.1016/j.brainres.2011.05.014

Ibanez, A; Riveros R; Hurtado E; Urquina, H; Cardona, J; Petroni, A; Barutta J, Lobos A, Baez S, Manes F. Facial and semantic emotional interference: Behavioral and cortical responses to the dual valence association task. *Behavioral and Brain Functions* 2011d, 7:8.

Ibañez, A; San Martin, R; Hurtado, E; Lopez, V. (2008a). ERP studies of cognitive processing during sleep. *International Journal of Psychology*, 44(4), 290 – 304.

Insel, T. R. (2010). The challenge of translation in social neuroscience: a review of oxytocin, vasopressin, and affiliative behavior. *Neuron*, 65(6), 768-779.

Ito, T.A., & Urland, G.R. 2005. The Influence of Processing Objectives on the Perception of Faces: An ERP Study of Race and Gender Perception. Cognitive, Affective, and Behavioral. *Neuroscience*, 5, 21–36.

Jacobs, J., & Kahana, M. J. (2010). Direct brain recordings fuel advances in cognitive electrophysiology. *Trends Cogn Sci*, 14(4), 162-171.

Jackson, P. L., Rainville, P., & Decety, J. (2006). To what extent do we share the pain of others? Insight from the neural bases of pain empathy. *Pain*, 125(1-2), 5-9.

Jeffreys, D.A. 1989. A Face-Responsive Potential Recorded from the Human Scalp. *Experimental Brain Research.*

Joyce C., & Rossion, B. 2005. The Face-Sensitive N170 and VPP Components Manifest the Same Brain Processes: The Effect of Reference Electrode Site, *Clin Neurophysiol*, 116, 2613-2631.

Kable, J. W. & Glimcher, P. W. The neurobiology of decision: consensus and controversy. *Neuron* 63, 733–745 (2009).

Kutas, M., & Federmeier, K.D. 2000. Electrophysiology Reveals Semantic Memory use in Language Comprehension. *Trends Cogn Sci.*, 4(12), 463–470.

Lachaux, J. P., Rudrauf, D., & Kahane, P. (2003). Intracranial EEG and human brain mapping. J Physiol Paris, 97(4-6), 613-628.

Ledoux, K., Camblin, C. C., Swaab, T. Y., & Gordon, P. C. (2006). Reading words in discourse: the modulation of lexical priming effects by message-level context. *Behav Cogn Neurosci Rev*, 5(3), 107-127.

Li, W., & Han, S. (2010). Perspective taking modulates event-related potentials to perceived pain. *Neurosci Lett*, 469(3), 328-332.

Lieberman, M. D., & Eisenberger, N. I. (2009). Neuroscience. Pains and pleasures of social life. *Science*, 323(5916), 890-891.

Luck, S.J., & Hillyard, S.A. 1994. Electrophysiological Correlates of Feature Analysis during Visual Search. *Psychophysiology*, 31, 291–308.

Mangun, G.R., Hillyard, S.A., & Luck, S.J. 1993. Electrocortical Substrates of Visual Selective Attention. In D. Meyer, & S. Kornblum (Eds.), *Attention and Performance*. (Vol. XIV, pp. 219–243). Cambridge. Massachusetts: MIT Press.

Miller G. 2006. Neuroscience. The Emotional Brain Weighs its Options. *Science*, 313, 600–1.

Nieuwenhuis, S., Yeung, N., Van Den Wildenberg, W., & Ridderinkhof, K.R. 2003. Electrophysiological Correlates of Anterior Cingulate Function in a Go/No-Go Task: Effects of Response Conflict and Trial Type Frequency. *Cognitive, Affective, and Behavioral Neuroscience*, 3, 17–26.

Ochsner, K. N. (2004). Current directions in social cognitive neuroscience. *Curr Opin Neurobiol*, 14(2), 254-258.

Paulmann, S., Pell, M. D., & Kotz, S. A. (2008). Functional contributions of the basal ganglia to emotional prosody: evidence from ERPs. *Brain Res*, 1217, 171-178.

Picton, T., & Hillyard, S. 1988. Endogenous Components of the Event-Related Brain Potential. In T. Picton (Ed.), *Human Event-Related Potentials: EEG Handbook* (pp. 361–426). Amsterdam: Elsevier.

Picton, T.W. 1992. The P300 Wave of the Human Eventrelated Potencial. *Clin. Neurophysiol. Lisse*, v. 9, n. 1, pp. 456–479.

Proverbio, A. M., Riva, F., & Zani, A. (2010). When neurons do not mirror the agent's intentions: sex differences in neural coding of goal-directed actions. *Neuropsychologia*, 48(5), 1454-1463.

Rodriguez-Fornells, A., Cunillera, T., Mestres-Misse, A., & de Diego-Balaguer, R. (2009). Neurophysiological mechanisms involved in language learning in adults. *Philos Trans R Soc Lond B Biol Sci*, 364(1536), 3711-3735.

Roopesh, B. N., Rangaswamy, M., Kamarajan, C., Chorlian, D. B., Stimus, A., Bauer, L. O., et al. (2009). Priming deficiency in male subjects at risk for alcoholism: the N4 during a lexical decision task. *Alcohol Clin Exp Res*, 33(12), 2027-2036.

Rangel, A. (2008). Consciousness meets neuroeconomics: what is the value of stimulus awareness in decision making? *Neuron*, 59(4), 525-527.

Rangel A, Camerer C, Montague, R (2008). A framework for studying the neurobiology of value-based decision making. *Nature Reviews Neuroscience*, 9, 545-556.

Rilling, J. K., & Sanfey, A. G. (2011). The neuroscience of social decision-making. *Annu Rev Psychol*, 62, 23-48.

Rushworth, M. F., Behrens, T. E., Rudebeck, P. H. & Walton, M. E. Contrasting roles for cingulate and orbitofrontal cortex in decisions and social behaviour. *Trends Cogn. Sci.* 11, 168–176 (2007).

Sadeh, B., Zhdanov, A., Podlipsky, I., Hendler, T., & Yovel, G. (2008). The validity of the face-selective ERP N170 component during simultaneous recording with functional MRI. *Neuroimage*, 42(2), 778-786.

San Martín, R; Manes, F, Hurtado, E, Isla, P; Ibáñez, A. (2010). Size and probability of rewards modulate the feedback error-related negativity associated with wins but not losses in a monetarily rewarded gambling task. *NeuroImage* 51, 1194–1204.

Sanfey, A. G. (2007). Social decision-making: insights from game theory and neuroscience. *Science*, 318(5850), 598-602.

Schupp, H. T., Cuthbert, B. N., Bradley, M. M., Cacioppo, J. T., Ito, T., & Lang, P. J. (2000). Affective picture processing: the late positive potential is modulated by motivational relevance. *Psychophysiology*, 37(2), 257-261.

Schupp, H.T., Junghöfer, M., Weike, A.I. & Hamm, A.O. 2004. The Selective Processing of Briefly Presented Affective Pictures: An ERP Analysis. *Psychophysiology*, 41, 441–449.

Schupp, H. T., Flaisch, T., Stockburger, J., & Junghofer, M. (2006). Emotion and attention: event-related brain potential studies. *Prog Brain Res*, 156, 31-51

Schwartz, T. J., Federmeier, K. D., Van Petten, C., Salmon, D. P., & Kutas, M. (2003). Electrophysiological analysis of context effects in Alzheimer's disease. *Neuropsychology*, 17(2), 187-201.

Singer, T., & Lamm, C. (2009). The social neuroscience of empathy. Ann N Y Acad Sci, 1156, 81-96.

Sitnikova, T., Kuperberg, G., & Holcomb, P. J. (2003). Semantic integration in videos of real-world events: an electrophysiological investigation. *Psychophysiology*, 40(1), 160-164.

Taylor, J. R., & Olichney, J. M. (2007). From amnesia to dementia: ERP studies of memory and language. Clin EEG *Neurosci*, 38(1), 8-17.

Van Petten, C., & Luka, B. J. (2006). Neural localization of semantic context effects in electromagnetic and hemodynamic studies. *Brain Lang*, 97(3), 279-293.

Verleger, R. 1998. Towards an Integration of P3 Research with Cognitive Neuroscience. *Behavioral and Brain Sciences* 21, 150–154.

Vuilleumier, P., & Pourtois, G. (2007). Distributed and interactive brain mechanisms during emotion face perception: evidence from functional neuroimaging. *Neuropsychologia*, 45(1), 174-194.

Walter, W., Cooper, R., Aldridge, V., McCallum, W., & Winter, A. 1964. Contingent Negative Variation: An Electric Sign of Sensori-Motor Association and Expectancy in the Human Brain. *Nature*, 203, 380–384.

Wassenaar, M., & Hagoort, P. (2005). Word-category violations in patients with Broca's aphasia: an ERP study. *Brain Lang*, 92(2), 117-137.

Woldorff, M.G., Gallen, C.C., Hampson, S.A., Hillyard, S.A., Pantev, C., Sobel, D., & Bloom, F.E. 1993. Modulation of early Sensory Processing in Human Auditory Cortex during Auditory Selective Attention. *Proc Natl Acad Sci U S A*. Sep 15; 90(18), 8722-6.

Yeung, N., Botvinick, M.M., & Cohen, J.D. 2004. The Neural Basis of Error Detection: Conflict Monitoring and the Error-Related Negativity. *Psychological Review*, 111, 931- 959.

Zaki, J., & Ochsner, K. (2009). The need for a cognitive neuroscience of naturalistic social cognition. *Ann N Y Acad Sci*, 1167, 16-30.

11

Deconstructing Central Pain with Psychophysical and Neuroimaging Studies

J.J. Cheng[1], D.S. Veldhuijzen[3], J.D. Greenspan[2] and F.A. Lenz[1]
[1]*Department of Neurosurgery, Johns Hopkins Hospital, Baltimore*
[2]*Department of Biomedical Sciences, University of Maryland Dental School,*
Program in Neuroscience, Baltimore
[3]*Division of Perioperative Care and Emergency Medicine,*
Rudolf Magus Institute of Neuroscience, Pain Clinic,
University Medical Center Utrecht, Utrecht,
[1,2]*USA*
[3]*Netherlands*

1. Introduction

The IASP has defined central pain as initiated or caused by a primary lesion or dysfunction of the central nervous system (CNS)" (Merskey, 1986). A more recent and specific definition describes central pain as "pain arising as a direct consequence of a lesion or disease affecting the central somatosensory system" (Treede et al., 2008). This definition recognizes that a disturbance of the central somatosensory system is the essential feature of central pain. A disturbance of this system applies to all central pain conditions, although they exhibit great variability across different etiologies. This chapter includes structural and functional imaging results, as well as the results of psychophysical studies, as they complement the imaging results. There is some overlap between the content of this chapter and our previous reviews of this topic (Veldhuijzen et al., 2007;Greenspan et al., 2008;Veldhuijzen et al., 2011).

2. Prevalence of sensory abnormalities in central pain?

Patients with central pain (CP) inevitably show stimulus-evoked sensory abnormalities which include negative symptoms such as hypoesthesia and hypoalgesia, as well as positive symptoms such as hyperalgesia Hyperalgesia is increased pain evoked by a stimulus which can be painful, such as deep pressure over a muscle which has been injured or bruised. Another positive symptom is allodynia which is pain evoked by a stimulus which is not normally painful, such as pain evoked by light touch following a sunburn.

When studied by quantitative sensory testing (QST, Table 1), patients with central post-stroke pain (CPSP) exhibit hypoesthesia for cold in 85-91% of patients, for warmth in 85-100%. Decreased sensation for pain (hypoalgesia) is found for cold pain in roughly 45% of patients, and for heat pain in 7-91% (Boivie et al., 1989;Leijon et al., 1989;Andersen et al., 1995;Vestergaard et al., 1995;Greenspan et al., 2004). As shown in Table 1, CPSP patients show decreased tactile sensibility in 27-52% of cases. These results demonstrate that decreased sensation or negative sensory signs vary widely across the CPSP patient population. Overall, these patients do not show sensory deficits for all types of thermal and

	(Ohara et al., 2004)	(Boivie et al., 1989;Leijon et al., 1989)	Clinic (Vestergaard et al., 1995) QST (Andersen et al., 1995).
Burning cold/cold pain	53% overall; 38%, burning & cold; 15%, hot and cold;	59%, 16/27	38%, 6/16 (freezing 3/16)
Mechanical pain	77% overall 33%, sharp/stab; 23%, pressure heavy; tight/ squeezing 7% each	Aching 30%, Pricking 30%, lacerating 26%.	86%, 23/27.
Pain rating	7.1 mean, 2.0 SD	2.5-7.9 mean by stroke location	3.3 median (0-7)
Touch – method	**Von Frey for threshold; brushes for allodynia**	**V Frey for threshold; Pin prick for hyperalgesia**	**V Frey hair, V Frey.**
Normal threshold	50%, 5/10	48%, 13/27.	54%, 6/11.
Hypoesthesia	50%, 5/10	52%, 14/27	27%, 3/11.
Allodynia/ hyperalgesia	54% 7/13.	16/27, 59% - hyperalgesia	1/11-hyperalgesia to rotating von Frey hair
Cool – method	**Peltier Medoc**	**Peltier Somedic, warm minus cool threshold**	**Peltier Somedic**
Normal threshold	15%, 2/13	0/27	9%, 1/11.
	85%, 11/13, 3 with equal bilateral hypoesthesia	Diff in cool-warm thresholds 17/27; larger change in cool 2/27	91%, 10/11.
Cold pain – method	**As above**		
Normal threshold	31%, 4/13	7% normal difference between cold & heat pain threshold	18%, 2/11-unaffected side lower
Hypoalgesia	46%, 6/13 (2 indeterminate)	93% abnormal difference between cold & heat pain threshold	45%, 5/11 (4/11-bilateral)
Allodynia	23%, 3/13	No abnormally sensitive thresholds, but 5/22 (23%) reported discomfort to metal at room temperature	0/11
Warm – method	**As above**		
Normal threshold	15%, 2/13	-	-
Hypoesthesia	85%, 11/13	Diff in cool-warm thresholds, 17/27; larger change in warm threshold 8/27	11/11

Heat pain – method	As above		
Normal	93%, 12/13	7% normal difference between cold & heat pain threshold	9%, 1/11.
Hypoalgesia	7%, 1/13 (2 indeterminate)	93% abnormal difference between cold & heat pain threshold	91%, 10/11.
Allodynia	0/13 (2 borderline)	No abnormally sensitive thresholds.	0/11

Table 1. Summary of QST and descriptors of CPSP. The fourth column included both clinical findings (n=16) (Vestergaard et al., 1995) and quantitative sensory testing (n=11) (Andersen et al., 1995). Similarly, the third column included both clinical (Leijon et al., 1989) and sensory testing results (both N=27) (Boivie et al., 1989). Another very large series could not included because quantitative sensory testing results were not described as population statistics, (Bowsher, 1997).

painful stimuli, but they do show decreased sensitivity to at least some submodality of thermal or noxious stimuli.

Another important observation is that some patients with injuries or disease of the central nervous system (CNS) may experience thermal hypoesthesia or hypoalgesia as a result of a CNS lesion without developing central pain. This has been demonstrated for patients with lesions of the spinal cord (Ducreux et al., 2006;Finnerup et al., 2003), and brain (Andersen et al., 1995;Garcia-Larrea et al., 2010).

In the case of cortical lesions, the results of a recent study demonstrate warm and cold hypoesthesia based on QST thresholds in all subjects with lesions of parietal or insular cortex or both (Veldhuijzen et al., 2009). The largest degree of thermal hypoesthesia by threshold measures was found in the subject with the largest lesion, which involved extensive parietal and insular lobar lesions (see also (Greenspan et al., 1999). Suprathreshold measures demonstrated that sensory loss for painful and nonpainful hot and cold modalities was maximal for the largest parietal lesions.

Subjects with relatively small lesions restricted to the posterior insula and retroinsula showed central pain and cold allodynia, based on thresholds and clinical assessment. Cold allodynia based on thresholds but not on clinical assessment were observed in patients with parietal lesions sparing the insula. Similarly, a study of two patients with lesions of the insula and adjacent cortical lobes confirmed normal heat pain thresholds but increased ratings of heat pain compared to controls (Starr et al., 2009). These results suggest that non-painful cold and heat sensations are jointly mediated by parietal and insular cortical structures, while thermal pain sensation is more robust, requiring larger cortical lesions of these same structures to produce hypoalgesia. In addition, these studies dramatically demonstrate that neither the presence nor the extent of abnormal thermal sensation nor cold allodynia following a CNS lesion predicts the presence or the characteristics of central pain syndromes.

The variability of negative and positive symptoms and signs in patients with central pain raises the possibility that the level of spontaneous pain is correlated with the extent of sensory loss in patients with central pain. Such a relationship has been reported among patients with central pain resulting from spinal cord injury (SCI) (Ducreux et al., 2006). Specifically, two differences were observed between syringomyelia patients with or without allodynia. Those with allodynia tended to have 1) lesser thermosensory deficits and 2) more asymmetrical thermosensory deficits than those without allodynia. The intensity of the spontaneous burning pain was correlated with the degree of thermal sensory loss. Additionally, thermal deficits were less severe in patients with cold allodynia compared to those with tactile allodynia. Therefore, the pattern of thermal sensory loss may differentially influence different features of central pain.

Another study of SCI secondary to syringomyelia compared diffusion tensor imaging (DTI) and electrophysiological potentials between patients with and without neuropathic pain and healthy controls (Hatem et al., 2010). Among those SCI patients with neuropathic pain, higher average daily pain intensity correlated with the extent of structural damage to the spinal cord tracts. Additionally, the number of intact nerve axons within the whole spinal cord was inversely correlated with deep spontaneous pain and dysaesthesias. Patients with both spontaneous and evoked pain had less structural spinal cord damage by morphological and electrophysiological criteria compared to patients with only spontaneous pain. Therefore, in patients with SCI there was strong evidence that the extent of structural lesions is strongly correlated with the expression of spontaneous and evoked pain, or hypersensitivity (Hatem et al., 2010).

Based on the sample of 30 central pain patients (mostly CPSP) evaluated with QST at our research center, we found no relationship between the extent of thermosensory loss (based on cool or warm thresholds), and the level of ongoing pain. Therefore, thermal hypoesthesia may manifest differently in patients with different etiologies of central pain.

3. Central pain and cold allodynia

Cold allodynia is often associated with central pain even though it is not found in the majority of patients with CPSP (Table 1). The expression of cold allodynia is variable, which suggests that there is more than one mechanism for cold allodynia in different patients. In our recent study of seven patients with isolated parietal and/or insular lesions, 4/7 patients had cold allodynia based on thresholds, but only two of these had central pain and clinical cold hyperalgesia based on increased ratings of a painful cold waterbath stimulus (Veldhuijzen et al., 2009). Overall, these results suggest that posterior insular/retroinsular lesions in isolation can lead to cold allodynia as assessed by clinical, threshold and suprathreshold measures.

The matter is further complicated by differences in cold allodynia measured by different QST techniques. Cold allodynia can be evoked by touching the patient with a cool object, such as metal, at room temperature. In this case, the obligatory tactile stimulus may contribute to allodynia sensation, particularly in subjects with tactile allodynia. During QST, cold allodynia is often measured by thresholds for cold pain using a probe which is held on the skin while the temperature decreases until the patient reports pain perception. Surprisingly, the pain with a cold object contact often does not correspond to the pain evoked by the contact probe at the same temperature.

These phenomena have been observed in an early study which reported that 5/22 central pain patients had clinical cold allodynia but none had cold allodynia as measured with a contact temperature probe (Boivie et al., 1989). A similar observation was made in a more recent study (see Table 1). In the same study, 2 patients showed increased sensitivity to cold pain by thresholds, which met experimental criteria for cold allodynia, but the patients did not exhibit cold allodynia during clinical exams.

3.1 Ongoing pain

No relation between the size or location of a lesion and the presence or intensity of central pain has been found, although CP requires an impairment of thermosensory pathways or nociceptive pathways or both (see Table 1) (Boivie et al., 1989;Leijon et al., 1989;Andersen et al., 1995;Vestergaard et al., 1995;Greenspan et al., 2004;Lewis-Jones et al., 1990). In addition, studies of patients with central pain secondary to SCI show that the spinothalamic tract is not differentially affected in pain-free patients as opposed to patients with ongoing central pain (Ducreux et al., 2006;Finnerup et al., 2003). Therefore, lesions involving the spinothalamic pathway and its cortical connections, while necessary, are not sufficient to explain the development of central pain.

In a large series of patients (n=270) investigated for somatosensory abnormalities following stroke, five subjects were identified that presented with central pain and pure thermoalgesic sensory loss contralateral to the cortical stroke. All of these patients had involvement of the posterior insula and inner parietal operculum. Lemniscal sensory modalities and somatosensory evoked potentials to non-noxious inputs were preserved, while thermal and pain sensations were profoundly altered, and laser-evoked potentials were abnormal in all (Garcia-Larrea et al., 2010).

The nature of neural abnormalities in central pain is poorly understood. It has been proposed that thalamic bursting (low-threshold spike or LTS pattern) occurs at a higher rate among neurons in the region of the Ventral caudal (Vc) nucleus in patients with central pain as opposed to those with movement disorders (Jeanmonod et al., 1996;Lenz et al., 1989;Lenz et al., 1994). Another report found no difference in the thalamic burst rate between patients with chronic pain as opposed to those with movement disorder (Radhakrishnan et al., 1999). In the latter report, most of the neuronal recordings were made outside Vc in patients with peripheral neuropathic pain rather than central pain. Thus, this latter report does not speak directly to the mechanism of central pain. Electrical stimulation in the area of Vc evoked pain more commonly in central pain patients with allodynia, versus those without allodynia (Lenz et al., 1998;Davis et al., 1996). Overall, these studies suggest that reorganization of the region of Vc contributes to the symptoms of central pain.

In a study of MR spectroscopy, concentrations of markers for neurons (N-acetyl aspartate, NA) and glial cells (myo-inositol, Ins) in the thalamus were significantly different between patients with versus without central pain after SCI (Pattany et al., 2002;Stanwell et al., 2010). NA concentrations and NA/Ins ratios were lower in patients with pain versus those without, while Ins concentrations were higher for pain patients. In addition, NA concentrations were inversely correlated with VAS pain intensity, and Ins was directly correlated with pain intensity in the pain group. These results suggest that in SCI patients, dysfunction or loss of thalamic neurons is greater among SCI patients with central pain than among those without.

A recent study of SCI patients used a sophisticated wavelet-based analysis of the entire MRS signal to identify differences between SCI patients and intact controls, and between SCI patients with versus without central pain (DiPiero et al., 1991;Hsieh et al., 1995;Iadarola et al., 1995). Signals from the thalamus best discriminated between SCI patients and intact controls, yet signals from regions of the anterior cingulate and prefrontal cortex, but not the thalamus, highly discriminated between SCI patients with versus without central pain. While such an approach cannot identify the specific molecular differences, it does reveal which brain regions exhibit neurochemical differences that relate specifically to neuropathic central pain.

Neuroimaging studies of CP patients have most often reported thalamic hypoactivity, but some have observed thalamic hyperactivity. PET (positron emission tomography) studies have found a decrease in thalamic cerebral blood flow (CBF) on the same side as the lesion in patients with central pain patients at rest (Ness et al., 1998). The spatial resolution of these studies does not permit identification of the specific thalamic nuclei which were involved. This decrease in activity could be reversed by stimulation of the motor cortex (Peyron et al., 1995), or therapeutic intravenous infusion of lidocaine (Cahana et al., 2004). A similar decrease in thalamic bloodflow has been reported in patients with central and peripheral neuropathic pain combined. Specifically, the thalamus opposite the affected body region had lower bloodflow than the thalamus on the same side as the affected region in patients with SCI and central pain (Lenz et al., 2010). However, a single photon emission CT (SPECT) study found bilateral increased thalamic metabolism associated with pain of high intensity, but decreased blood flow associated with pain of low intensity (Cesaro et al., 1991).

Finally, PET results from CP patients show decreased thalamic bloodflow in both medial and lateral thalamus. Both SPECT and PET studies demonstrate increased thalamic activity contralateral to stimulation of the allodynic sites compared to non-allodynic sites in CPSP patients with or without unilateral allodynia (Lenz et al., 2010). The brain metabolic and bloodflow differences estimated by PET or SPECT reflect both inhibitory and excitatory synaptic activity. Therefore, decreased thalamic bloodflow in patients with CP might reflect decreased inhibitory synaptic activity, which may be related to loss of neurons, as suggested by the MR spectroscopy study reviewed above (Fukumoto et al., 1999). This decrease in bloodflow could occur despite the increased spontaneous thalamic firing rates, since spontaneous activity may not be reflected in metabolic or bloodflow imaging studies of the brain.

It is also possible these results are due to adaptive changes in the thalamus following the inciting lesion. For example, in patients with complex regional pain syndrome a SPECT study found increased thalamic bloodflow in patients with symptoms at 3 to 7 months after the injury, while decreased bloodflow occurred with long-term symptoms (24–36 months after) (Fukumoto et al., 1999).

Finally, ongoing pain in patients with CP might be related to changes in the opiodergic intrinsic modulatory system. These patients show decreased binding of the non-selective opioid binding ligand, diprenorphine, versus healthy controls, which indicate higher levels of binding sites occupied by opioids originating in the brain's intrinsic opioid system (Willoch et al., 2004). These reductions in opioid receptor binding within the "medial nociceptive system" were most pronounced in the dorsolateral prefrontal cortex (Brodmann area 10), anterior cingulate cortex (Brodmann area 24), insular cortex, and the medial thalamus. There were also reductions in binding in the lateral nociceptive system including the inferior parietal cortex (Brodmann area 40). Similar but more extensive decreases in binding were found in a study which included parietal cortex, cingulate and midbrain gray matter; these decreases were independent of the lesion locus which caused CP (Head and Holmes, 1911).

3.2 Mechanisms of cold allodynia in patients with central pain

An often cited hypothesis of cold allodynia suggests that it is the result of disinhibition of the medial nociceptive system following disruption of the lateral nociceptive system (Lenz et al., 2010). An approximate version of this hypothesis was proposed long ago (Head and Holmes, 1911), but the more recent version proposes that the medial system (ACC and medial thalamus) is critical to the mechanism of both central pain and cold allodynia.

This hypothesis was tested by a PET study which reported the bloodflow activity resulting from cutaneous stimulation with a cool, tactile stimulus (ice in a plastic container) in patients with central pain due to lateral medullary stroke (Wallenberg) syndrome (Peyron et al., 1998). This stimulus produced differential activation of structures contralateral to the affected side but not when it was applied to the unaffected side. These structures included: the primary sensory and motor cortex (contralateral to stimulation), the lateral thalamus (contralateral to stimulation), inferior parietal lobule (bilateral), and the frontal inferior gyrus. Notably, allodynic stimulation failed to evoke responses in medial thalamus or the portion of the ACC associated with pain. This study, then, did not support the model of disinhibition of the medial nociceptive processing system, but rather supported an amplification of the lateral nociceptive processing system as a basis for central pain allodynia.

A single subject PET study of a patient with central pain resulting from an infarct of the thalamus revealed a dramatic increase in sensory and motor cortical activation contralateral to allodynic cold stimulation of the affected hand (Kim et al., 2007). These increases may indicate disruption of a modulatory effect of the insula upon sensorimotor cortex which occurs in the normal brain. A study of two patients with large insular lesions but without central pain found that activation of S1 cortex ipsilateral to the lesioned insula was dramatically increased in response to painful heat stimulation (Starr et al., 2009).

Cold allodynia was associated with BOLD (blood oxygen level dependent) activation in the posterior insula, ACC, bilateral anterior insula, inferior parietal cortex, and supplementary motor cortex contralateral to the stimulus, and in the ipsilateral frontal gyrus of patients with syringomyelia (Ducreux et al., 2006). Brain activation in response to cold allodynic stimulation was much greater than usually evoked by the normally innocuous stimulus, and was comparable to the activation evoked by painful stimuli in controls without sensory abnormality. As noted above, a PET study of patients with Wallenburg strokes did not find activation of the ACC in response to stimuli which produced allodynia (Peyron et al., 1998), although such activation is often found in response to acute pain stimuli in healthy controls (Apkarian et al., 2005;Lenz et al., 2010). A combined PET and fMRI study of a unique patient with strokes of both the ACC and parietal cortex demonstrated cold allodynia, in the absence of hyperactivity in the remaining ACC (Peyron et al., 2000).

In contrast, one fMRI study of a patient with CPSP resulting from a stroke of the postero-lateral thalamus and adjacent internal capsule found activation of the ACC, the posterior parietal cortex, and the putamen during allodynia evoked by a cool stimulus (Seghier et al., 2005). Another fMRI study examined cold allodynia in normal controls evoked by cutaneous application of menthol, which rendered the skin hypersensitive to normally non-painful cold stimuli (Seifert and Maihofner, 2007). Stimulation of the sensitized skin was compared with the same intensity evoked by a normal cold pain stimulus. The pain evoked during allodynia resulted in more activation in dorso-lateral prefrontal cortex, bilateral anterior insula, and in parts of the brainstem. This range of results limits our ability to understand the mechanism of cold allodynia in terms of structures in the brain, particularly the ACC.

3.3 Mechanisms of tactile allodynia in patients with central pain

Tactile hypoesthesia and allodynia are common features of central pain as measured by use of von Frey hairs and camel hair brushes. Hypoesthesia for tactile sensation are associated with lesions of the dorsal columns, while such sensory loss is not found with lesions of the STT which spare the dorsal columns (Finnerup et al., 2007).

One recent study provided the first evidence that A-beta fibers are involved in dynamic mechanical allodynia (Landerholm and Hansson, 2010) In a portion of the central pain patients, dynamic allodynia occurred during a compression nerve block transitioning to a sensation of dysethesia. The remaining patients transitioned directly to the absence of allydynia following the block. In a subset of patients with central pain, concurrent changes in cold, but not warm, perception were found indicating A-delta involvement as well.

In contrast, tactile allodynia was more often associated with normal tactile thresholds than with tactile hypoesthesia in a study of CPSP patients (Hofbauer et al., 2006). Therefore, tactile allodynia may be the result of abnormal forebrain processing of signals transmitted through a relatively intact dorsal column – medial lemniscal system. This is consistent with reports of dysesthesias, which can be evoked by activation of afferents projecting through the dorsal column – medial lemniscal pathway in patients with post-stroke dysesthesias, a variation of CPSP (Triggs and Beric, 1994).

Cortical activation associated with tactile allodynia has been examined in experimental allodynia and peripheral neuropathic pain. A study of experimental allodynia resulting from application of capsaicin treatment in normal volunteers found that S1 and S2 activation occurred during nonpainful stimulation using von Frey filaments (Lorenz et al., 2002). When stimulating the area with mechanical allodynia, significant activation was found in the prefrontal cortex, as well as middle and inferior frontal gyri. There was no activation of the ACC.

In a patient with peripheral neuropathic pain after a peroneal nerve injury ongoing burning pain and tactile allodynia were observed; tactile stimuli evoked a deep pain, despite decreased tactile sensation (Hofbauer et al., 2006). Tactile allodynic sensations of the involved foot were compared with brush stimulation of the non-involved foot, and were associated with higher BOLD signals in S2, ipsilateral anterior insula, and ACC. Increased BOLD signals in S1 or ipsilateral posterior insula were not associated with stimulation of the involved foot, although such increased signals were observed after stimulation of the non-involved foot.

In a group of patients with complex regional pain syndrome, mechanical stimulation of the involved side evoked hyperalgesia and larger than control BOLD signals in several pain-related brain regions, including contralateral S1, bilateral S2, bilateral insula, inferior parietal lobule, and widespread ACC (Maihofner and Handwerker, 2005). Allodynia to a moving brush stimulus has also been studied in patients with traumatic peripheral nerve injury of the extremities, who suffered from ongoing pain and tactile allodynia (Witting et al., 2006). In these patients, allodynia in the affected limb yielded higher bloodflow than in the non-affected limb in contralateral orbitofrontal cortex and ipsilateral anterior insular cortex. Brushing of normal skin in the mirror image of the allodynic area produced a distinctly different pattern with increased bloodflow in contralateral S1 and posterior parietal cortex.

One imaging study has examined BOLD activation by tactile allodynia in patients with central pain secondary to syringomyelia (Ducreux et al., 2006). Tactile allodynia evoked by repeated brushing with a soft brush produced a pattern of brain activation distinct from that produced in normal controls with the same brushing, or with cold allodynic stimulation in these same patients. In all groups, activation was observed in the contralateral S1 and S2, and in parietal association areas. Tactile allodynia specific BOLD activation was elicited in the contralateral thalamus, bilateral middle frontal gyrus, and supplementary motor area, but was not observed in the insula or in the anterior and middle cingulate cortexes.

4. Conclusions

Based upon the data available today, it is not possible to draw any more than tentative conclusions. A frequent observation from PET and SPECT studies is that of thalamic hypometabolism in the painful resting state. At the same time, allodynic stimulation can evoke a stronger thalamic signal than normal. Both observations can be explained by a partially denervated thalamus and by a major disruption of GABA-mediated inhibition (Rausell et al., 1992). There is also some evidence that dysfunction of the thalamic nucleus Vc is involved in the mechanism of central pain (Montes et al., 2005;Kim et al., 2007).

The cortical regions associated with central pain can vary considerably among studies and symptoms of central pain. A recent study has suggested that CPSP occurred only in individuals with lesions including posterior insula/retroinsula, which spare the anterior and posterior parietal cortex (Veldhuijzen et al., 2009). Evidence from neuroimaging studies suggests that the parietal lobe is involved in the mechanism of CPSP and CPSP-associated allodynia in subjects with strokes of the lateral medulla (Wallenberg syndrome)(Peyron et al., 1998), and the thalamic nucleus Vc which projects to the parietal cortex (Kim et al., 2007). In both studies, a combined cold and mechanical cutaneous stimulus produced allodynia, and was associated with intense bloodflow activation of contralateral sensorimotor (frontal and parietal) cortex. In addition, pain sensations are evoked in subjects with CPSP by electrical stimulation of S1 cortex (Katayama et al., 1994;Nguyen et al., 2000;Brown and Barbaro, 2003) or of thalamic nucleus Vc, which projects to it (Lenz et al., 1998;Davis et al., 1996). Lesions of parietal cortex can dramatically relieve pain in subjects with CPSP resulting from thalamic lesions (Soria and Fine, 1991;Helmchen et al., 2002;Canavero and Bonicalzi, 2007). Consideration of these observations suggests the hypothesis that a network of insular and sensorimotor cortex is specifically disrupted in central pain, leading to increased activity in sensorimotor cortex, particularly with respect to the expression of allodynia.

5. Acknowledgement

This work was supported by the National Institutes of Health – National Institute of Neurological Disorders and Stroke (NS38493 and NS40059 to FAL NS-39337 to JDG). We thank C. Cordes and L. H. Rowland for excellent technical assistance.

6. References

Andersen P, Vestergaard K, Ingeman-Nielsen M, Jensen TS (1995) Incidence of post-stroke central pain. *Pain,* 61, pp. 187-193.

Apkarian AV, Bushnell MC, Treede R-D, Zubieta JK (2005) Human brain mechanisms of pain perception and regulation in health and disease. *European Journal of Pain,* 9, pp. 463-484.

Boivie J, Leijon G, Johansson I (1989) Central post-stroke pain--a study of the mechanisms through analyses of the sensory abnormalities. *Pain,* pp. 37:173-185.

Bowsher D (1997) Central pain: clinical and physiological characteristics. J Neurol Neurosurg Psychiatry 61:62-69.

Brown JA, Barbaro NM (2003) Motor cortex stimulation for central and neuropathic pain: current status. *Pain,* pp. 104:431-435.

Cahana A, Carota A, Montadon ML, Annoni JM (2004) The long-term effect of repeated intravenous lidocaine on central pain and possible correlation in positron emission tomography measurements. *Anesth Analg,* 98, pp. 1581-4, table.

Canavero S, Bonicalzi V (2007) *Central Pain Syndrome: Pathophysiology, diagnosis and management.* NY, NY.: Cambridge Press.

Cesaro P, Mann MW, Moretti JL, Defer G, Roualdes B, Nguyen JP, Degos JD (1991) Central pain and thalamic hyperactivity: a single photon emission computerized tomographic study. *Pain* 47, pp. 329-336.

Davis KD, Kiss ZHT, Tasker RR, Dostrovsky JO (1996) Thalamic stimulation-evoked sensations in chronic pain patients and nonpain (movement disorder) patients. *J Neurophysiol* 75, pp. 1026-1037.

DiPiero V, Jones AKP, Iannotti F, Powell M, Lenzi GL, Frackowiak RSJ (1991) Chronic pain: A PET study of the central effects of percutaneous high cervical cordotomy. *Pain* 46, pp. 9-12.

Ducreux D, Attal N, Parker F, Bouhassira D (2006) Mechanisms of central neuropathic pain: a combined psychophysical and fMRI study in syringomyelia. *Brain* 129, pp. 963-976.

Finnerup NB, Johannesen IL, Fuglsang-Frederiksen A, Bach FW, Jensen TS (2003) Sensory function in spinal cord injury patients with and without central pain. *Brain* 126, pp. 57-70.

Finnerup NB, Sorensen L, Biering-Sorensen F, Johannesen IL, Jensen TS (2007) Segmental hypersensitivity and spinothalamic function in spinal cord injury pain. *Exp Neurol* 207, pp. 139-149.

Fukumoto M, Ushida T, Zinchuk VS, Yamamoto H, Yoshida S (1999) Contralateral thalamic perfusion in patients with reflex sympathetic dystrophy syndrome. *Lancet* 354, pp. 1790-1791.

Garcia-Larrea L, Perchet C, Creac'h C, Convers P, Peyron R, Laurent B, Mauguiere F, Magnin M (2010) Operculo-insular pain (parasylvian pain): a distinct central pain syndrome. *Brain* 133, pp. 2528-2539.

Greenspan JD, Lee RR, Lenz FA (1999) Pain sensitivity alterations as a function of lesion location in the parasylvian cortex. *Pain* 81, pp. 273-282.

Greenspan JD, Ohara S, Sarlani E, Lenz FA (2004) Allodynia in patients with post-stroke central pain (CPSP) studied by statistical quantitative sensory testing within individuals. *Pain* 109, pp. 357-366.

Greenspan JD, Treede RD, Tasker RR, Lenz FA (2008) Central pain states. In: *Bonica's Management of Pain* (Fishman SM, Ballantyne JC, Rathmell JC, eds), pp 357-384. NY:NY: Lippincott, Williams and Wilkens.

Hatem SM, Attal N, Ducreux D, Gautron M, Parker F, Plaghki L, Bouhassira D (2010) Clinical, functional and structural determinants of central pain in syringomyelia. *Brain* 133, pp. 3409-3422.

Head H, Holmes G (1911) Sensory disturbances from cerebral lesions. *Brain* 34, pp. 102-254.

Helmchen C, Lindig M, Petersen D, Tronnier V (2002) Disappearance of central thalamic pain syndrome after contralateral parietal lobe lesion: implications for therapeutic brain stimulation. *Pain.* 98, pp. 325-330.

Hofbauer RK, Olausson HW, Bushnell MC (2006) Thermal and tactile sensory deficits and allodynia in a nerve-injured patient: a multimodal psychophysical and functional magnetic resonance imaging study. *Clin J Pain*, 22, pp. 104-108.

Hsieh JC, Belfrage M, Stone-Elander S, Hansson P, Ingvar M (1995) Central representation of chronic ongoing neuropathic pain studied by positron emission tomography. *Pain,* 63, pp. 225-236.

Iadarola MJ, Max MB, Berman KF, Byas-Smith MG, Coghill RC, Gracely RH, Bennett GJ (1995) Unilateral decrease in thalamic activity observed with PET in patients with chronic neuropathic pain. *Pain,* 63, pp. 55-64.

Jeanmonod D, Magnin M, Morel A (1996) Low-threshold calcium spike bursts in the human thalamus. Common physiopathology for sensory, motor and limbic positive symptoms. *Brain* 119, pp. 363-375.

Katayama Y, Tsubokawa T, Yamamoto T (1994) Chronic motor cortex stimulation for central deafferentation pain: experience with bulbar pain secondary to Wallenberg syndrome. *Stereotact Funct Neurosurg* 62, pp. 295-299.

Kim JH, Greenspan JD, Coghill RC, Ohara S, Lenz FA (2007) Lesions limited to the human thalamic principal somatosensory nucleus (ventral caudal) are associated with loss of cold sensations and central pain. *J Neurosci* 27, pp. 4995-5004.

Landerholm AH, Hansson PT (2010) Mechanisms of dynamic mechanical allodynia and dysesthesia in patients with peripheral and central neuropathic pain. *Eur J Pain*.

Leijon G, Boivie J, Johansson I (1989) Central post-stroke pain-neurological symptoms and pain characteristics. *Pain*, 36, pp. 13-25.

Lenz FA, Casey KL, Jones EG, Willis WDJr (2010) *The Human Pain System: Experimental and Clinical Perspectives*. NY, NY: Cambridge University Press.

Lenz FA, Gracely RH, Baker FH, Richardson RT, Dougherty PM (1998) Reorganization of sensory modalities evoked by microstimulation in region of the thalamic principal sensory nucleus in patients with pain due to nervous system injury. *J Comp Neurol* 399, pp. 125-138.

Lenz FA, Kwan HC, Dostrovsky JO, Tasker RR (1989) Characteristics of the bursting pattern of action potentials that occurs in the thalamus of patients with central pain. *Brain Res* 496, pp. 357-360.

Lenz FA, Kwan HC, Martin R, Tasker R, Richardson RT, Dostrovsky JO (1994) Characteristics of somatotopic organization and spontaneous neuronal activity in the region of the thalamic principal sensory nucleus in patients with spinal cord transection. *J Neurophysiol* 72, pp. 1570-1587.

Lewis-Jones H, Smith T, Bowsher D, Leijon G (1990) Magnetic Resonance Imaging In 36 Cases Of Central Post-Stroke Pain (CPSP).*Pain*. pp S278.

Lorenz J, Cross D, Minoshima S, Morrow T, Paulson P, Casey K (2002) A unique representation of heat allodynia in the human brain. *Neuron* 35, pp. 383-393.

Maihofner C, Handwerker HO (2005) Differential coding of hyperalgesia in the human brain: a functional MRI study. *Neuroimage* 28, pp. 996-1006.

Merskey H (1986) Classification of chronic pain. *Pain* S1-S220.

Montes C, Magnin M, Maarrawi J, Frot M, Convers P, Mauguiere F, Garcia-Larrea L (2005) Thalamic thermo-algesic transmission: ventral posterior (VP) complex versus VMpo in the light of a thalamic infarct with central pain. *Pain* 113, pp. 223-232.

Ness TJ, San Pedro EC, Richards JS, Kezar L, Liu HG, Mountz JM (1998) A case of spinal cord injury-related pain with baseline rCBF brain SPECT imaging and beneficial response to gabapentin. *Pain* 78, pp. 139-143.

Nguyen JP, Lefaucheur JP, Le Guerinel C, Eizenbaum JF, Nakano N, Carpentier A, Brugieres P, Pollin B, Rostaing S, Keravel Y (2000) Motor cortex stimulation in the treatment of central and neuropathic pain. *Arch Med Res*, 31, pp. 263-265.

Ohara S, Weiss N, Hua S, Anderson W, Lawson C, Greenspan JD, Crone NE, Lenz FA (2004) Allodynia due to forebrain sensitization demonstrated by thalamic microstimulation. In: Hyperalgesia: molecular mechanisms and clinical implications (Brune K, Handwerker HO, eds), pp 353-371. Seattle: IASP Press.

Pattany PM, Yezierski RP, Widerstrom-Noga EG, Bowen BC, Martinez-Arizala A, Garcia BR, Quencer RM (2002) Proton magnetic resonance spectroscopy of the thalamus in patients with chronic neuropathic pain after spinal cord injury. *Am J Neuroradiol* 23, pp. 901-905.

Peyron R, Garcia-Larrea L, Deiber MP, Cinotti L, Convers P, Sindou M, Mauguiere F, Laurent B (1995) Electrical stimulation of precentral cortical area in the treatment of central pain: electrophysiological and PET study. *Pain* 62, pp. 275-286.

Peyron R, Garcia-Larrea L, Gregoire MC, Convers P, Lavenne F, Veyre L, Froment JC, Mauguiere F, Michel D, Laurent B (1998) Allodynia after lateral-medullary (Wallenberg) infart: a PET study. *Brain* 121, pp. 345-356.

Peyron R, Garcia-Larrea L, Gregoire MC, Convers P, Richard A, Lavenne F, Barral FG,
    Mauguiere F, Michel D, Laurent B (2000) Parietal and cingulate processes in central
    pain. A combined positron emission tomography (PET) and functional magnetic
    resonance imaging (fMRI) study of an unusual case. *Pain,* 84, pp. 77-87.
Radhakrishnan V, Tsoukatos J, Davis KD, Tasker RR, Lozano AM, Dostrovsky JO (1999) A
    comparison of the burst activity of lateral thalamic neurons in chronic pain and
    non-pain patients. *Pain,* 80, pp. 567-575.
Rausell E, Cusick CG, Taub E, Jones EG (1992) Chronic deafferentation in monkeys
    differentially affects nociceptive and nonnociceptive pathways distinguished by
    specific calcium-binding proteins and down-regulates gamma-aminobutyric acid
    type A receptors at thalamic levels. *Proc Natl Acad Sci U S A* 89, pp. 2571-2575.
Seghier ML, Lazeyras F, Vuilleumier P, Schnider A, Carota A (2005) Functional magnetic
    resonance imaging and diffusion tensor imaging in a case of central poststroke
    pain. *J Pain* 6, pp. 208-212.
Seifert F, Maihofner C (2007) Representation of cold allodynia in the human brain--a
    functional MRI study. *Neuroimage* 35, pp. 1168-1180.
Soria ED, Fine EJ (1991) Disappearance of thalamic pain after parietal subcortical stroke.
    Pain. 44, pp. 285-288.
Stanwell P, Siddall P, Keshava N, Cocuzzo D, Ramadan S, Lin A, Herbert D, Craig A, Tran
    Y, Middleton J, Gautam S, Cousins M, Mountford C (2010) Neuro magnetic
    resonance spectroscopy using wavelet decomposition and statistical testing
    identifies biochemical changes in people with spinal cord injury and pain.
    Neuroimage 53, pp. 544-552.
Starr CJ, Sawaki L, Wittenberg GF, Burdette JH, Oshiro Y, Quevedo AS, Coghill RC (2009)
    Roles of the insular cortex in the modulation of pain: insights from brain lesions. *J
    Neurosci* 29, pp. 2684-2694.
Treede RD, Jensen TS, Campbell JN, Cruccu G, Dostrovsky JO, Griffin JW, Hansson P,
    Hughes R, Nurmikko T, Serra J (2008) Neuropathic pain: redefinition and a grading
    system for clinical and research purposes. *Neurology,* 70, pp. 1630-1635.
Triggs WJ, Beric A (1994) Dysaesthesiae induced by physiological and electrical activation of
    posterior column afferents after stroke. *J Neurol Neurosurg Psychiatry,* 57, pp. 1077-1080.
Veldhuijzen DS, Greenspan JD, Coghill RC, Treede RD, Kim JH, Ohara S, Lenz FA (2007)
    Imaging central pain syndromes. *Curr Pain Headache Rep* 11, pp. 183-189.
Veldhuijzen DS, Greenspan JD, Kim JH, Lenz FA (2009) Altered pain and thermal sensation
    in subjects with isolated parietal and insular cortical lesions. *Eur J Pain* 14:e535-e1-
    e535-e11.
Veldhuijzen DS, Lenz FA, Lagraize SC, Greenspan JD (2011) What (if anything) can
    Neuroimaging tell us about Central Pain? In: *Chronic Pain Syndromes.* (Kruger L,
    Light AR, eds), NY, NY.
Vestergaard K, Nielsen J, Andersen G, Ingeman-Nielsen M, Arendt-Nielsen L, Jensen TS
    (1995) Sensory abnormalities in consecutive unselected patients with central post-
    stroke pain. *Pain* 61, pp. 177-186.
Willoch F, Schindler F, Wester HJ, Empl M, Straube A, Schwaiger M, Conrad B, Tolle TR
    (2004) Central poststroke pain and reduced opioid receptor binding within pain
    processing circuitries: a [11C]diprenorphine PET study. *Pain'* 108, pp. 213-220.
Witting N, Kupers RC, Svensson P, Jensen TS (2006) A PET activation study of brush-
    evoked allodynia in patients with nerve injury pain. *Pain,* 120, pp. 145-154.

12

EEG-Biofeedback as a Tool to Modulate Arousal: Trends and Perspectives for Treatment of ADHD and Insomnia

B. Alexander Diaz, Lizeth H. Sloot,
Huibert D. Mansvelder and Klaus Linkenkaer-Hansen
*Department of Integrative Neurophysiology, Center for Neurogenomics and
Cognitive Research (CNCR), Neuroscience Campus Amsterdam,
VU University Amsterdam, Amsterdam
The Netherlands*

1. Introduction

EEG-biofeedback (EBF) is a method to provide information about a person's brain state using real-time processing of electroencephalographic data (Budzynski, 1973; Morin, 2006). The idea behind EBF training is that by giving the participant access to a physiological state she will be able to modulate this state in a desired direction. As such EBF makes use of a brain-computer interface (BCI), in itself a field of study that has seen rapidly growing interest over recent years (Felton et al., 2007; Kübler, Kotchoubey et al., 2001; Leuthardt et al., 2006; Schalk et al., 2007). There is a distinction between using BCI to gain control over an external device or to use it to modify the internal state of the user. The former has seen fascinating applications in facilitating control of prosthetics (Nicolelis, 2003) or in offering new channels of communication to the paralysed (Birbaumer et al., 1999; Krusienski et al., 2006; Krusienski et al., 2008). EEG biofeedback belongs to the latter category as it aims to provide a means for the user to modify her own cognition or behaviour through feedback on specific EEG characteristics (Fig. 1). EBF therapy should, after repeated training, result in improved brain states or an effective internalized strategy to invoke such a brain state.

EEG-biofeedback (EBF) was first used in operant conditioning studies on cats in the 1960s. By rewarding the generation of the sensori-motor rhythm (SMR, Table 1), cats learned to increase SMR by suppression of voluntary movement (Roth et al., 1967; Sterman et al., 1969; Sterman & Wyrwicka, 1967; Wyrwicka & Sterman, 1968). Interestingly, a lasting effect of the biofeedback training became apparent when the same cats were later used in a dose-response study of an epileptogenic compound in which they showed significantly elevated seizure thresholds (Sterman, 1977; Sterman et al., 1969). These serendipitous findings motivated the use of biofeedback in research on humans with epilepsy (Sterman, 2006). Because the EEG is altered in several other disorders, biofeedback research has expanded to a range of clinical disorders including addiction (Passini et al., 1977; Peniston & Kulkosky, 1989; Saxby & Peniston, 1995), anxiety (Angelakis et al., 2007), attention-deficit/hyperactivity disorder, autism (Coben & Padolsky, 2007; Pineda et al., 2008), depression (Baehr et al., 1997; Hammond, 2005), post-traumatic stress disorder (Peniston & Kulkosky, 1991), and sleep disorders (Cortoos et al., 2009). More recently, research has explored the potential of biofeedback to enhance normal cognition, e.g. to improve attention (Egner et al., 2002; Gruzelier et al., 2006), working memory (Hoedlmoser et al., 2008; Vernon et al., 2003), or athletic performance (Egner & Gruzelier, 2003; Vernon, 2005).

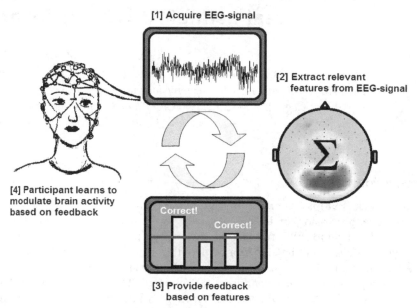

Fig. 1. The concept of EEG-biofeedback. The EEG is recorded [1], a suitable EEG-biomarker is extracted [2] and made available to the participant and correct changes in brain activity are rewarded by, e.g., a visual stimulus indicating success [3]. With repetition, this enables the participant to learn what strategies to employ in order to change brain activity in the desired direction [4].

In spite of the many studies using EBF to improve a clinical condition, the concept awaits a solid theoretical framework and the efficacy of EBF therapy requires further validation to gain widespread acceptance. Nevertheless, EBF holds the prospects to become an alternative to pharmaceutical intervention, where side-effects and dependency are prominent risks. An efficient EBF protocol that enables learning with a moderate number of sessions, will not only be more cost-effective but may bear additional psychological benefits such as avoiding certain stigmata (requiring psychiatric consultation or medication) and giving the participant more control over his/her own treatment. It is also conceivable that the mechanism with which EBF training exerts its therapeutic action is distinct from drug treatment as has been observed, e.g., when comparing neurobiological changes following successful treatment of depression using either cognitive behavioural therapy (CBT) or medication (Kumari, 2006).This would raise the perspective that EBF could be of help to those patients that do not respond to medication.

In this chapter, we focus on two disorders that share a characteristic arousal component, which EEG-biofeedback therapy attempts to modulate: attention-deficit hyperactivity disorder (ADHD) and insomnia.

Band	Frequency range (Hz)	Hallmark
δ	0.1–4	Sleep (stages N3-N4)
θ	4–8	Drowsiness, Sleep (stages N1-N2)
α	8–13	Relaxed wakefulness, cortical idling
σ	12–14	Spindle range (N2)
SMR	12–15	Sensorimotor rhythm
β	13–30	Cognitive effort, alertness

Table 1. All EEG bands from delta to beta have proven relevant for EBF in ADHD and insomnia.

ADHD has been described as a disorder of decreased CNS arousal and cortical inhibition, partially explaining the symptom normalizing effect psychostimulants have in the treatment of ADHD (Satterfield et al., 1974). These arousal deficits become manifest in lowered skin conductance levels (Barry et al., 2009; Raine et al., 1990; Satterfield et al., 1974), EEG deviations (e.g. increased theta but less beta activity) (Barry et al., 2003a; Barry et al., 2003b; Clarke et al., 2002; Clarke et al., 2001) and are related to CNS dopamine systems and associated genes (Li et al., 2006).

Insomniacs in contrast, exhibit elevated (cognitive) arousal effectively delaying the transition from wakefulness to sleep or resulting in frequent awakenings, oftentimes directly related to persistent (psychological) stressors (Bonnet, 2010; Bonnet & Arand, 1997; Bonnet & Arand, 2005; Cortoos et al., 2006; Drake et al., 2004; Drummond et al., 2004; Jansson & Linton, 2007; Nofzinger, 2004; Perlis, 2001). Brain areas involved in sleep regulation, arousal and attention are closely related (Brown et al., 2001) possibly explaining the observation that 50% of ADHD children also have difficulties falling asleep and 20% report recurring severe sleep problems (Ball et al., 1997; Stein, 1999). The association between arousal and sleep has classically been described using the EEG, where elevated arousal is associated with beta and gamma (>30 Hz) activity, whereas decreases in arousal are associated with enhanced delta and theta band activity (Alkire et al., 2008; Rechtschaffen & Kales, 1968; Steriade et al., 1993).

Here we propose that for EBF to have a therapeutic effect it is required that (1) EEG can index (disease-)relevant states of the brain, (2) one can learn to modulate these brain states, (3) training the modulation of brain states causes (lasting and desired) changes to the brain, and (4) EBF-related changes to the brain have cognitive and/or behavioral correlates. In the following, ADHD and insomnia are treated as case examples of disorders that have been proposed to benefit from EEG-biofeedback therapy. We present the evidence that EBF has a therapeutic effect on these disorders and outline trends and perspectives by reviewing recent progress in the design of EBF for pre-clinical research.

2. EEG-biofeedback in ADHD

Attention deficit/ hyperactivity disorder (ADHD) is a psychiatric disorder, characterized by symptoms of inattention and/or impulsivity and hyperactivity. These symptoms frequently co-exist with emotional, behavioural and learning deficits such as conduct disorder and oppositional defiant disorder, anxiety disorders and major depressive disorder (Barry et al., 2003). Prevalence in school-aged children is fairly high (3–12%) (Brown et al., 2001) and 30–50% of these children will continue to experience symptoms into adulthood (Barry et al., 2003; Monastra, 2005). DSM-IV criteria allow the distinction of three ADHD subtypes: (1) the predominantly inattentive type, (2) the predominantly hyperactive-impulsive type and (3) the combined type, which exhibits symptoms of both inattention and hyperactivity-impulsivity (DSM-IV-TR; American Psychiatric Association, 2000).

Pharmacological intervention based on psychostimulant medication leads to a reduction of ADHD symptoms by increasing CNS arousal (Satterfield et al., 1974), but lacks long-term efficacy (Faraone & Buitelaar, 2010; Faraone & Glatt, 2010; Molina et al., 2009) and introduces adverse effects in 20-50% of the patients (Charach et al., 2004; Efron et al., 1997; Goldstein & Goldstein, 1990). Still, 35–45% of the patients with an "inattentive" type of ADHD and 10–30% of those diagnosed as "combined" type do not respond to medication, limiting the effectiveness of pharmaceutical intervention (Barkley, 1998; Hermens et al., 2006; Swanson et al., 1993). EEG biofeedback therapy for ADHD is one proposed alternative treatment and aims at restoring CNS arousal imbalances by training participants to suppress EEG rhythms associated with underarousal and enhance those rhythms associated with attention (J. F. Lubar & Shouse, 1976; Monastra et al., 2005; Thompson & Thompson, 1998).

2.1 Training duration and feedback

An EBF training session consists of repeated training blocks of typically 3 minutes, each starting with a measure of baseline activity, like 5 minutes eyes-closed rest (J. O. Lubar & Lubar, 1984), within the specified frequency band in order to establish a target threshold value (Table 2). The participant will then attempt to match or exceed this value during a subsequent feedback trial by modulating activity within the set frequency band. The participant need not be aware of the underlying parameter(s) and is merely instructed to meet/exceed the threshold. Participants are encouraged to find their own optimal strategy to alter the brain activity. When the participant successfully exceeds the threshold, e.g., for 0.5 s (Monastra, 2005), a reward signal indicating success (e.g. a bonus point that can be traded for money or toys) is presented to reinforce learning. ADHD patients prefer smaller and immediate rewards to delayed, but larger ones (Loo & Barkley, 2005; Marco et al., 2009; Tripp & Alsop, 2001) and as the ADHD population largely consists of children, feedback protocols often involve video games where success is rewarded instantly (Drechsler et al., 2007; Leins et al., 2007).

2.2 Target brain activity

Spontaneous (resting-state) EEG profiles of ADHD children differ significantly from those of normally developing children, especially increased theta/beta ratio but also lowered alpha band activity has been reported (Barry & Clarke, 2009; Barry et al., 2003; Barry et al., 2009; Barry et al., 2003; Clarke et al., 2002; Clarke et al., 2001).

The increased theta/beta ratio has been proposed as a characteristic biomarker for CNS underarousal (Mann et al., 1992), whereas the SMR has been classically described as reflecting motor inhibition (Sterman & Friar, 1972; Sterman et al., 1970). The vast majority of EBF studies has been inspired by a two-phase protocol of Lubar et al. (1984), in which participants where first trained to increase their SMR and later to inhibit theta activity while simultaneously increasing beta activity (Beauregard & Levesque, 2006; Carmody et al., 2000; Fuchs et al., 2003; Gevensleben et al., 2009; Heywood & Beale, 2003; Holtmann et al., 2009; Kaiser, 1997; Kaiser & Othmer, 2000; Kropotov et al., 2005; La Vaque et al., 2002; Leins et al., 2007; Levesque et al., 2006; Linden et al., 1996; J.F. Lubar et al., 1995; Monastra et al., 2002; Rossiter, 2004; Rossiter, 1998; Rossiter & La Vaque, 1995; Strehl et al., 2006; Thompson & Thompson, 1998).

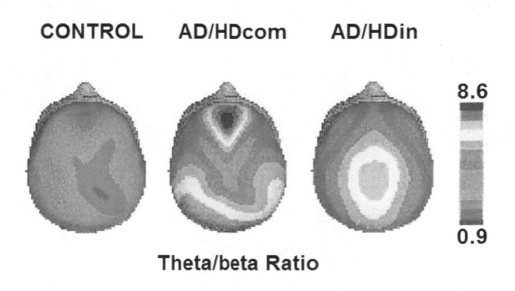

Fig. 2. Brain activity profiles in children with ADHD differ from healthy controls. Theta/beta-band activity ratio is strongly elevated in ADHD, but differs in spatial localization between combined (AD/HDcom) and inattentive (AD/HDin) subtypes. (From: Barry et al., 2003.).

In recent years, however, an interesting new target for EBF has been found in the form of slow cortical potentials (SCPs). These slow event-related DC shifts represent excitation thresholds of large neuronal assemblies and training ADHD patients to increase SCPs robustly improves symptoms of ADHD (Doehnert et al., 2008; Drechsler et al., 2007; Gevensleben et al., 2009; Heinrich et al., 2007; Kropotov et al., 2005; Leins et al., 2007; Siniatchkin et al., 2000; Strehl et al., 2006).

Study	Control P/R/B[*1]	N (m)	Age	Electrodes /Ref	Freq.	Stim/ Reward	#Ses./ Dur.
Monastra et al., 2002	-/-/-	[1] 49(40) [2] 51 (43)	[1] 10.0± 3.7 [2] 10.0± 3.1	CPz & Cz/A2	β ↑ θ ↓	Visual & auditory /Money	43 (34– 50) / 30–40 min
Fuchs et al., 2003	-/-/-	[1] 12(12) [2] 22(21)	[1] 9.6±1.2 [2] 9.8±1.3	C3 or C4/A1+A2	SMR↑ /β ↑ θ ↓	Visual & auditory /Points	36 / 30-60 min
Rossiter, 2004	-/-/-	[1] 31(21) [2] 31(22)	[1] 16.7±12.5 [2] 16.6±12.7	C3/A2 or C4/A1	β ↑ θ ↓	Visual & auditory	40 or >60 /30 or 36 min
Lévesque et al., 2006	+/+/-	[1] 5(5) [2] 14(11)	[1] 10.2±0.8 [2] 10.2±1.3	Cz/A1	SMR↑ θ ↓	Visual & auditory (video game)	40 / 60 min
Drechsler et al., 2007	-/-/-	[1] 13(10) [2] 17(13)	[1] 11.2±1.0 [2] 10.5±1.3	Cz/A1+A2	SCP↑/↓	Visual /Points	2x15 /2x45 min
Leins et al., 2007	-/+/+	[1] 16(13) [2] 16(13)	[1] 9.16±1.43 [2] 9.16±1.53	[1] CF3,CF4/ A1+A2 [2] Cz/A1+A2	[1] β ↑ θ ↓ [2] SCP↑/↓	Visual /Points	30 /60 min
Doehnert et al., 2008	-/-/-	[1] 12(10) [2] 14(12)	[1] 11.4±0.9 [2] 10.8±1.3	Cz/A1+A2	SCP↑/↓	Visual /Points	2x15 /2x45 min
Gevensleben et al., 2009	-/+/-	[1] 35(26) [2] 59 (51)	[1] 9.3± 1.16 [2] 9.8± 1.25	Cz/A1+A2	β ↑ θ ↓ SCP↑/↓	Visual	2x9 /2x 50 min

[*1] P/R/B= Placebo/Randomized/Blind (- = no, + = yes). N(m): Number of participants (males), Freq.: Target frequency ↑/↓ (increase/decrease) of EBF condition(s).

Table 2. EBF therapy focused at treating ADHD is an active field of research.

2.3 Efficacy of EEG-biofeedback in the treatment of ADHD

The first study of EBF in ADHD (J. F. Lubar & Shouse, 1976) reported improved attention and normalized levels of arousal, together with improved grades and achievement scores for the (eight) children under treatment. Subsequent studies have reported similarly positive results, showing improvements of behaviour, attention and impulsivity (Alhambra et al., 1995; Carmody et al., 2000; Drechsler et al., 2007; Gevensleben et al., 2010; Gevensleben et al., 2009; Heinrich et al., 2004; Kaiser & Othmer, 2000; Kropotov et al., 2005; Leins et al., 2007; Linden et al., 1996; J.F. Lubar et al., 1995; J. F. Lubar, 1991; Rossiter, 1998; Rossiter & La Vaque, 1995; Strehl, et al., 2006; Thompson & Thompson, 1998; Doehnert et al., 2008). Efficacy of EBF is comparable to psychostimulant medication and group (CBT) therapy programs with effects lasting 6 months and longer (Fuchs et al., 2003; Gani et al., 2009; Gevensleben et al., 2010; Kaiser, 1997; Leins et al., 2007; Linden et al., 1996; J.F. Lubar et al., 1995; Monastra et al., 2002; Rossiter & La Vaque, 1995; Thompson & Thompson, 1998). Overall, EBF treatment results in clinical improvement in about 75% of the cases, without any reported adverse effects so far (Leins et al., 2007; Monastra et al., 2005).

It should be noted, however, that the use of the theta/beta ratio as marker of general arousal has been questioned, because it does not correlate with skin conductance level (R.J. Barry & Clarke, 2009; R.J. Barry et al., 2009). Similarly, SCPs are no direct correlates of arousal but rather represent attentional processes (Siniatchkin et al., 2000). This raises the interesting notion that in ADHD, EBF may not restore or modulate arousal systems per se, but compensate underarousal by strengthening cognitive functions that have been negatively affected by the arousal dysfunction.

3. EBF as treatment of insomnia

Insomnia is a most pervasive disorder, affecting about 15% of the general population while 6% meet clinical (DSM-IV) criteria (Ohayon, 2002) and interferes with cognition, quality of life, job performance and represents a multi-billion dollar burden on healthcare providers (Daley et al., 2009; Ebben & Spielman, 2009; Edinger et al., 2004). Insomnia can be subdivided into primary and co-morbid insomnia with the most salient symptoms being difficulty initiating and/or maintaining sleep (Espie, 2007). Causes of primary insomnia include physiological, cognitive and behavioural factors (Espie, 2007). Symptoms and duration are related to severity and persistence of stressors (Morin et al., 2006).

To better understand the possible therapeutic targets of insomnia, the so-called "3P model" has been proposed (Ebben & Spielman, 2009). This model specifies three categories of factors influencing the risk at developing or worsening insomnia: predisposing, precipitating and perpetuating factors. The first category constitutes genetic factors or personality traits, such as increased basal level of anxiety or hyperarousal (Drake et al., 2004), whereas precipitating events represent work and educational stress together with health and emotional problems (Bastien et al., 2004). Finally, perpetuating factors, such as continuous stress and poor sleep hygiene, may cause the actual transition to chronic insomnia and complete the vicious circle.

Pharmacological treatment of insomnia with sedative-hypnotic agents has seen a steady decline over the past (Aldrich, 1992; Walsh & Schweitzer, 1999), because of side effects, discontinuation discomfort, and the risk of developing drug tolerance or dependency (Ebben & Spielman, 2009; Walsh & Schweitzer, 1999). Alternative treatment options that have been met with success are cognitive-behavioural therapy (CBT) (Ebben & Spielman, 2009; Espie, 1999; Morin et al., 1999; Morin et al., 1994; Murtagh & Greenwood, 1995; Siebern & Manber, 2010) or treatments

increasing body temperature (e.g., physical exercise, hot bath before bed), which has recently been shown to hasten sleep onset (Van Someren, 2006). Whereas CBT causes sustained improvements and reduces sleep complaints, one fifth of the patients does not respond to the intervention (Cortoos et al., 2010; Harvey & Payne, 2002; Morin, 2006). EBF therapy for insomnia could be a safer alternative to medication and may offer treatment where CBT fails.
The EEG profile of insomniacs (Fig. 3) consists of increased levels of beta activity especially during the sleep-onset period and early sleep stages (Merica et al., 1998). These observations may be interpreted as evidence of cognitive hyperarousal, which is in line with the often reported 'racing thoughts' of insomniacs (Bastien et al., 2003; Buysse et al., 2008; Buysse et al., 2008; Freedman, 1986; Harvey & Payne, 2002; Jacobs et al., 1993; Lamarche & Ogilvie, 1997; Merica, et al., 1998; Merica & Gaillard, 1992; Nofzinger et al., 1999; Perlis et al., 2001). In addition, elevated levels of alpha activity at sleep onset (Besset et al., 1998; Krystal et al., 2002) as well as a decrease in delta activity during non-REM sleep (Merica et al., 1998; Merica & Gaillard, 1992) have been reported. Furthermore, it has been demonstrated that insomniacs produce less spontaneous waking SMR activity than controls (P. Hauri, 1981; Krystal et al., 2002). One interesting aspect about the SMR is that it lies in the same frequency range as sleep spindles (Sterman, et al., 1970). Spindles are the hallmark waveform of stage 2 sleep, and their occurrence is reduced in insomniacs (Besset et al., 1998), possibly resulting in lighter and more fragmented sleep (Glenn & Steriade, 1982; Perlis et al., 2001).

3.1 Training duration and feedback
Protocols for EEG-biofeedback in insomnia are quite similar in many respects to the ones used in the treatment of ADHD, e.g. patients usually receive feedback and reward in the form of auditory and/or visual stimuli and are encouraged to search for their own

Study	Conds.	Control P/R/B[*1)]	N (m)	Age	Electrodes /Ref	Freq.	Stim/ Reward	#Ses./ Dur.
Hauri,1981	[1] EBF+EMG [2] EBF [3] EMG [4] Control	-/+/-	[1]12 [2]12 [3]12 [4]12	Total: 41.3±14.6	C3 /A2	$\theta \uparrow$ SMR$\uparrow$	Visual	24.8 (15-62) / 60 min
Hauri et al.,1982	[1] EBF(θ) [2] EBF(SMR)	-/+/-	[1]8(5) [2]8(5)	50.1 47.4	T7&C3/A2	$\theta \uparrow$ SMR$\uparrow$	Visual	25.4/ 60 min 27.8/60 min
Berner et al., 2006	EBF/Sham	+/+/+	11(4)	20.8±2.8	Cz / FCz	$\sigma \uparrow$	Visual & Auditory	1 / 4x10 min
Hoedlmoser et al., 2008	[1] EBF [2] Sham	+/+/+	[1]16(?) [2]11(?) Total: 27(13)	Total: 23.6±2.7	C3 /A2	SMR$\uparrow$	Visual & Auditory	10/ 24 min
Cortoos et al., 2009	[1] EBF [2] EMG [3] Control	-/+/-	[1] 9(6) [2] 8(5) [3]12(7)	41.5±9.5 43.8±9.5 44.4±7.8	FPz & Cz /A2	SMR$\uparrow$ $\theta \downarrow$ $\beta \downarrow$	Visual	20/ 20 min

[*1)] **P/R/B**= Placebo/Randomized/Blind (- = no, + = yes). **N(m)**: Number of participants (males), **Freq.**: Target frequency $\uparrow/\downarrow$ (increase/decrease), ? = data unavailable

Table 3. Overview of EBG group studies aimed at improving sleep.

individual strategies (Berner et al., 2006; Cortoos et al., 2009; Hauri et al., 1982; Hoedlmoser et al., 2008). Training sessions (Table 3) are usually blocked (e.g., 3 minute intervals) during which a threshold of activity expressed as a percentage of, or within a predefined band around the baseline, must be maintained for 250–500 ms (Berner et al., 2006; Cortoos et al., 2010; Hoedlmoser et al., 2008).

3.2 Target brain activity

Insomniacs differ from good sleepers in terms of their EEG profile (Fig. 3), especially exhibiting large spectral decreases in the lower frequency bands (delta, theta) (Merica et al., 1998) and attenuated sigma activity, corresponding to less occurrences of sleep spindles (Besset et al., 1998). These findings have led to the design of EBF therapies aimed at either increasing theta activity, due to its close relationship with drowsiness and early sleep stages, or SMR activity, as this rhythm overlaps with the sigma range and is believed to stimulate sleep spindle occurrence which in turn is key to further progression into deeper sleep stages

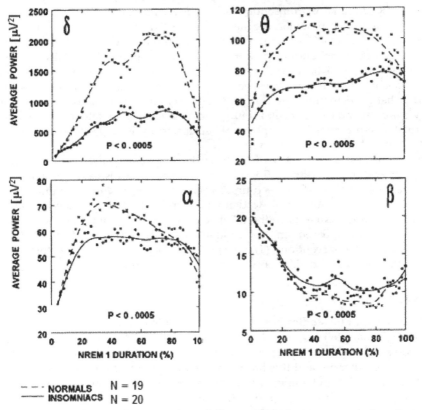

--- NORMALS   N = 19
——— INSOMNIACS N = 20

Fig. 3. Insomniacs and normal sleepers have different EEG during stage 1 sleep. Insomniacs (solid line) have reduced delta, theta and alpha activity, but higher levels of beta activity compared to normal sleepers (dashed line) during early stages of sleep. Y-axis: average power over all participants in specific frequency band. X-axis: normalized duration of sleep stage 1, each of the 50 dots marks a 2% interval. From: Merica et al., 1998.

(Berner et al., 2006; Budzynski, 1973; Hauri, 1981; Sittenfeld, 1972; Steriade, 2003). The application of either protocol depends on the insomnia sub-population: theta feedback (enhancement training) is used for patients with difficulty initiating sleep, whereas SMR/sigma feedback is best used on patients that have problems maintaining sleep. The importance of disentangling insomnia subtypes is further illustrated by the studies of Hauri et al. (1981,1982). Even though all participants showed a trend towards improvement, the experimental groups (i.e. theta feedback, SMR feedback) did not differ, which could be attributed to participants having received treatment unsuitable to the underlying symptoms (Hauri, 1981; et al., 1982).

3.3 Efficacy of EEG-biofeedback in the treatment of insomnia
A pioneering case study used theta training to treat an insomnia patient and observed a near doubling of theta activity by the end of the 11-week (one session per week) EBF training, together with vastly decreased sleep-onset latency (from 54 to 16 minutes), an increase in total sleep time and a halving in intrusive thoughts (Bell, 1979). Recent studies have compared SMR training with pseudo-EBF training and reported positive results with respect to the total sleep time and the sleep latency (Berner et al., 2006; Hoedlmoser et al., 2008). Cortoos et al. (2009) compared electromyography (EMG) biofeedback, aimed at reducing muscle tension and relaxation, with an EBF protocol of SMR increase and simultaneous theta-, and beta-band suppression. Both groups showed decreases in sleep latency (-8.5 and -12.3 minutes respectively) and time awake after sleep onset. It is noteworthy that participants were trained to apply electrodes and initiate training in their home environment and experimental control was established remotely through the internet, making this "tele-neurofeedback" protocol an interesting example of fusing established knowledge with advanced technology.

In contrast to the case of ADHD where subjective ratings largely define outcome measures (Table 2), efficacy and validity of EBF-therapy for insomniacs is easier to assess through objective measures such as total sleep time, sleep-onset latency and the number of nightly awakenings. In 1998, the American Academy of Sleep Medicine recommended biofeedback in general, including EMG-biofeedback, as treatment for insomnia and classified it as "probably efficacious", based on the Guidelines for Evaluation of Clinical Efficacy of Psychophysiological Interventions (Table 3). In the update of 1999–2004, this rating was maintained (Morgenthaler et al., 2006; Morin et al., 2006; Morin et al., 1999).

4. Conclusion

The methodology of EBF studies has often been subject to criticism (Kline et al., 2002; Loo & Barkley, 2005; Pelham & Waschbusch, 2006; Ramirez et al., 2001; Rickles et al., 1982). While some concerns are undoubtedly warranted, much effort has been put in establishing strict guidelines for EBF therapy and this has been met with positive results (Arns et al., 2009; La Vaque et al., 2002). Double-blind, randomised and placebo controlled experiments are unfortunately not always an option. Blinding requires a control condition that is indistinguishable from the treatment condition, which is often technically not feasible. Randomisation, while powerful, is only useful when the target sample is either well-known or homogenous to avoid samples being treated with inadequate protocols (Hauri, 1981; Hauri et al., 1982). Finally, a placebo condition, especially in the case of ADHD, is problematic from an ethical viewpoint, as denying patients a standard and efficacious treatment (i.e., medication) is in conflict with the Declaration of Helsinki (Vernon et al., 2004). Employing sham (random frequency) feedback (Hoedlmoser et al., 2008; Logemann et al., 2010) is therefore not always an option when treating patients. Thus, apart from reaching certain endpoints of treatment, the further validation of EBF therapy is likely to depend on the observation of complimentary physiological changes, e.g., obtained from neuroimaging experiments or other biomarker assays (Frank & Hargreaves, 2003).

Motivation and cognitive strategies are also important aspects to consider (Bregman & McAllister, 1982; Meichenbaum, 1976). If participants are motivated and rewarded for their success they will put effort into the therapy, whereas lack thereof leads to frustration and possibly resignation (Huang et al., 2006). Good methodology can compensate for possible expectancy effects, i.e., improved symptoms like decreases in sleep onset latency induced by the sheer hope of becoming better through therapy (Hauri et al., 1982). However, providing sham feedback, which lacks obvious rewards, bears the risk of the participant becoming unmotivated, ceasing effort and thus confounding the comparison between control and experimental condition (Logemann et al., 2010). In addition, the instructions given to participants in the EBF studies reviewed here do not go beyond the direction to meet some specified criterion, i.e., increasing an onscreen bar towards a target value. The general idea is that participants need to search for their own strategies to modulate their brain activity. In our view, this is unfortunate, because good instructions/guidance can increase participant compliance and speed of learning (Weinert et al., 1989). While individual strategies are likely to vary greatly, an opportunity for future research presents itself in the collection of these strategies and finding patterns that may be useful to guide participants towards success more efficiently. Interestingly, Gevensleben et al. (2009) report on having queried individual strategies of their participants (albeit without further analysis), making future compilation of strategies feasible.

Technological advances have made it possible to record high-density EEG data from several hundred electrodes at once (Dornhege et al., 2006). However, current EBF studies seldom record from more than two active electrodes (Tables 2 and 3). With ongoing developments towards ever more powerful and cost-effective computational equipment, it is feasible that future research should focus on the opportunities these advances can offer EBF, possibly in combination with tools from the field of BCI (e.g., more sophisticated algorithms, spatial filtering allowing feedback on localized anatomical structures and less artefacts). Despite some (methodological) issues that have subjected the field to scepticism, recent developments give rise to optimism, as stricter guidelines are increasingly being adhered to and new avenues continue to be explored (e.g., SCP feedback and tele-neurofeedback as in Cortoos et al., 2009). Overall, from the studies reviewed here we conclude that EBF is a promising tool for treating disorders of arousal, which offers many opportunities for future research.

5. References

Aldrich, M. S. (1992). Sleep disorders. *Curr Opin Neurol Neurosurg, 5*(2), 240-246.

Alhambra, M. A., Fowler, T. P., & Alhambra, A. A. (1995). EEG biofeedback: A new treatment option for ADD/ADHD. *Journal of Neurotherapy, 1*(2), 39-43.

Alkire, M. T., Hudetz, A. G., & Tononi, G. (2008). Consciousness and anesthesia. *Science, 322*(5903), 876-880.

Angelakis, E., Stathopoulou, S., Frymiare, J. L., Green, D. L., Lubar, J. F., & Kounios, J. (2007). EEG neurofeedback: a brief overview and an example of peak alpha frequency training for cognitive enhancement in the elderly. *The Clinical Neuropsychologist, 21*(1), 110-129.

Arns, M., de Ridder, S., Strehl, U., Breteler, M., & Coenen, A. (2009). Efficacy of neurofeedback treatment in ADHD: the effects on inattention, impulsivity and hyperactivity: a meta-analysis. *Clin EEG Neurosci, 40*(3), 180-189.

Baehr, E., Rosenfeld, J. P., & Baehr, R. (1997). The clinical use of an alpha asymmetry protocol in the neurofeedback treatment of depression: two case studies. *Journal of Neurotherapy, 2*, 10-23.

Ball, J., Tiernan, M., Janusz, J., & Furr, A. (1997). Sleep patterns among children with attention-deficit hyperactivity disorder: a reexamination of parent perceptions. *Journal of pediatric psychology, 22*(3), 389.

Barkley, R. A. (1998). *Attention-deficit hyperactivity disorder: a handbook of diagnosis and treatment (2nd ed.)*. New York: Guilford.

Barry, R. J., & Clarke, A. R. (2009). Spontaneous EEG oscillations in children, adolescents, and adults: Typical development, and pathological aspects in relation to AD/HD. *Journal of Psychophysiology, 23*(4), 157.

Barry, R. J., Clarke, A. R., & Johnstone, S. J. (2003). A review of electrophysiology in attention-deficit/hyperactivity disorder: I. Qualitative and quantitative electroencephalography. *Clin Neurophysiol, 114*(2), 171-183.

Barry, R. J., Clarke, A. R., Johnstone, S. J., McCarthy, R., & Selikowitz, M. (2009). Electroencephalogram [theta]/[beta] Ratio and Arousal in Attention-Deficit/ Hyperactivity Disorder: Evidence of Independent Processes. *Biological Psychiatry, 66*(4), 398-401.

Barry, R. J., Johnstone, S. J., & Clarke, A. R. (2003). A review of electrophysiology in attention-deficit/hyperactivity disorder: II. Event-related potentials. *Clinical Neurophysiology, 114*(2), 184-198.

Bastien, C. H., LeBlanc, M., Carrier, J., & Morin, C. M. (2003). Sleep EEG power spectra, insomnia, and chronic use of benzodiazepines. *Sleep, 26*(3), 313-317.

Bastien, C. H., Vallieres, A., & Morin, C. M. (2004). Precipitating factors of insomnia. *Behav Sleep Med, 2*(1), 50-62.

Beauregard, M., & Levesque, J. (2006). Functional magnetic resonance imaging investigation of the effects of neurofeedback training on the neural bases of selective attention and response inhibition in children with attention-deficit/hyperactivity disorder. *Appl Psychophysiol Biofeedback, 31*(1), 3-20.

Bell, J. S. (1979). The use of EEG theta biofeedback in the treatment of a patient with sleep-onset insomnia. *Biofeedback Self Regul, 4*(3), 229-236.

Berner, I., Schabus, M., Wienerroither, T., & Klimesch, W. (2006). The significance of sigma neurofeedback training on sleep spindles and aspects of declarative memory. *Appl Psychophysiol Biofeedback, 31*(2), 97-114.

Besset, A., Villemin, E., Tafti, M., & Billiard, M. (1998). Homeostatic process and sleep spindles in patients with sleep-maintenance insomnia: effect of partial (21 h) sleep deprivation. *Electroencephalogr Clin Neurophysiol, 107*(2), 122-132.

Birbaumer, N., Ghanayim, N., Hinterberger, T., Iversen, I., Kotchoubey, B., Kübler, A., et al. (1999). A spelling device for the paralysed. *Nature, 398*(6725), 297-298.

Bonnet, M. H. (2010). Hyperarousal and insomnia. *Sleep medicine reviews, 14*(1).

Bonnet, M. H., & Arand, D. (1997). Physiological activation in patients with sleep state misperception. *Psychosomatic medicine, 59*(5), 533.

Bonnet, M. H., & Arand, D. L. (2005). Impact of motivation on Multiple Sleep Latency Test and Maintenance of Wakefulness Test measurements. *Journal of Clinical Sleep Medicine: JCSM: Official Publication of the American Academy of Sleep Medicine, 1*(4), 386.

Bregman, N. J., & McAllister, H. A. (1982). Motivation and Skin Temperature Biofeedback: Yerkes Dodson Revisited. *Psychophysiology, 19*(3), 282-285.

Brown, R. T., Freeman, W. S., Perrin, J. M., Stein, M. T., Amler, R. W., Feldman, H. M., et al. (2001). Prevalence and assessment of attention-deficit/hyperactivity disorder in primary care settings. *Pediatrics, 107*(3), E43.

Budzynski, T. H. (1973). Biofeedback procedures in the clinic. *Semin Psychiatry, 5*(4), 537-547.

Buysse, D., Hall, M., Strollo, P., Kamarck, T., Owens, J., Lee, L., et al. (2008). Relationships between the Pittsburgh Sleep Quality Index (PSQI), Epworth Sleepiness Scale (ESS), and clinical/polysomnographic measures in a community sample. *Journal of Clinical Sleep Medicine: JCSM: Official Publication of the American Academy of Sleep Medicine, 4*(6), 563.

Buysse, D. J., Germain, A., Hall, M. L., Moul, D. E., Nofzinger, E. A., Begley, A., et al. (2008). EEG Spectral Analysis in Primary Insomnia: NREM Period Effects and Sex Differences. *Sleep, 31*(12), 1673.

Carmody, D. P., Radvanski, D. C., Wadhwani, S., Sabo, M. J., & Vergara, L. (2000). EEG biofeedback training and attention-deficit/hyperactivity disorder in an elementary school setting. *Journal of Neurotherapy, 4*(3), 5-27.

Charach, A., Ickowicz, A., & Schachar, R. (2004). Stimulant treatment over five years: adherence, effectiveness, and adverse effects. *Journal of the American Academy of Child & Adolescent Psychiatry, 43*(5), 559-567.

Clarke, A., Barry, R., McCarthy, R., Selikowitz, M., & Brown, C. (2002). EEG evidence for a new conceptualisation of attention deficit hyperactivity disorder. *Clinical Neurophysiology, 113*(7), 1036-1044.

Clarke, A. R., Barry, R. J., McCarthy, R., & Selikowitz, M. (2001). Age and sex effects in the EEG: differences in two subtypes of attention-deficit/hyperactivity disorder. *Clinical Neurophysiology, 112*(5), 815-826.

Coben, R., & Padolsky, I. (2007). Assessment-guided neurofeedback for Autistic Spectrum Disorder. *Journal of Neurotherapy, 11*(1), 5-23.

Cortoos, A., De Valck, E., Arns, M., Breteler, M. H., & Cluydts, R. (2009). An Exploratory Study on the Effects of Tele-neurofeedback and Tele-biofeedback on Objective and Subjective Sleep in Patients with Primary Insomnia. *Appl Psychophysiol Biofeedback*.

Cortoos, A., De Valck, E., Arns, M., Breteler, M. H., & Cluydts, R. (2010). An exploratory study on the effects of tele-neurofeedback and tele-biofeedback on objective and subjective sleep in patients with primary insomnia. *Appl Psychophysiol Biofeedback, 35*(2), 125-134.

Cortoos, A., Verstraeten, E., & Cluydts, R. (2006). Neurophysiological aspects of primary insomnia: implications for its treatment. *Sleep Med Rev, 10*(4), 255-266.

Daley, M., Morin, C. M., LeBlanc, M., Grégoire, J. P., & Savard, J. (2009). The economic burden of insomnia: direct and indirect costs for individuals with insomnia syndrome, insomnia symptoms, and good sleepers. *Sleep, 32*(1), 55.

Doehnert, M., Brandeis, D., Straub, M., Steinhausen, H. C., & Drechsler, R. (2008). Slow cortical potential neurofeedback in attention deficit hyperactivity disorder: is there neurophysiological evidence for specific effects? *J Neural Transm, 115*(10), 1445-1456.

Dornhege, G., Blankertz, B., Krauledat, M., Losch, F., Curio, G., & Muller, K. R. (2006). Combined optimization of spatial and temporal filters for improving brain-computer interfacing. *Biomedical Engineering, IEEE Transactions on, 53*(11), 2274-2281.

Drake, C., Richardson, G., Roehrs, T., Scofield, H., & Roth, T. (2004). Vulnerability to stress-related sleep disturbance and hyperarousal. *Sleep, 27*(2), 285-291.

Drechsler, R., Straub, M., Doehnert, M., Heinrich, H., Steinhausen, H. C., & Brandeis, D. (2007). Controlled evaluation of a neurofeedback training of slow cortical potentials in children with Attention Deficit/Hyperactivity Disorder (ADHD). *Behav Brain Funct, 3*, 35.

Drummond, S., Brown, G. G., Salamat, J. S., & Gillin, J. C. (2004). Increasing task difficulty facilitates the cerebral compensatory response to total sleep deprivation. *Sleep, 27*(3), 445-451.

Ebben, M. R., & Spielman, A. J. (2009). Non-pharmacological treatments for insomnia. *J Behav Med, 32*(3), 244-254.

Edinger, J. D., Bonnet, M. H., Bootzin, R. R., Doghramji, K., Dorsey, C. M., Espie, C. A., et al. (2004). Derivation of research diagnostic criteria for insomnia: report of an American Academy of Sleep Medicine Work Group. *Sleep, 27*(8), 1567-1596.

Efron, D., Jarman, F., & Barker, M. (1997). Side effects of methylphenidate and dexamphetamine in children with attention deficit hyperactivity disorder: a double-blind, crossover trial. *Pediatrics, 100*(4), 662.

Egner, T., & Gruzelier, J. H. (2003). Ecological validity of neurofeedback: modulation of slow wave EEG enhances musical performance. *Neuroreport, 14*(9), 1221-1224.

Egner, T., Strawson, E., & Gruzelier, J. H. (2002). EEG signature and phenomenology of alpha/theta neurofeedback training versus mock feedback. *Applied Psychophysiology and Biofeedback, 27*(4), 261-270.

Espie, C. A. (1999). Cognitive behaviour therapy as the treatment of choice for primary insomnia. *Sleep Med Rev, 3*(2), 97-99.

Espie, C. A. (2007). Understanding insomnia through cognitive modelling. *Sleep Med, 8 Suppl 4*, S3-8.

Faraone, S. V., & Buitelaar, J. (2010). Comparing the efficacy of stimulants for ADHD in children and adolescents using meta-analysis. *Eur Child Adolesc Psychiatry, 19*(4), 353-364.

Faraone, S. V., & Glatt, S. J. (2010). A comparison of the efficacy of medications for adult attention-deficit/hyperactivity disorder using meta-analysis of effect sizes. *The Journal of clinical psychiatry, 71*(6), 754.

Felton, E. A., Wilson, J. A., Williams, J. C., & Garell, P. C. (2007). Electrocorticographically controlled brain-computer interfaces using motor and sensory imagery in patients with temporary subdural electrode implants. *Journal of neurosurgery, 106*(3), 495-500.

Frank, R., & Hargreaves, R. (2003). Clinical biomarkers in drug discovery and development. *Nature Reviews Drug Discovery, 2*(7), 566-580.

Freedman, R. R. (1986). EEG power spectra in sleep-onset insomnia. *Electroencephalogr Clin Neurophysiol, 63*(5), 408-413.

Fuchs, T., Birbaumer, N., Lutzenberger, W., Gruzelier, J. H., & Kaiser, J. (2003). Neurofeedback treatment for attention-deficit/hyperactivity disorder in children: a comparison with methylphenidate. *Appl Psychophysiol Biofeedback, 28*(1), 1-12.

Gani, C., Birbaumer, N., & Strehl, U. (2009). Long term effects after feedback of slow cortical potentials and of theta-beta-amplitudes in children with attentiondeficit/ hyperactivity disorder (ADHD). *International Journal of Bioelectromagnetics, 10*, 209-232.

Gevensleben, H., Holl, B., Albrecht, B., Schlamp, D., Kratz, O., Studer, P., et al. (2010). Neurofeedback training in children with ADHD: 6-month follow-up of a randomised controlled trial. *Eur Child Adolesc Psychiatry, 19*(9), 715-724.

Gevensleben, H., Holl, B., Albrecht, B., Vogel, C., Schlamp, D., Kratz, O., et al. (2009). Is neurofeedback an efficacious treatment for ADHD? A randomised controlled clinical trial. *Journal of Child Psychology and Psychiatry, 50*(7), 780-789.

Glenn, L. L., & Steriade, M. (1982). Discharge rate and excitability of cortically projecting intralaminar thalamic neurons during waking and sleep states. *J Neurosci, 2*(10), 1387-1404.

Goldstein, S., & Goldstein, M. (1990). *Managing attention disorders in children: A guide for practitioners.* New York: Wiley.

Gruzelier, J., Egner, T., & Vernon, D. (2006). Validating the efficacy of neurofeedback for optimising performance. *Progress in Brain Research, 159*, 421-431.

Hammond, D. C. (2005). Neurofeedback treatment of depression and anxiety. *Journal of Adult Development, 12*, 131-137.

Harvey, A., & Payne, S. (2002). The management of unwanted pre-sleep thoughts in insomnia: distraction with imagery versus general distraction. *Behaviour Research and Therapy, 40*(3), 267-277.

Hauri, P. (1981). Treating psychophysiologic insomnia with biofeedback. *Arch Gen Psychiatry, 38*(7), 752-758.

Hauri, P. J., Percy, L., Hellekson, C., Hartmann, E., & Russ, D. (1982). The treatment of psychophysiologic insomnia with biofeedback: a replication study. *Biofeedback Self Regul, 7*(2), 223-235.

Heinrich, H., Gevensleben, H., Freisleder, F. J., Moll, G. H., & Rothenberger, A. (2004). Training of slow cortical potentials in attention-deficit/hyperactivity disorder: evidence for positive behavioral and neurophysiological effects. *Biol Psychiatry, 55*(7), 772-775.

Heinrich, H., Gevensleben, H., & Strehl, U. (2007). Annotation: neurofeedback - train your brain to train behaviour. *J Child Psychol Psychiatry, 48*(1), 3-16.

Hermens, D. F., Rowe, D. L., Gordon, E., & Williams, L. M. (2006). Integrative neuroscience approach to predict ADHD stimulant response. *Expert Rev Neurother, 6*(5), 753-763.

Heywood, C., & Beale, I. (2003). EEG biofeedback vs. placebo treatment for attention-deficit/hyperactivity disorder: a pilot study. *J Atten Disord, 7*(1), 43-55.

Hoedlmoser, K., Pecherstorfer, T., Gruber, G., Anderer, P., Doppelmayr, M., Klimesch, W., et al. (2008). Instrumental conditioning of human sensorimotor rhythm (12-15 Hz) and its impact on sleep as well as declarative learning. *Sleep, 31*(10), 1401-1408.

Holtmann, M., Grasmann, D., Cionek-Szpak, E., Hager, V., Panzer, N., & Beyer, A. (2009). Spezifische wirksamkeit von Neurofeedback auf die Impulsivitat bei ADHS - Literaturuberblick und ergebnisse einer prospective, kontrollierten Studie. *Kindheit und Entwicklung, 18*, 95-104.

Huang, H., Wolf, S. L., & He, J. (2006). Recent developments in biofeedback for neuromotor rehabilitation. *Journal of NeuroEngineering and Rehabilitation, 3*(1), 11.

Jacobs, G. D., Benson, H., & Friedman, R. (1993). Home-based central nervous system assessment of a multifactor behavioral intervention for chronic sleep-onset insomnia. *Behavior Ther, 24*, 159-174.

Jansson, M., & Linton, S. J. (2007). Psychological mechanisms in the maintenance of insomnia: arousal, distress, and sleep-related beliefs. *Behav Res Ther, 45*(3), 511-521.

Kaiser, D. A. (1997). Efficacy of Neurofeedback on adults with Attention Defecit and Related disorders: EEG Spectrum Inc.

Kaiser, D. A., & Othmer, S. (2000). Effects of neurofeedback on variables of attention in a large multi-center trial. *Journal of Neurotherapy, 4*(1), 5-15.

Kline, J. P., Brann, C. N., & Loney, B. R. (2002). A cacophony in the brainwaves: a critical appraisal of neurotherapy for attention-deficit disorders. *The Scientific Review of Mental Health Practice, 1,* 44-54.

Kropotov, J. D., Grin-Yatsenko, V. A., Ponomarev, V. A., Chutko, L. S., Yakovenko, E. A., & Nikishena, I. S. (2005). ERPs correlates of EEG relative beta training in ADHD children. *Int J Psychophysiol, 55*(1), 23-34.

Krusienski, D. J., Sellers, E. W., Cabestaing, F., Bayoudh, S., McFarland, D. J., Vaughan, T. M., et al. (2006). A comparison of classification techniques for the P300 speller. *Journal of Neural Engineering, 3,* 299.

Krusienski, D. J., Sellers, E. W., McFarland, D. J., Vaughan, T. M., & Wolpaw, J. R. (2008). Toward enhanced P300 speller performance. *Journal of neuroscience methods, 167*(1), 15-21.

Krystal, A. D., Edinger, J. D., Wohlgemuth, W. K., & Marsh, G. R. (2002). NREM sleep EEG frequency spectral correlates of sleep complaints in primary insomnia subtypes. *Sleep, 25*(6), 630.

Kübler, A., Kotchoubey, B., Kaiser, J., Wolpaw, J. R., & Birbaumer, N. (2001). Brain–computer communication: Unlocking the locked in. *Psychological Bulletin, 127*(3), 358.

Kumari, V. (2006). Do psychotherapies produce neurobiological effects? *Acta neuropsychiatrica, 18*(2), 61-70.

La Vaque, T. J., Hammond, D. C., Trudeau, D., Monastra, V. J., J., P., & Lehrer, P. (2002). Template for developing guidelines for the evaluation of the clinical efficacy of psychophysiological interventions. *Applied Psychophysiology and Biofeedback, 27,* 273-281.

Lamarche, C. H., & Ogilvie, R. D. (1997). Electrophysiological changes during the sleep onset period of psychophysiological insomniacs, psychiatric insomniacs, and normal sleepers. *Sleep(New York, NY), 20*(9), 724-733.

Leins, U., Goth, G., Hinterberger, T., Klinger, C., Rumpf, N., & Strehl, U. (2007). Neurofeedback for children with ADHD: a comparison of SCP and Theta/Beta protocols. *Appl Psychophysiol Biofeedback, 32*(2), 73-88.

Leuthardt, E. C., Miller, K. J., Schalk, G., Rao, R. P. N., & Ojemann, J. G. (2006). Electrocorticography-based brain computer interface-the Seattle experience. *Neural Systems and Rehabilitation Engineering, IEEE Transactions on, 14*(2), 194-198.

Levesque, J., Beauregard, M., & Mensour, B. (2006). Effect of neurofeedback training on the neural substrates of selective attention in children with attention-deficit/hyperactivity disorder: a functional magnetic resonance imaging study. *Neurosci Lett, 394*(3), 216-221.

Li, D., Sham, P. C., Owen, M. J., & He, L. (2006). Meta-analysis shows significant association between dopamine system genes and attention deficit hyperactivity disorder (ADHD). *Human molecular genetics, 15*(14), 2276.

Linden, M., Habib, T., & Radojevic, V. (1996). A controlled study of the effects of EEG biofeedback on cognition and behavior of children with attention deficit disorder and learning disabilities. *Applied Psychophysiology and Biofeedback, 21*(1), 35-49.

Logemann, H. N. A., Lansbergen, M. M., Van Os, T. W. D. P., Bocker, K. B. E., & Kenemans, J. L. (2010). The effectiveness of EEG-feedback on attention, impulsivity and EEG: A sham feedback controlled study. *Neuroscience Letters, 479,* 49-53.

Loo, S. K., & Barkley, R. A. (2005). Clinical utility of EEG in attention deficit hyperactivity disorder. *Appl Neuropsychol, 12*(2), 64-76.

Lubar, J., Swartwood, M., Swartwood, J., & O'Donnell, P. (1995). Evaluation of the effectiveness of EEG neurofeedback training for ADHD in a clinical setting as measured by changes in TOVA scores, behavioral ratings, and WISC-R performance. *Applied Psychophysiology and Biofeedback, 20*(1), 83-99.

Lubar, J. F. (1991). Discourse on the development of EEG diagnostics and biofeedback for attention-deficit/hyperactivity disorders. *Applied Psychophysiology and Biofeedback, 16*(3), 201-225.

Lubar, J. F., & Shouse, M. N. (1976). EEG and behavioral changes in a hyperkinetic child concurrent with training of the sensorimotor rhythm (SMR). *Applied Psychophysiology and Biofeedback, 1*(3), 293-306.

Lubar, J. F., Swartwood, M. O., Swartwood, J. N., & O'Donnell, P. H. (1995). Evaluation of the effectiveness of EEG neurofeedback training for ADHD in a clinical setting as measured by changes in T.O.V.A. scores, behavioral ratings, and WISC-R performance. *Biofeedback Self Regul, 20*(1), 83-99.

Lubar, J. O., & Lubar, J. F. (1984). Electroencephalographic biofeedback of SMR and beta for treatment of attention deficit disorders in a clinical setting. *Applied Psychophysiology and Biofeedback, 9*(1), 1-23.

Mann, C. A., Lubar, J. F., Zimmerman, A. W., Miller, C. A., & Muenchen, R. A. (1992). Quantitative analysis of EEG in boys with attention-deficit-hyperactivity disorder: controlled study with clinical implications. *Pediatr Neurol, 8*(1), 30-36.

Marco, R., Miranda, A., Schlotz, W., Melia, A., Mulligan, A., Müller, U., et al. (2009). Delay and reward choice in ADHD: An experimental test of the role of delay aversion. *Neuropsychology, 23*(3), 367.

Meichenbaum, D. (1976). Cognitive factors in biofeedback therapy. *Applied Psychophysiology and Biofeedback, 1*(2), 201-216.

Merica, H., Blois, R., & Gaillard, J. M. (1998). Spectral characteristics of sleep EEG in chronic insomnia. *Eur J Neurosci, 10*(5), 1826-1834.

Merica, H., & Gaillard, J. (1992). The EEG of the sleep onset period in insomnia: a discriminant analysis. *Physiology & behavior, 52*(2), 199-204.

Molina, B. S., Hinshaw, S. P., Swanson, J. M., Arnold, L. E., Vitiello, B., & Jensen, P. S. (2009). The MTA at 8 years: propsective follow-up of children treated for combined-type ADHD in a multisite study. *Journal of American Academy of Child and Adolescent Psychiatry, 48*, 484-500.

Monastra, V. J. (2005). Electroencephalographic biofeedback (neurotherapy) as a treatment for attention deficit hyperactivity disorder: rationale and empirical foundation. *Child Adolesc Psychiatr Clin N Am, 14*(1), 55-82, vi.

Monastra, V. J., Lynn, S., Linden, M., Lubar, J. F., Gruzelier, J., & LaVaque, T. J. (2005). Electroencephalographic biofeedback in the treatment of attention-deficit/hyperactivity disorder. *Appl Psychophysiol Biofeedback, 30*(2), 95-114.

Monastra, V. J., Monastra, D. M., & George, S. (2002). The effects of stimulant therapy, EEG biofeedback, and parenting style on the primary symptoms of attention-deficit/hyperactivity disorder. *Applied Psychophysiology and Biofeedback, 27*(4), 231-249.

Morgenthaler, T., Kramer, M., Alessi, C., Friedman, L., Boehlecke, B., Brown, T., et al. (2006). Practice parameters for the psychological and behavioral treatment of insomnia: an update. An American Academy of Sleep Medicine report. *Sleep, 29*(11), 1415-1419.

Morin, C., Hauri, P., Espie, C., Spielman, A., Buysse, D., & Bootzin, R. (1999). Nonpharmacologic treatment of chronic insomnia. An American Academy of Sleep Medicine review. *Sleep, 22*(8), 1134-1156.

Morin, C. M. (2006). Combined therapeutics for insomnia: should our first approach be behavioral or pharmacological? *Sleep Med, 7 Suppl 1,* S15-19.

Morin, C. M., Bootzin, R. R., Buysse, D. J., Edinger, J. D., Espie, C. A., & Lichstein, K. L. (2006). Psychological and behavioral treatment of insomnia: update of the recent evidence (1998-2004). *Sleep, 29*(11), 1398-1414.

Morin, C. M., Culbert, J. P., & Schwartz, S. M. (1994). Nonpharmacological interventions for insomnia: a meta-analysis of treatment efficacy. *Am J Psychiatry, 151*(8), 1172-1180.

Morin, C. M., Hauri, P. J., Espie, C. A., Spielman, A. J., Buysse, D. J., & Bootzin, R. R. (1999). Nonpharmacologic treatment of chronic insomnia. *Sleep(New York, NY), 22*(8), 1134-1156.

Murtagh, D. R., & Greenwood, K. M. (1995). Identifying effective psychological treatments for insomnia: a meta-analysis. *J Consult Clin Psychol, 63*(1), 79-89.

Nicolelis, M. A. L. (2003). Brain–machine interfaces to restore motor function and probe neural circuits. *Nature Reviews Neuroscience, 4*(5), 417-422.

Nofzinger, E. A. (2004). What can neuroimaging findings tell us about sleep disorders? *Sleep Medicine, 5,* S16-S22.

Nofzinger, E. A., Nowell, P. D., Buysee, D. J., Vasco, R. C., Thase, M. E., E., F., et al. (1999). Towards a neurobiology of sleep disturbance in primary insomnia and depression: a comparison of subjective, visually scored, period amplitude, and power spectral density sleep measures. *Sleep, 22*(1), S99.

Ohayon, M. M. (2002). Epidemiology of insomnia: what we know and what we still need to learn. *Sleep Med Rev, 6*(2), 97-111.

Passini, F. T., Watson, C. G., Dehnel, L., Herder, J., & Watkins, B. (1977). Alpha wave biofeedback training therapy in alcoholics. *Journal of Clinical Psychology, 33*(1), 292-299.

Pelham, W. E., & Waschbusch, D. A. (2006). Attention-deficit hyperactivity disorder (ADHD). *Practitioner's Guide to Evidence-Based Psychotherapy*, 93-100.

Peniston, E. G., & Kulkosky, P. J. (1989). Alpha-theta brainwave training and beta-Endorphin levels in alcholics. *Alcoholism: Clinical and Experimental Research, 13*(2), 271-279.

Peniston, E. G., & Kulkosky, P. J. (1991). Alpha-theta brainwave neurofeedback for Vietnam veterans with combat-related post-traumatic stress disorder. *Medical Psychotherapy, 4,* 47-60.

Perlis, M. L. (2001). Response to "Do increases in beta EEG activity uniquely reflect insomnia?" (C. H. Bastein and M. H. Bonnet). *Sleep Med Rev, 5*(5), 379-383.

Perlis, M. L., Merica, H., Smith, M. T., & Giles, D. E. (2001). Beta EEG activity and insomnia. *Sleep Med Rev, 5*(5), 363-374.

Perlis, M. L., Smith, M. T., Andrews, P. J., Orff, H., & Giles, D. E. (2001). Beta/Gamma EEG activity in patients with primary and secondary insomnia and good sleeper controls. *Sleep(New York, NY), 24*(1), 110-117.

Pineda, J. A., Brang, D., Hecht, E., Edwards, L., Carey, S., Bacon, M., et al. (2008). Positive behavioral and electrophysiological changes following neurofeedback training in children with autism. *Research in Autism Spectrum Disorders, 2,* 557-581.

Raine, A., Venables, P. H., & Williams, M. (1990). Relationships between central and autonomic measures of arousal at age 15 years and criminality at age 24 years. *Archives of General Psychiatry, 47*(11), 1003.

Ramirez, P. M., Desantis, D., & Opler, L. A. (2001). EEG Biofeedback Treatment of ADD. *Annals of the New York Academy of Sciences, 931*(1), 342-358.

Rechtschaffen, A., & Kales, A. (1968). A manual of standardized terminology, techniques and scoring system for sleep stages of human subjects.

Rickles, W. H., Onoda, L., & Doyle, C. C. (1982). Task force study section report. *Applied Psychophysiology and Biofeedback, 7*(1), 1-33.

Rossiter, T. (2004). The effectiveness of neurofeedback and stimulant drugs in treating AD/HD: part II. Replication. *Appl Psychophysiol Biofeedback, 29*(4), 233-243.

Rossiter, T. R. (1998). Patient-directed neurofeedback for AD/HD. *Journal of Neurotherapy, 2*(4), 54-64.

Rossiter, T. R., & La Vaque, T. J. (1995). A comparison of EEG biofeedback and psychostimulants in treating attention deficit/hyperactivity disorders. *Journal of Neurotherapy, 1*(1), 48-59.

Roth, S. R., Sterman, M. B., & Clemente, C. C. (1967). Comparison of EEG correlates of reinforcement, internal inhibition, and sleep. *Electroencephalography and Clinical Neurophysiologie, 23*, 509-520.

Satterfield, J. H., Cantwell, D. P., & Satterfield, B. T. (1974). Pathophysiology of the hyperactive child syndrome. *Archives of General Psychiatry, 31*(6), 839.

Saxby, E., & Peniston, E. G. (1995). Alpha-theta brainwave neurofeedback training: an effective treatment for male and female alcoholics with depressive symptoms. *Journal of Clinical Psychology, 51*(5), 685-693.

Schalk, G., Kubanek, J., Miller, K., Anderson, N., Leuthardt, E., Ojemann, J., et al. (2007). Decoding two-dimensional movement trajectories using electrocorticographic signals in humans. *Journal of Neural Engineering, 4*, 264.

Siebern, A. T., & Manber, R. (2010). Insomnia and its effective non-pharmacologic treatment. *Med Clin North Am, 94*(3), 581-591.

Siniatchkin, M., Kropp, P., & Gerber, W. D. (2000). Neurofeedback--the significance of reinforcement and the search for an appropriate strategy for the success of self-regulation. *Appl Psychophysiol Biofeedback, 25*(3), 167-175.

Sittenfeld, P. (1972). *The control of the EEG theta rhythm.* Chicago: Aldine.

Stein, M. A. (1999). Unravelling sleep problems in treated and untreated children with ADHD. *Journal of Child and Adolescent Psychopharmacology, 9*(3), 157-168.

Steriade, M. (2003). The corticothalamic system in sleep. *Front Biosci, 8*, d878-899.

Steriade, M., Contreras, D., Curro Dossi, R., & Nunez, A. (1993). The slow (< 1 Hz) oscillation in reticular thalamic and thalamocortical neurons: scenario of sleep rhythm generation in interacting thalamic and neocortical networks. *Journal of Neuroscience, 13*(8), 3284.

Sterman, M., & Friar, L. (1972). Suppression of seizures in an epileptic following sensorimotor EEG feedback training. *Electroencephalography and Clinical Neurophysiology, 33*(1), 89-95.

Sterman, M. B. (1977). *Effects of sensorimotor EEG feedback training on sleep and clinical manifestations of epilepsy.* New York: Plenum.

Sterman, M. B., Howe, R. D., & MacDonald, L. R. (1970). Facilitation of spindle-burst sleep by conditioning of electroencephalographic activity while awake. *Science, 167*, 1146-1148.

Sterman, M. B., LoPresti, R. W., & Fairchild, M. D. (1969). Electroencephalographic and behavioral studies of monomethylhydrazine toxicity in the cat. *Technical Report AMRL-TR-69-3, Wright-Patterson Air Force Base, Ohio, Air Systems Command*.

Sterman, M. B., & Wyrwicka, W. (1967). EEG correlates of sleep: Evidence for seperate forebrain substrates. *Brain Research, 49*, 558-576.

Strehl, U., Leins, U., Goth, G., Klinger, C., Hinterberger, T., & Birbaumer, N. (2006). Self-regulation of slow cortical potentials: a new treatment for children with attention-deficit/hyperactivity disorder. *Pediatrics, 118*(5), e1530-1540.

Swanson, J., McBurnett, T., Wigal, T., Pfiffner, L., Lerner, M., & Williams, L. (1993). Effect of stimulant medication on children with attention deficit disorder: A "review of reviews". *Exceptional Children, 60*, 154-162.

Thompson, L., & Thompson, M. (1998). Neurofeedback combined with training in metacognitive strategies: effectiveness in students with ADD. *Appl Psychophysiol Biofeedback, 23*(4), 243-263.

Tripp, G., & Alsop, B. (2001). Sensitivity to reward delay in children with attention deficit hyperactivity disorder (ADHD). *Journal of Child Psychology and Psychiatry, 42*(5), 691-698.

Van Someren, E. J. (2006). Mechanisms and functions of coupling between sleep and temperature rhythms. *Prog Brain Res, 153*, 309-324.

Vernon, D. (2005). Can neurofeedback training enhance performance? An evaluation of the evidence with implications for future research. *Applied Psychophysiology and Biofeedback, 30*(4), 347-364.

Vernon, D., Egner, T., Cooper, N., Compton, T., Neilands, C., Sheri, A., et al. (2003). The effect of training distinct neurofeedback protocols on aspects of cognitive performance. *International Journal of Psychophysiology, 47*(1), 75-85.

Vernon, D., Frick, A., & Gruzelier, J. (2004). Neurofeedback as a treatment for ADHD: A methodological review with implications for future research. *Journal of Neurotherapy, 8*(2), 53-82.

Walsh, J. K., & Schweitzer, P. K. (1999). Ten-year trends in the pharmacological treatment of insomnia. *Sleep, 22*(3), 371-375.

Weinert, F. E., Schrader, F. W., & Helmke, A. (1989). Quality of instruction and achievement outcomes. *International Journal of Educational Research, 13*(8), 895-914.

Wyrwicka, W., & Sterman, M. B. (1968). Instrumental conditioning of sensorimotor cortex EEG spindles in the waking cat. *Physiology and Behavior, 3*, 703-707.

Permissions

The contributors of this book come from diverse backgrounds, making this book a truly international effort. This book will bring forth new frontiers with its revolutionizing research information and detailed analysis of the nascent developments around the world.

We would like to thank Dr. Peter Bright, for lending his expertise to make the book truly unique. He has played a crucial role in the development of this book. Without his invaluable contribution this book wouldn't have been possible. He has made vital efforts to compile up to date information on the varied aspects of this subject to make this book a valuable addition to the collection of many professionals and students.

This book was conceptualized with the vision of imparting up-to-date information and advanced data in this field. To ensure the same, a matchless editorial board was set up. Every individual on the board went through rigorous rounds of assessment to prove their worth. After which they invested a large part of their time researching and compiling the most relevant data for our readers. Conferences and sessions were held from time to time between the editorial board and the contributing authors to present the data in the most comprehensible form. The editorial team has worked tirelessly to provide valuable and valid information to help people across the globe.

Every chapter published in this book has been scrutinized by our experts. Their significance has been extensively debated. The topics covered herein carry significant findings which will fuel the growth of the discipline. They may even be implemented as practical applications or may be referred to as a beginning point for another development. Chapters in this book were first published by InTech; hereby published with permission under the Creative Commons Attribution License or equivalent.

The editorial board has been involved in producing this book since its inception. They have spent rigorous hours researching and exploring the diverse topics which have resulted in the successful publishing of this book. They have passed on their knowledge of decades through this book. To expedite this challenging task, the publisher supported the team at every step. A small team of assistant editors was also appointed to further simplify the editing procedure and attain best results for the readers.

Our editorial team has been hand-picked from every corner of the world. Their multi-ethnicity adds dynamic inputs to the discussions which result in innovative outcomes. These outcomes are then further discussed with the researchers and contributors who give their valuable feedback and opinion regarding the same. The feedback is then collaborated with the researches and they are edited in a comprehensive manner to aid the understanding of the subject.

Apart from the editorial board, the designing team has also invested a significant amount of their time in understanding the subject and creating the most relevant covers. They scrutinized every image to scout for the most suitable representation of the subject and create an appropriate cover for the book.

The publishing team has been involved in this book since its early stages. They were actively engaged in every process, be it collecting the data, connecting with the contributors or procuring relevant information. The team has been an ardent support to the editorial, designing and production team. Their endless efforts to recruit the best for this project, has resulted in the accomplishment of this book. They are a veteran in the field of academics and their pool of knowledge is as vast as their experience in printing. Their expertise and guidance has proved useful at every step. Their uncompromising quality standards have made this book an exceptional effort. Their encouragement from time to time has been an inspiration for everyone.

The publisher and the editorial board hope that this book will prove to be a valuable piece of knowledge for researchers, students, practitioners and scholars across the globe.

List of Contributors

Bernardo Dell'Osso, Cristina Dobrea, Maria Carlotta Palazzo, Laura Cremaschi, Chiara Arici, Beatrice Benatti and A. Carlo Altamura
Department of Psychiatry, University of Milan, Fondazione IRCCS Cà Granda, Ospedale Maggiore Policlinico, Milano, Italy

Masahiro Kawasaki
Rhythm-based Brain Computation Unit, RIKEN, BSI-TOYOTA Collaboration Center, Japan

Massimo Silvetti and Tom Verguts
Ghent University, Belgium

Nicolas Bourdillon and Stéphane Perrey
Movement To Health (M2H), Montpellier-1 University, Euromov, France

Arlette Streri
Paris Descartes University/LPP UMR 8158 CNRS, Paris, France

Edouard Gentaz
Pierre Mendès-France University/LPNC UMR 5105 CNRS, Grenoble, France

S.M. Golaszewski
Department of Neurology and Neuroscience Institute, Paracelsus Medical University Salzburg, Austria
Karl Landsteiner Institute for Neurorehabilitation and Space Neurology Vienna, Austria

M. Christova and E. Gallasch
Institute of Physiology, Medical University Graz, Austria

M. Seidl and E. Trinka
Department of Neurology and Neuroscience Institute, Paracelsus Medical University Salzburg, Austria

F. Gerstenbrand
Department of Neurology, Medical University Innsbruck, Austria
Karl Landsteiner Institute for Neurorehabilitation and Space Neurology Vienna, Austria

A.B. Kunz
Department of Neurology and Neuroscience Institute, Paracelsus Medical University Salzburg, Austria
Karl Landsteiner Institute for Neurorehabilitation and Space Neurology Vienna, Austria

R. Nardone
Department of Neurology and Neuroscience Institute, Paracelsus Medical University Salzburg, Austria
Department of Neurology, F. Tappeiner Hospital Meran, Italy

Junning Li and Z. JaneWang
Department of Electrical and Computer Engineering

Martin J. McKeown
Department of Medicine (Neurology), Pacific Parkinson's Research Centre, University of British Columbia, Canada

Chiung-Chih Chang
Department of Neurology, Taiwan
Department of Biological Science, National Sun Yet-sen University, Taiwan

Ya-Ting Chang, Wen-Neng Chang and Nai-Ching Chen
Department of Neurology, Chang Gung Memorial Hospital, Kaohsiung Medical Center and Chang Gung University College of Medicine, Taiwan

Chun-Chung Lui and Chen-Chang Lee
Radiology, Chang Gung Memorial Hospital, Kaohsiung Medical Center and Chang Gung University College of Medicine, Taiwan

Shu-Hua Huang
Nuclear Medicine, Chang Gung Memorial Hospital, Kaohsiung Medical Center and Chang Gung University College of Medicine, Taiwan

Chao Suo and Michael J. Valenzuela
Regenerative Neuroscience Group, School of Psychiatry & Brain and Ageing Research Program, University of New South Wales, Australia

Agustin Ibanez
Laboratory of Experimental Psychology and Neuroscience (LPEN), Institute of Cognitive Neurology (INECO), Buenos Aires, Argentina
National Scientific and Technical Research Council (CONICET), Buenos Aires, Argentina
Laboratory of Cognitive Neuroscience, Universidad Diego Portales, Santiago, Chile
Institute of Neuroscience, Favaloro University, Buenos Aires, Argentina

Phil Baker and Alvaro Moya
Laboratory of Experimental Psychology and Neuroscience (LPEN), Institute of Cognitive Neurology (INECO), Buenos Aires, Argentina

J.J. Cheng and F.A. Lenz
Department of Neurosurgery, Johns Hopkins Hospital, Baltimore, USA

J.D. Greenspan
Department of Biomedical Sciences, University of Maryland Dental School, Program in Neuroscience, Baltimore, USA

D.S. Veldhuijzen
Division of Perioperative Care and Emergency Medicine, Rudolf Magus Institute of Neuroscience, Pain Clinic, University Medical Center Utrecht, Utrecht, Netherlands

B. Alexander Diaz, Lizeth H. Sloot, Huibert D. Mansvelder and Klaus Linkenkaer-Hansen
Department of Integrative Neurophysiology, Center for Neurogenomics and Cognitive Research (CNCR), Neuroscience Campus Amsterdam, VU University Amsterdam, Amsterdam, The Netherlands